WOMEN'S HEALTH AND MENOPAUSE

Medical Science Symposia Series

Volume 17

The titles published in this series are listed at the end of this volume.

Women's Health and Menopause

New Strategies – Improved Quality of Life

Edited by

R.A. Lobo
Department of Obstetrics and Gynecology, Columbia University, New York, New York, U.S.A.

P.G. Crosignani
First Department of Obstetrics and Gynecology, University of Milan, Milan, Italy

R. Paoletti
Department of Pharmacological Sciences, University of Milan, Milan, Italy

and

F. Bruschi (Assistant Editor)
First Department of Obstetrics and Gynecology, University of Milan, Milan, Italy

KLUWER ACADEMIC PUBLISHERS
DORDRECHT / BOSTON / LONDON

Fondazione Giovanni Lorenzini, Medical Science Foundation, Milan, Italy
Giovanni Lorenzini Medical Foundation, Houston, Texas, U.S.A.

Library of Congress Cataloging-in-Publication Data

International Symposium on Women's Health in Menopause (4th : 2001 : Washington, D.C.)
Women's health and menopause : new strategies--improved quality of life / edited by R.A. Lobo ... [et al.].
p. ; cm. -- (Medical science symposia series ; v. 17)
Includes bibliographical references and index.
ISBN 1-4020-7149-3 (hardback : alk. paper)
1. Menopause--Congresses. 2. Middle aged women--Health and hygiene--Congresses. I. Lobo, Rogerio A. II. Title. III. Series.
[DNLM: 1. Menopause--Congresses. 2. Estrogen Replacement Therapy--Congresses. 3. Osteoporosis, Postmenopausal--prevention & control--Congresses. 4. Women's Health--Congresses. WP 580 I615w 2002]
RG186 .I578 2001
618.1'75052--dc21

2002072997

ISBN 1-4020-7149-3

Published by Kluwer Academic Publishers,
P.O. Box 17, 3300 AA Dordrecht, The Netherlands.

Sold and distributed in North, Central and South America
by Kluwer Academic Publishers,
101 Philip Drive, Norwell, MA 02061, U.S.A.

In all other countries, sold and distributed
by Kluwer Academic Publishers,
P.O. Box 322, 3300 AH Dordrecht, The Netherlands.

Printed on acid-free paper

Printed in the United States of America.

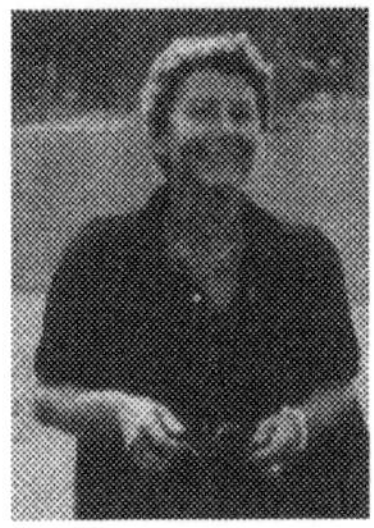

In memoriam

FIORENZA BRUSCHI

Dr. Fiorenza Bruschi, a clinician at the First Department of Obstetrics and Gynecology of the University of Milan (Italy), died suddenly on March 13, 2002 at the age of 46.

Her untimely death interrupted a brilliant career as a devoted physician and researcher in the field of phospho-calcic and lipid metabolism, and cardiovascular diseases in pre- and postmenopausal women; at the time of her death, she was the director of the Menopause Unit of the First Department of Obstetrics and Gynecology at the University of Milan. Her interest and expertise in the field of women's health had been evidenced in her role as member of the International Advisory Board for the series of *International Symposia on WOMEN'S HEALTH AND MENOPAUSE* (1993, 1996, 1998, and 2001) and as Assistant Editor of the *Proceedings* of the most recent symposium held in Washington, D.C. in May 2001. Her intense hospital and research activity did not detract her from tutoring on an individual basis many young and capable collaborators, who are now continuing her work. Her many friends around the world shall remember her as a individual with a rich and warm personality, always interested in culture, in learning, and in sharing her knowledge. They will ensure that her work, interrupted by her untimely death, will continue.

P.G. Crosignani *R.A. Lobo* *R. Paoletti*

Contents

PREFACE

The number of people over 65 is growing very quickly. This number will double in 50 years and due to increased life expectancy the majority of senior citizens will be women. As expected the projected increase in the elderly population, is more pronounced in the less developed regions of the world.

In 1950 the median age of the world population was 29; today it is 38 years of age and in 2050 in many European countries it is projected to be 52-54. In 1950, 5% of the global population was aged 65 and over, by 2050, the number of elderly in Europe is projected to increase to 28%. The most rapid growth will take place in the ages 80 and over. By 2050 their number is projected to increase to 100 million from the present 11 million in China and to 47 million from the present 6 million in India. Humankind is aging rapidly. Population aging already has and in the next future will continue to have great implications.

For instance, in the coming years few countries will be able to provide specialized care for their large population of aged individuals. This crisis will occur despite the vast range of resources today available, despite so much knowledge and such powerful technologies. One reason lies in our need for institutional reform since many institutions are designed for a population structure that in fact no longer exists. But significant changes, major reforms, and constructive revolutions are always difficult and risky.

Let me remind you the tale of Galileo. In 1612 he was professor of physics in Padua when he submitted for publication the manuscript "Sidereus nuncius" setting out his new astronomical theory. The two referees who read the paper rejected the manuscript suggesting drastic changes. After another four years the editor-in-chief of the journal, Cardinal Bellarmino, rejected the paper apparently for three reasons: small numbers, several biases, and wrong statistics. Sixteen years later, Galileo laid the foundations for modern astronomy, publishing the "Dialogo sopra i massimi sistemi del mondo." As a consequence he was suddenly sentenced to prison for life and in order to survive he was obliged to abjure his theory.

We see this as a good example of how, despite its intrinsic risks, science was in the past, still is today, and again will be in the future the only pragmatic answer to human needs.

The program of the *4th International Symposium on WOMAN'S HEALTH AND MENOPAUSE,* promoted and organized by the Giovanni Lorenzini Medical Foundation (Milan, Italy and Houston, Texas) and held in Washington, D.C. on May 19-23, 2001, has been focused on the new strategies able to improve the quality of life, having in mind the main age-related degenerative processes occurring after the menopause: cardiovascular disease, cancer, fractures, and dementia. This extensive analysis has also been the goal of the International Position Paper on Women's Health and Menopause: A Comprehensive Approach, prepared over the last 3 years by the National Institutes of Health and the Giovanni Lorenzini Medical Foundation. A summary of selected portions of the document have been included in this volume of proceedings.

In addition, the different sections of the book illustrate the most recent biological information on the "new" estrogen receptors as well as the updated and critical vision on the controversial role of HRT in widening the therapeutic options for menopausal and postmenopausal women.

The comprehensive approach of the book offers to researchers and practicing clinicians, an easy access to critical opinions and documented judgements of scientific authorities in the fast moving field of women's health and menopause.

The editors wish to express their gratitude to the Giovanni Lorenzini Medical Foundation, the speakers, the participants, and the sponsors who have made this Symposium and this volume possible.

The Editors

List of Contributors

Fadi Abushahin, *Department of Obstetrics and Gynecology and Center for Research in Reproductive Biology, Yale University, New Haven, Connecticut 06520-8063, U.S.A.*

Nigel K. Arden, *MRC Environmental Epidemiology Unit, University of Southampton, Southampton General Hospital, Southampton SO16 6YD, U.K.*

Takeshi Aso, *Comprehensive Reproductive Medicine, Graduate School, Tokyo Medical and Dental University, 1-5-45 Yushima, Bunkyo-ku, Tokyo 113, Japan*

Etienne-Emile Baulieu, *INSERM U488, 80 rue du Général Leclerc, 94276 Le Kremlin Bicêtre Cedex, France*

Lucia Becherini, *Department of Internal Medicine, University of Florence, Florence, Italy*

Silvia Belcredito, *Center of Excellence on Neurodegenerative Diseases and Department of Pharmacological Science, University of Milan, Via Balzaretti, 9, 20133 Milan, Italy*

F. Bernardi, *Department of Reproductive Medicine and Child Development, Division of Obstetrics and Gynecology, University of Pisa, Via Roma 35, 56100 Pisa, Italy*

John Bidmead, *Department of Urogynecology, Kings College Hospital, London, U.K.*

Maria Luisa Brandi, *Department of Internal Medicine, University of Florence, Florence, Italy*

K.M. Brett, *National Center for Health Statistics/Centers for Disease, Control and Prevention, Rockville, Maryland, U.S.A.*

Louise A. Brinton, *Environmental Epidemiology Branch, Division of Cancer Epidemiology and Genetics, National Cancer Institute, Executive Plaza South, Rm. 7068, MSC 7234, Bethesda, Maryland 20892-7234, U.S.A.*

D. Browne, *Office of Women's Health, Department of Health and Human Services, Washington, D.C., U.S.A.*

Curt W. Burger, *Department of Obstetrics and Gynecology, Erasmus University Medical Centre Rotterdam, PO Box 2040, 3000 CA, Rotterdam, The Netherlands*

Henry Burger, *Prince Henry's Institute of Medical Research, Monash Medical Centre, Clayton, Victoria, Australia*

Linda Cardozo, *Department of Urogynecology, Kings College Hospital, London, U.K*

Richard O. Cannon III, *National Institutes of Health, Building 10 Room 7B-15, 10 Center Drive MSC 1650, Bethesda, Maryland 20892-1650, U.S.A.*

K.K. Chapman, *U.S. Food and Drug Administration, Rockville, Maryland, U.S.A.*

Y. Chong, *National Center for Health Statistics/Centers for Disease, Control and Prevention, Rockville, Maryland, U.S.A.*

C. M. Clancy, *Agency for Healthcare Research and Quality, Rockville, Maryland, U.S.A.*

Colin Clyne, *Prince Henry's Institute of Medical Research, Melbourne, Australia*

Aila Collins, *Department of Clinical Neuroscience, Karolinska Hospital, Stockholm, Sweden*

Peter Collins, *Imperial College School of Medicine, National Heart and Lung Institute, London, U.K.*

Ginger D. Constantine, *Wyeth-Ayerst Research, P.O. Box 42528, Philadelphia, Pennsylvania 19101-2528, U.S.A.*

Cyrus Cooper, *MRC Environmental Epidemiology Unit, Southampton General Hospital, Southampton SO16 6YD, U.K.*

C. Cornell, *Centers for Disease Control & Prevention, National Institutes of Health, Bethesda, Maryland and University of Alabama at Birmingham, Birmingham, Alabama, U.S.A.*

PierGiorgio Crosignani, *1st Department of Obstetrics and Gynecology, University of Milan, Via della Commenda 12, 20122 Milan, Italy*

Susan Davis, *The Jean Halles Foundation, Research Unit, 173 Carinish Road, Clayton, Victoria 3168, Australia*

Lorraine Dennerstein, *Office for Gender and Health, Department of Psychiatry, The University of Melbourne, Royal Melbourne Hospital, Charles Connibere Building, Parkville, Victoria 3050, Australia*

Elaine M. Dennison, *MRC Environmental Epidemiology Unit, University of Southampton, Southampton General Hospital, Southampton SO16 6YD, U.K.*

Alberto Falchetti, *Department of Internal Medicine, University of Florence, Florence, Italy*

Loretta P. Finnegan, *Office of Research on Women's Health, National Institutes of Health, Department of Health and Human Services, Bethesda, Maryland, U.S.A.*

A. Fugh-Berman, *Office of Women's Health, Department of Health and Human Services, Washington, D.C., U.S.A.*

J. C. Gallagher, *Creighton University Medical Center, St. Joseph's Hospital, 601 North 30th St, Suite 6712, Omaha, Nebraska 68131, U.S.A.*

Marco Gambacciani, *Department of Reproductive Medicine and Child Development, Division of Obstetrics and Gynecology, University of Pisa, Pisa, Italy*

I. Ross Garrett, *Medicine/Endocrinology #7877, University of Texas Health Science Center, 7703 Floyd Curl Drive, San Antonio, Texas 78229-3900, U.S.A.*

Luigi Gennari, *Department of Internal Medicine, University of Florence, Florence, Italy*

Andrea R. Genazzani, *Department of Reproductive Medicine and Child Development, Division of Obstetrics and Gynecology, University of Pisa, Via Roma 35, 56100 Pisa, Italy*

Christine Goertz, *National Center for Complementary and Alternative Medicine, National Institutes of Health, Bethesda, Maryland, U.S.A.*

David J. Gordon, *National Heart, Lung, and Blood Institute, 6701 Rockledge Drive, Suite 9044, Bethesda, Maryland 20892-7940, U.S.A.*

J.Y. Groff, *Centers for Disease Control and Prevention, National Institutes of Health, Bethesda, Maryland and University of Alabama at Birmingham, Birmingham, Alabama, U.S.A.*

M.L. Gross, *Agency for Healthcare Research and Quality, Rockville, Maryland, U.S.A.*

Jan-Åke Gustafsson, *Departments of Medical Nutrition and Biosciences, Karolinska Institute, S-141 86 Huddinge, Sweden*

Gloria Gutierrez, *Medicine/Endocrinology #7877, University of Texas Health Science Center, 7703 Floyd Curl Drive, San Antonio, Texas 78229-3900, U.S.A.*

Victor W. Henderson, *Departments of Geriatrics and Neurology, Donald W. Reynolds Center on Aging, University of Arkansas for Medical Sciences, 4301 W. Markham Street, Slot 810, Little Rock, Arkansas 72201 U.S.A.*

Susan L. Hendrix, *Wayne State University School of Medicine, Hutzel Hospital, Department of Obstetrics and Gynecology, 4707 St. Antoine Boulevard, Detroit, Michigan 48201-1427, U.S.A.*

C. Herman, *Centers for Disease Control & Prevention, National Institutes of Health, Bethesda, Maryland and University of Alabama at Birmingham, Birmingham, Alabama, U.S.A.*

David M. Herrington, *Department of Internal Medicine/Cardiology, Wake Forest University School of Medicine, Medical Center Boulevard, Winston-Salem, North Carolina 27157, U.S.A.*

K.A. Hollinger, *U.S. Food and Drug Administration, Rockville, Maryland, U.S.A.*

C. Hunter, *Office of Women's Health, Department of Health and Human Services, Washington, D.C., U.S.A.*

Melinda L. Irwin, *The Fred Hutchinson Cancer Research Center, 1100 Fairview Ave North MP-900, Seattle, Washington, 98109-1024, U.S.A.*

Muhammad K. Javaid, *MRC Environmental Epidemiology Unit, University of Southampton, Southampton General Hospital, Southampton SO16 6YD, U.K.*

Karen Johnson, *Department of Preventive Medicine, University of Tennessee, Memphis, Tennessee, U.S.A.*

J. Kaczmarczyk, *Office of Women's Health, Department of Health and Human Services, Washington, D.C., U.S.A.*

N. Keenan, *Office of Women's Health, Department of Health and Human Services, Washington, D.C., U.S.A.*

Peter Kenemans, *Department of Obstetrics and Gynecology, Free University Medical Centre, PO Box 7057, 1007 MB, Amsterdam, The Netherlands*

Karen Potvin Klein, *Department of Internal Medicine/Cardiology, Wake Forest University School of Medicine, Medical Center Boulevard, Winston-Salem, North Carolina 27157, U.S.A.*

Krista Kotz, *Kotz Health Policy Consulting, 174 Glorietta Boulevard, Orinda, California 94611, U.S.A.*

Peter R. Kowey, *Jefferson Medical College, Philadelphia, Pennsylvania and Division of Cardiovascular Disease, Lankenau Hospital and the Mainline Health System, Wynnewood, Pennsylvania, U.S.A.*

Carlo La Vecchia, *Istituto di Ricerche Farmacologiche "Mario Negri," Via Eritrea 62, 20157 Milan, Italy and Istituto di Statistica Medica e Biometria, Università degli Studi di Milano, Via Venezian 1, 20133 Milan, Italy*

Marianne J. Legato, *Partnership for Women's Health, Columbia University, New York, NewYork, U.S.A.*

Philippe Lehert, *Office for Gender and Health, Department of Psychiatry, The University of Melbourne, Victoria, Australia and Statistical Department, Faculty of Economics, FUCAM, Mons, Belgium*

Jeanne Leventhal Alexander, *Kaiser Permanente Oakland, Psychiatry Department, 3900 Broadway, Oakland, California 94611, U.S.A.*

C.E. Lewis, *Centers for Disease Control and Prevention, National Institutes of Health, Bethesda, Maryland and University of Alabama at Birmingham, Birmingham, Alabama, U.S.A.*

M. Liut, *Department of Reproductive Medicine and Child Development, Division of Obstetrics and Gynecology, University of Pisa, Via Roma 35, 56100 Pisa, Italy*

Rogerio A. Lobo, *Sloane Hospital for Women, Columbia-Presbyterian Medical Center, New York, New York, U.S.A.*

Susan Love, *UCLA Medical School, Los Angeles, California, U.S.A.*

M. Luisi, *Department of Reproductive Medicine and Child Development, Division of Obstetrics and Gynecology, University of Pisa, Via Roma 35, 56100 Pisa, Italy*

Adriana Maggi, *Center of Excellence on Neurodegenerative Diseases and Department of Pharmacological Science, University of Milan, Via Balzaretti, 9, 20133 Milan, Italy*

JoAnn E. Manson, *Brigham and Women's Hospital, Harvard Medical School, Boston, Massachusetts, U.S.A.*

S. Mark, *Office of Women's Health, Department of Health and Human Services, Washington, D.C., U.S.A.*

Laura Masi, *Department of Internal Medicine, University of Florence, Florence, Italy*

H. McCreath, *Centers for Disease Control & Prevention, National Institutes of Health, Bethesda, Maryland and University of Alabama at Birmingham, Birmingham, Alabama, U.S.A.*

R. McKeown, *Centers for Disease Control and Prevention, National Institutes of Health, Bethesda, Maryland and University of Alabama at Birmingham, Birmingham, Alabama, U.S.A.*

Anne McTiernan, *The Fred Hutchinson Cancer Research Center, 1100 Fairview Ave North MP-900, Seattle, Washington, 98109-1024, U.S.A.*

Clara Meda, *Center of Excellence on Neurodegenerative Diseases and Department of Pharmacological Science, University of Milan, Via Balzaretti, 9, 20133 Milan, Italy*

M.A. Miller, *U.S. Food and Drug Administration, Rockville, Maryland, U.S.A.*

Patrizia Monteleone, *Department of Reproductive Medicine and Child Development, Division of Obstetrics and Gynecology, University of Pisa, Pisa, Italy*

Gil Mor, *Department of Obstetrics and Gynecology, Yale University, School of Medicine, 333 Cedar St. FMB 202, New Haven, Connecticut 06520, U.S.A.*

Gregory R. Mundy, *Medicine/Endocrinology #7877, University of Texas Health Science Center, 7703 Floyd Curl Drive, San Antonio, Texas 78229-3900, U.S.A.*

Frederick Naftolin, *Department of Obstetrics and Gynecology and Center for Research in Reproductive Biology, Yale University, New Haven, Connecticut 06520-8063, U.S.A.*

Rodolfo Paoletti, *Institute of Pharmacological Sciences, University of Milan, Via Balzaretti 9, Milan, Italy*

Fabio Parazzini, *Istituto di Recerche Farmacologiche Mario Negri, Milan, Italy*

Trevor M. Penning, *Department of Pharmacology, University of Pennsylvania School of Medicine, 3620 Hamilton Walk, Philadelphia, PA 19104-6084, U.S.A.*

James H. Pickar, *Wyeth-Ayerst Research, P.O. Box 42528, Philadelphia, Pennsylvania 19101-2528, U.S.A.*

M. Pieri, *Department of Reproductive Medicine and Child Development, Division of Obstetrics and Gynecology, University of Pisa, Via Roma 35, 56100 Pisa, Italy*

Vivian W. Pinn, *Office of Research on Women's Health, National Institutes of Health, Department of Health and Human Services, Bethesda, Maryland, U.S.A.*

Bertram Pitt, *Division of Cardiology, Department of Internal Medicine, University of Michigan Medical Center, Ann Arbor, Michigan, U.S.A.*

L. Pulley, *Centers for Disease Control & Prevention, National Institutes of Health, Bethesda, Maryland and University of Alabama at Birmingham, Birmingham, Alabama, U.S.A.*

Susan M. Resnick, *Laboratory of Personality and Cognition, National Institute on Aging, National Institutes of Health, Baltimore, Maryland, U.S.A.*

D. Richter, *Centers for Disease Control & Prevention, National Institutes of Health, Bethesda, Maryland and University of Alabama at Birmingham, Birmingham, Alabama, U.S.A.*

B. Lawrence Riggs, *Mayo Clinic and Mayo Foundation, Division of Endocrinology, Metabolism and Nutrition, Department of Internal Medicine, 200 First Street SW, North 6 Plummer, Rochester, Minnesota 55905, U.S.A.*

Paulo Rinaudo, *Department of Obstetrics and Gynecology and Center for Research in Reproductive Biology, Yale University, New Haven, Connecticut 06520-8063, U.S.A.*

Jacques E. Rossouw, *National Heart, Lung, and Blood Institute, Women's Health Initiative, NIH, 6705 Rockledge Drive, 1 Rockledge Center, Suite 300, MSC 7966, Bethesda, Maryland 28892-7966, U.S.A.*

Gary Rubin, *Prince Henry's Institute of Medical Research, Melbourne, Australia*

Irma H. Russo, *Breast Cancer Research Laboratory, Fox Chase Cancer Center, 7701 Burholme Ave., Philadelphia, Pennsylvania 19111, U.S.A.*

Jose Russo, *Breast Cancer Research Laboratory, Fox Chase Cancer Center, 7701 Burholme Ave., Philadelphia, Pennsylvania 19111, U.S.A.*

Göran Samsioe, *Department of Obstetrics and Gynecology, Lund University Hospital, S-221 85 Lund, Sweden*

Costante Donati Sarti, *Ospedale Policlinico, Division of Obstetrics and Gynecology, University of Perugia, Perugia, Italy*

H.P.G. Schneider, *Department of Obstetrics and Gynecology, University of Muenster, Germany*

Barbara B. Sherwin, *McGill University, Departments of Psychology and Obstetrics and Gynecology, 1205 Dr. Penfield Ave., Montreal, Quebec Canada H3A 1B1*

Evan R Simpson, *Prince Henry's Institute of Medical Research and the Department of Biochemistry and Molecular Biology, Monash University, Melbourne, Australia*

MaryFran Sowers, *Department of Epidemiology, School of Public Health, University of Michigan, 109 Observatory, Ann Arbor, Michigan 48109-2029, U.S.A.*

Caroline Speed, *Prince Henry's Institute of Medical Research, Melbourne, Australia*

M. Stomati, *Department of Reproductive Medicine and Child Development, Division of Obstetrics and Gynecology, University of Pisa, Via Roma 35, 56100 Pisa, Italy*

Eddie Sze, *Department of Obstetrics and Gynecology and Center for Research in Reproductive Biology, Yale University, New Haven, Connecticut 06520-8063, U.S.A.*

Edward A. Trott, *Wyeth-Ayerst Research, P.O. Box 42528, Philadelphia, Pennsylvania 19101-2528, U.S.A.*

Yvonne T. van der Schouw, *Julius Center for General Practice and Patient Oriented Research, University Medical Center Utrecht, Room D 01.335, PO Box 85500, 3508 GA Utrecht, The Netherlands*

Gijs A. van Unnik, *Department of Obstetrics and Gynecology, Free University Medical Centre, PO Box 7057, 1007 MB, Amsterdam, The Netherlands*

Elisabetta Vegeto, *Center of Excellence on Neurodegenerative Diseases and Department of Pharmacological Science, University of Milan, Via Balzaretti, 9, 20133 Milan, Italy*

Karen Walker-Bone, *MRC Environmental Epidemiology Unit, University of Southampton, Southampton General Hospital, Southampton SO16 6YD, U.K.*

Nanette K. Wenger, *Emory University School of Medicine, 69 Butler Street S.E., Atlanta, 30303 Georgia, U.S.A.*

S.F. Wood, *U.S. Food and Drug Administration, Rockville, Maryland, U.S.A.*

Herbert Yu, *Department of Epidemiology and Public Health, Yale University, School of Medicine, 60 College Street, P.O. Box 208034, New Haven, Connecticut 06520-8034, U.S.A.*

Estrogen Receptor β — A Multifaceted Player

Jan-Åke Gustafsson

Introduction

Since the discovery of ERβ in 1995 [1], our report on this finding at a Keystone meeting in April 1996, and publication of the data a couple of months later [2], several hundred papers on this novel receptor have appeared. There are many reasons why ERβ has attracted so much attention.

At the time of its discovery it was generally thought that there existed only one estrogen receptor and this view affected most of the thinking in the field. For example, pharmaceutical ambitions to develop new and better-targeted hormone replacement therapeutics were restricted by the dogma of one single hormone binding site on one single receptor. Furthermore, based on the premise that a single molecule mediated all the effects of estrogen, the many contradictory effects of estrogens in the body were difficult to explain. In addition, estrogens were known to affect tissues, e.g. regions in the brain, where no ERα was detectable by immunohistochemical methods. The sudden and unexpected appearance of ERβ on the scene, like *a deus ex machina*, caused somewhat of a catharsis in the field and offered explanations to old enigmas and controversies. At the same time, the possibilities of new and exciting developments revitalized the whole field of estrogen action.

During these recent few years a significant amount of new knowledge has been generated and this short review will briefly summarize some of the most important insights gained.

ERβ and Reproduction

One of the astounding facts regarding ERβ is that it appears to be involved in such a great variety of biological functions, consistent with its widespread distribution in the body. It is clear that these diverse functions cannot solely be ascribed to gender and reproductive functions but reflect a much more general role of ERβ. Nevertheless, one of the obvious phenotypes of female mice in which ERβ has been deleted (ERβKO mice) is a severe reproductive disturbance manifested as drastic reduction in number and size of litters [3,4]. This is not surprising since the levels of ERβ in ovarian granulosa cells are among the highest in the body and deletion of this receptor results in follicular arrest, atretic follicles, and significantly reduced ovulation.

Interestingly and importantly, these changes appear to be unrelated to the hypothalamo-pituitary axis since ERβKO mice have normal levels of pituitary hormones in their blood. This is in distinct contrast to the situation in ERαKO mice where the severe ovarian phenotype (hyperemic ovaries and complete infertility) is essentially normalized following reduction of the elevated LH levels in these animals. Accordingly, in the ovary itself, ERβ seems to be the more dominant ER isoform even though ERα also appears to play some role.

The exact function of ERβ in the granulosa cells of the ovary has not yet been defined; its levels are highest at the beginning of the estrus cycle and tend to fall towards the end of follicular development [5]. This cyclic variation in ERβ expression in granulosa cells has turned out to be true for several species. One potentially important aspect of ERβ function in the granulosa cells is its capacity to downregulate the androgen receptor (AR) in these cells. AR has several roles in the recruitment of primordial follicles as well as in their further differentiation to preovulatory follicles. Treatment with the antiandrogen flutamide normalizes the ERβKO ovarian phenotype and the treated mice have an increased number of pregnancies [4]. This situation is reminiscent of the human disease polycystic ovarian (PCO) disorder where fertility may be restored with antiandrogen treatment and where the patients suffer from several signs of hyperandrogenism. Our lab as well as those of others are currently investigating whether a deficiency in ERβ function and an ensuing AR hyperactivity might be involved in the etiology of this disease.

ERβ and Prostate

One of the dogmas of endocrinology that has changed as a result of the sudden appearance on the scene of ERβ is that estrogen receptors are more important in females than in males. Clearly, ERβ is very prominent in the male urogenital tract and in the prostate epithelium (the tissue from which ERβ was first cloned), the level of ERβ is higher than in any other tissue in males [2]. Prostate stroma contains small amounts of ERα but there is no ERα in the normal prostate epithelium. Deletion of ERβ results in hyperplasia of the prostate with increased expression of Ki67 and cyclin A, indicating that ERβ has an antiproliferative effect in the prostate [6]. One mechanism for this effect might be the upregulated AR levels seen in the ERβKO prostate. Interestingly, treatment of normal mice with ERβ ligand results in reduced AR levels in the prostate. This is yet another example of crosstalk between ERβ and AR where ERβ downregulates AR.

Much speaks in favor of an important role of ERβ in controlling prostate growth. The dominant ERβ ligand in the prostate is 5α-androstane-3β,17β-diol (3β-Adiol), a metabolite of 5α-dihydrotestosterone (DHT). In this metabolic pathway, testosterone is converted to DHT by 5α-reductase in the prostate and further metabolized to 3β-Adiol, an ERβ agonist. The binding of 3β-Adiol to ERβ leads to downregulation of AR and decreased growth. This pathway provides a negative feedback for androgen stimulation of prostatic growth. Very interestingly, 3β-Adiol is specifically inactivated by a tissue specific cytochrome P-450, CYP 7B, expressed in the prostate and central nervous system (CNS) but not in the liver [7-9]. Preliminary data indicate that this enzyme is upregulated in the prostate during conditions of increased growth of the gland, consistent with a role of 3β-Adiol (via ERβ) as a balancing force against prostate growth.

In view of the presence of this pathway in the prostate, the use of inhibitors of 5α-reductase to inhibit prostate growth, can be questioned. One may well ask whether the use of these inhibitors to prevent prostate cancer development in healthy high risk male subjects, would not result in decreased formation of 3β-Adiol and hence an increased risk for prostate growth. From this perspective it may be a more logical strategy to treat high risk subjects with ERβ ligands. Perhaps the commonly held layman's view that prostatic disease may be alleviated by consumption of certain plants could be related to the high concentration of phytoestrogens in these plants. Many phytoestrogens are known to be excellent ligands for ERβ and it may be that the alleged beneficial effects of the plant derivatives on the prostate may be related to their stimulatory effects on ERβ function in the gland.

ERβ and Uterus

An antiproliferative effect of ERβ is also apparent in tissues other than in the prostate. In the immature uterus ERα mediates the proliferative action of estradiol-17β whereas ERβ counteracts this effect [10]. This interesting antagonism between ERβ and ERα is seen also in several estrogen regulated systems and has led to the idea of the yin-yang principle in which ERβ and ERα are two equal opposing forces which balance each other. Accordingly, ERβ-/- mice often display a paradoxical hyper-responsiveness to estrogen since the remaining ER isoform, ERα, can exert its actions in the absence of an inhibitory influence from ERβ. This is illustrated in the immature uterus of ERβKO mice which responds to estrogen by growing faster than corresponding wild type mouse (wt) uteri.

ERβ and Spleen

Another example of ERβ's antiproliferative action is seen in the spleen; female ERβKO mice show rapidly growing spleens which are significantly larger than female wt spleens by 6 months of age. Apparently it is mainly the B lymphocytes which are responsible for this growth. These B cells are not normal and eventually invade the liver as these animals grow older. Our working hypothesis is that the growth of B lymphocytes is driven by ERα in these cells and that lack of antiproliferative ERβ leads to uncontrolled cellular growth.

ERβ and Breast Cancer

One exciting issue, which is being explored, is whether the balance between ERα and ERβ in terms of growth control also applies to mammary gland and breast cancer. The field has been somewhat impeded by a few early publications which reported lack of ERβ in mammary gland but it now seems clear from work in several laboratories that ERβ is a major ER in both normal and malignant breast tissue. Indeed, several variants of ERβ are present in this tissue. For instance, in the rat mammary gland, ERβ18aa ins (an isoform with 18 amino acids inserted into the LBD, creating a receptor with much reduced affinity for estradiol-17β) reaches levels equal to those of ERβwt [11]. It appears that ERβ18aa ins is more efficient than ERβwt in heterodimerizing with ERα, thereby reducing the biological activity of ERα. A similar role may be exerted by ERβcx (an isoform where the wt exon 9 has been switched for another exon creating a receptor isoform with lack of binding ability) in the human; this ERβ variant very efficiently shuts down ERα activity. Indeed, our recent data indicate that the explanation for the existence of the ERα positive, PR (progesterone receptor) negative breast tumors, which are generally resistant towards antihormone therapy, is their presence of ERβcx. Accordingly, one would expect that presence of ERβcx in human breast cancer would be a bad prognostic sign. Although this has not yet been proven we have recently shown that solid breast cancers analyzed immunohistochemically demonstrate colocalization of cyclin A/Ki67 proliferation markers with ERβ but not with ERα; since the ERβ antibody we have used in this study recognizes total ERβ (wt plus isoforms), an exciting possibility is that the ERβ immunoreactivity in these tumor samples mainly or solely represents ERβcx [12]. If this turns out to be correct, new pharmaceutical possibilities to treat these antihormone-resistant breast cancer patients can be envisioned, e.g. interventions designed to change the ERβwt/ERβcx ratio in tumors. Clearly, a more complete understanding of estrogen regulation of growth of breast cancer cells necessitates a detailed knowledge of ERβ and its isoforms in breast cancer tissue.

ERβ and CNS

An organ where ERβ appears to be of great physiological importance is the CNS. Surprisingly and dramatically, mice of both sexes show severe loss of neurons in several brain regions upon deletion of ERβ. In some areas of the CNS this is associated with a remarkable overgrowth of astroglia [13]. Furthermore, ERβKO mice are much more vulnerable to treatment with the neurotoxic agent kainic acid. Finally, ERβKO mice are slower learners in the water maze test than wt counterparts. All these observations point to an important role of ERβ in brain function, giving further support to the notion that estrogens play a vital role in maintaining the integrity of the CNS. The specific and differential distribution of the two ER isoforms in the brain indicates that isoform specific ER ligands could be of great potential interest as psychoactive drugs.

Conclusion

In conclusion, investigation into estrogen signaling has undergone a dramatic renaissance and yet many more surprises are to expected as ER-KO and aromatase KO mice are studied further. Perhaps the multitude of physiological events regulated by estrogens and ERs is related to an alleged, very early role of ER as the precursor of all other nuclear receptors implying that ligands to this ancient ER used to have paramount and general regulatory tasks in these ancestral organisms, a situation that may in part have survived in more developed animals.

Acknowledgments

This study was made possible through grants from the Swedish Cancer Fund and KaroBio AB.

References

1. The ER beta cDNA sequence and protein is protected through patents (international patent application WO97/09348). Granted patents: EP0792292 (Europe), US 5,978,710 (US), 3131649 (Japan), 2,201,098 (Canada) 715528 (Australia), 263137 (Korea).
2. Kuiper GGJM, Enmark E, Pelto-Huikko M, Nilsson S, Gustafsson, J-Å. Cloning of a novel estrogen receptor expressed in rat prostate and ovary. Proc Natl Acad Sci USA 1996;93: 5925-30.
3. Krege JH, Hodgin JB, Couse JF, et al. Generation and reproductive phenotypes of mice lacking estrogen receptor β. Proc Natl Acad Sci USA 1998;95:15677-82.
4. Cheng G, Weihua Z, Mäkinen S, et al. A role for the androgen receptor in follicular atresia of estrogen receptor beta knockout mouse ovary. Biol Reprod 2002;66:77-84.
5. Byers M, Kuiper GGJM, Gustafsson JÅ, Park-Sarge O-K. Estrogen receptor-β mRNA expression in rat ovary: Down-regulation by gonadotropins. Mol Endocrinol 1997;11:172-82.
6. Weihua Z, Mäkelä S, Andersson LC, et al. A role for estrogen receptor β in the regulation of growth of the ventral prostate. Proc Natl Acad Sci USA 2001;98;6330-35.
7. Sundin M, Warner M, Haaparanta T, Gustafsson J-Å. Isolation and catalytic activity of cytochrome P-450 from ventral prostate of control rats. J Biol Chem 1987;262:12293-97.
8. Warner M, Strömstedt M Möller L, Gustafsson J-Å. Distribution and regulation of 5α-androstane-3β,17β-diol hydroxylase in the rat central nervous system. Endocrinology 1989;124:2699-2706.
9. Rose, K., Allan, A., Gauldie, S., et al. Neurosteroid hydroxylase CYP7B vivid reporter activity in dentate gyrus of gene-targeted mice and abolition of a widespread pathway of steroid and oxysterol hydroxylation. J Biol Chem 2001;276:23937-44.
10. Weihua Z, Saji S, Mäkinen S, et al. Estrogen receptor (ER) β, a modulator of ERα in the uterus. Proc Natl Acad Sci USA 2000;97:5936-41.
11. Saji S, Sakaguchi H, Andersson S, Warner M, Gustafsson J-Å. (2001). Quantitative analysis of estrogen receptor proteins in rat mammary gland. Endocrinol 2001;142:3177-86.
12. Jensen EV, Cheng G, Palmieri C, et al. Estrogen receptors and proliferation markers in primary and recurrent breast cancer. Proc Natl Acad Sci USA 2001;98,:15197-202.
13. Wang L, Andersson S, Warner M, Gustafsson J-Å. Morphological abnormalities in the brains of estrogen receptor β knockout mice. Proc Natl Acad Sci USA 2001;98:2792-96.

ANDROPAUSE AT THE BEGINNING OF THE NEW CENTURY: A FEW REMARKS ON HORMONES AND AGING OF MEN

Etienne-Emile Baulieu

Introduction

In a woman's life, a remarkable event occurs when she is approximately 50 years old, now as well as a century ago when longevity was much shorter: ovulation stops, and therefore fertility. Consequently, estradiol, the archetypal estrogen, decreases to a very low level in the blood – lower (naturally in absence of replacement administration) than it is in men and even aging men (Table 1). In women, hormone replacement therapy, mainly with estrogen, produces recognized benefits for several estrogen deficit-associated physical impairments. In the twentieth century, the discoveries of sex hormones, of their main mechanism of action at the gene expression level via nuclear receptors, and of the synthesis of synthetic active derivatives and preparations permitting relatively easy utilization (including specific estrogen receptor modulators (SERMs), have had many positive effects on the lives of menopausal and postmenopausal women.

The question arises with regard to men, whose mean life expectancy, particularly in industrialized countries, is several years shorter than that of women, not even reaching 80 years of age for approximately 50% of men: what is the effect of a decrease in sex hormones and what can be done to alleviate the symptoms? Clearly the second part of a man's life is not as hormonally standardized and selective as in that of a woman. Some decline of the testicular endocrine function is always there [1,2]: the decrease of blood testosterone (Figure 1) and its active metabolite 5α-dihydrotestosterone (DHT) (Figure 2) although globally incomplete is variable according to individual, whose several other health parameters may be deficient while fertility, though certainly decreased, is far from eliminated. However, although many sperm characteristics are preserved [3], Sertoli cells are functionally diminished. What is functionally a problem in terms of quality of life has been summarized under the heading of "climacteric" symptoms (Table 2) [4-6] which are very similar to those of women with an emphasis on the decrease of sex life components – from diminished sexual desire to several forms of impotence. If the hormonal status of menopause, including pre- and perimenopausal symptoms, may occur within in a few months, there is a long period – many years – during which a "Partial Androgen Deficiency in Aging Men," the so-called PADAM, progresses, although the precise criteria have not yet been established. It follows that it is particularly difficult to decide if the observed physical (and mental) changes in aging men are dependent on hormonal modifications, or whether the androgen deficit is a consequence of age. Thus, one may predict that androgen substitution is difficult to rationalize and its potential beneficial effects relatively uncertain. Nevertheless, PADAM is increasingly recognized as important for health and quality of life issues. To give approximative values to the hormonal deficit, one may cite the mean level observed in 75-year-old men as two-thirds that of young men, with sexual dysfunction in young men as being observed when testosterone is ≤ 3 ng/ml (≤ 10 nmoles). The bioavailable testosterone is lower in 25 % of aged men than the lowest normal young values.

Table 1. Aging Males. Body Composition versus Hormones [7]

	Young	Middle-aged	Elderly
Age (y)	~27	~42	~75
Weight (kg)	74	81	74
Height (cm)	180	177	168
BMI	23	26	27
Total fat (kg)	13	21	29
Testosterone (ng/ml)	6	5	5
Free Testo (pg/ml)	150	130	81
SBP (nmol/l)	36	33	53
E2 (pg/ml)	25	22	24
IGF-1 (ng/dl)	230	176	122
Insulin (µU/ml)	7	9	8

Hormones

The basis of any scientific reasoning is to be found in publications carefully measuring hormonal and other behavioral and physical parameters. Circulating (plasma) testosterone, specifically of testicular origin, decreases each year of approx. 0.5 to 1 % between 40 and 70 years, and this decrease of circulating testosterone is associated to (and probably responsible for) modest LH increase [8,9], with attenuation of secretory burst amplitude suggesting hypothalamic defect [10,11]. In Figure 3, the global decrease of blood testosterone in aging people may be observed, with a decrease of the diurnal rhythm of unknown pathophysiological interest [12].

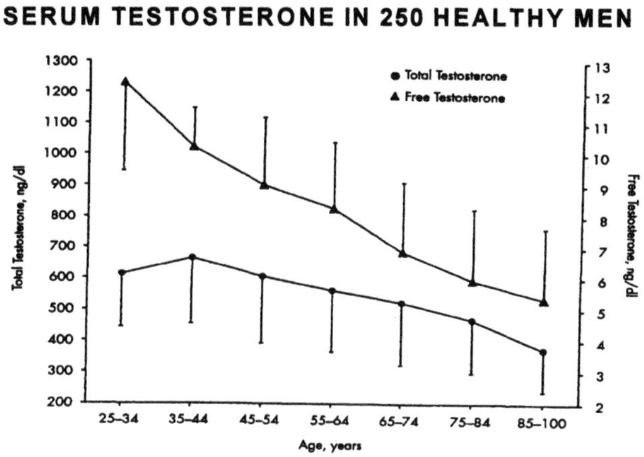

Figure 1. Serum testosterone in 250 healthy men [13].

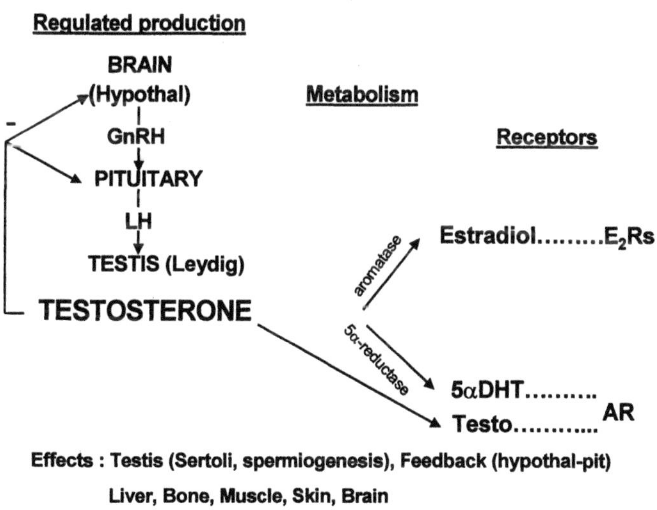

Figure 2. A schematic global view of testosterone biology.

Table 2. Aging Men: "Climacteric" Symptoms [14]

Psvchological	Somato-vegetative	Sexual
Discouraged	Joint complaints	Decreased potency
Depressed	Sweating	Decreased erectibility
Irritable	Need for more sleep	Decreased libido
Anxious	Sleep disturbance	Decreased beard growth
Nervous	Decreased well-being	"Passed zenith of life"
	Weakness	
	Exhaustion	

SERUM TESTOSTERONE IN NORMAL (17) AND OLD (12) MEN

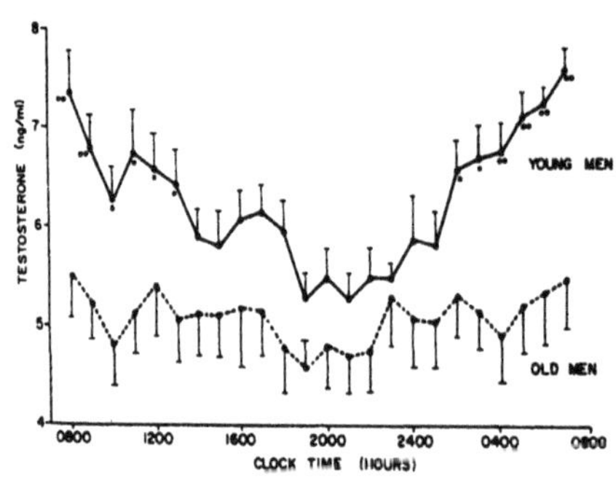

Figure 3. Serum testoterone in normal (17) and old (12) men [12].

Measurement of blood testosterone should be further interpreted for several reasons:

1) General metabolism. Testosterone is metabolized to at least 2 active steroids, DHT and estradiol (Figure 2). DHT is formed mostly in liver, skin, kidney, and prostate. DHT is more active than testosterone at the cellular level, and an overall index of androgenicity should take its level in consideration. However, there is no known condition where a significant change of the testosterone/DHT ratio in blood is observed in aging as compared to the young values and thus would be of biological importance.

Testosterone (and clearly not DHT) is metabolized in part to estradiol. In aging men the level of circulating testosterone in most cases is still sizable, and probably the reason for estradiol levels in men being equal or superior to that of found in untreated aged women. In aging men, the precursors (testosterone and dehydroepiandrosterone sulfate DHEAS) of estradiol decrease, but fat tissues increase, in such a way that the blood level of this estrogen is approximately maintained. The relatively lower testosterone/estradiol ratio in older men is possibly important physiologically. Estradiol is mostly formed in fat, muscle, but also in liver, kidney, and brain.

2) Binding in blood modifies testosterone activity. In plasma, testosterone is partly bound (order of magnitude: 30-50 %) to a high affinity protein which also binds DHT and estradiol (but not DHEA(S)), called sex steroid binding plasma protein (SBP) [15], testosterone-estradiol binding globulin (TeBG), or sex hormone binding protein (SHBG). The rest of testosterone is mostly bound to albumin with weak affinity (order of magnitude: 40-50 %), and in small amount (approximately 2 %) is unbound ("free fraction"). The two last fractions are considered as directly bioavailable (and conveniently measurable [16], Figure 4), because of easier transfer from plasma to target cells. SBP, synthesized in liver, increases with age (approximately 1 % each year between 40 and 70) and this could be due to low growth hormone and/or IGF-I levels [17], and thus the bioavailable testosterone decreases with age even more so than total testosterone itself. It is possible, but not strictly demonstrated that abnormal SBP synthesis is involved in changes of active circulating testosterone.

3) Autocrine testosterone. Testosterone can be formed from inactive precursors. DHEA(S) and Δ_4-androstenedione secreted by adrenals and testis may be transformed to testosterone (and DHT) within androgen responsive cells (expressing androgen receptor), and thus the most active androgens escape to blood measurement. For this reason, a measure of 5αandrostane-3α,17βdiol (a "direct metabolite of testosterone [18] in form of circulating 3α,5αandrostanediol glucuronide [ADG]) may be informative even it could be produced in nonandrogen responsive cells and thus not an androgen index.

4) DHEA(S) secretion rates observed physiologically (that is < 30 mg/d in > 60 years old men) do not contribute significantly to blood testosterone levels in men (order of magnitude: ≤ 1 ng/ml, and thus practically < 10 % of total serum testosterone).

The activity of testosterone does not depend only on circulating levels of the hormones, but also on events occurring at the target cell levels. There is no definitive demonstration that age-related change of testosterone metabolism may be involved in testosterone activity, such as less 5α-reductase activity leading to less DHT, or more inactivating metabolism to reduced compounds (e.g. ADG) provoking decreasing biologically active androgens.

Another possibility is that there is a regulatory change of the androgen receptor such as a decrease of its expression in aging; however, this has not been proven thus far. Interestingly, shorter polymorphic CAG repeat length in exon 1 of the androgen receptor (AR) is associated with higher transcription activation and may modulate the age-related decline of testosterone [19].

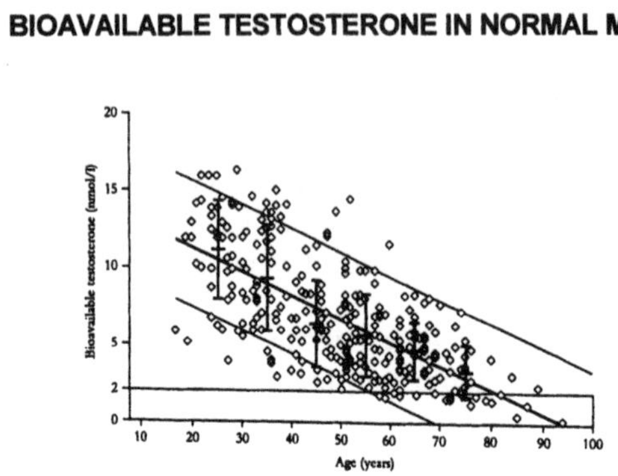

Figure 4. Bioavailable testosterone in normal men [16].

DHEA(S)

In most men as in most women, there is a profound decrease of DHEA(S) correlated with age ([20], Figure 5). DHEA(S) means DHEA itself, that is the unconjugated form in a few ng/ml concentration, and DHEAS, its ester-sulfate form, principally of adrenal secretion origin and ~ 500 times more abundant. In men older than 60 years of age, normal values still are in the µg/ml range. Both forms are decreased in aging. As indicated in Figure 6, DHEAS has to be hydrolyzed to become DHEA which itself is metabolized to testosterone. From pharmacokinetic studies of DHEA replacement administration in which 25 mg or 50 mg/d of DHEA were orally administered, we found that circulating DHEA's half-size life is much longer when it is given orally than after intravenous injection of (radioactive) DHEA. Circulating DHEA after oral administration in fact derives from both DHEA which has escaped from hepatic and gut sulfation and from hydrolysis of newly formed DHEAS [21]. While oral 50 mg DHEA restores testosterone level in aging women to "young" values, the increase (~ 1 ng/ml as indicated above) is not significant in men ([22], Table 3, Figure 7). As testosterone has been shown to induce only modest increases in prostate volume, it is still undetermined whether testosterone-DHT possibly formed in the prostate may be deleterious. However, prostate cancer currently should be considered an absolute contraindication of DHEA supplementation, in light of its properties as an androgen-sensitive tumor.

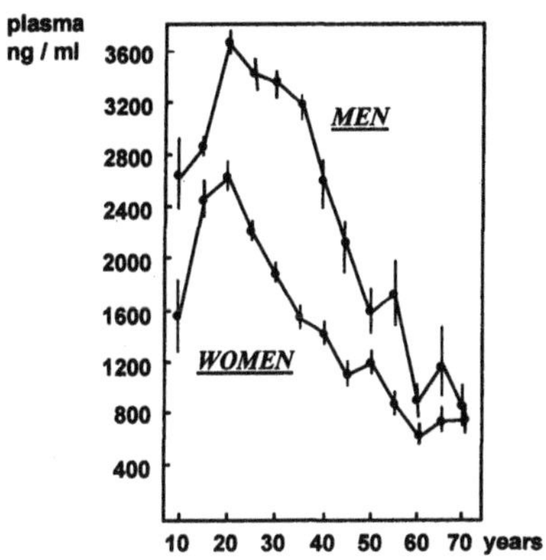

Figure 5. Blood DHEAS and aging [20].

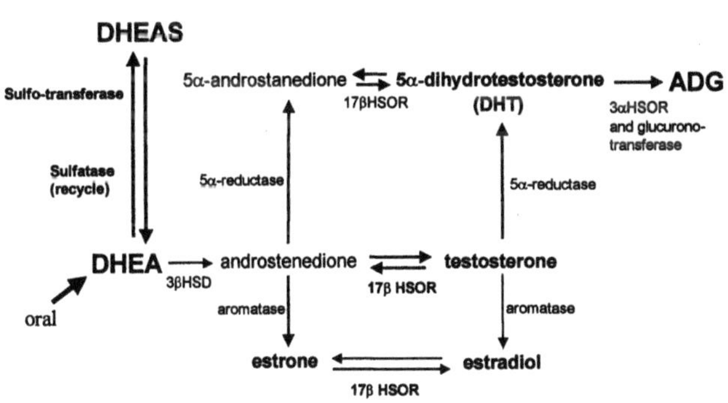

Figure 6. Metabolism of DHEA [21].

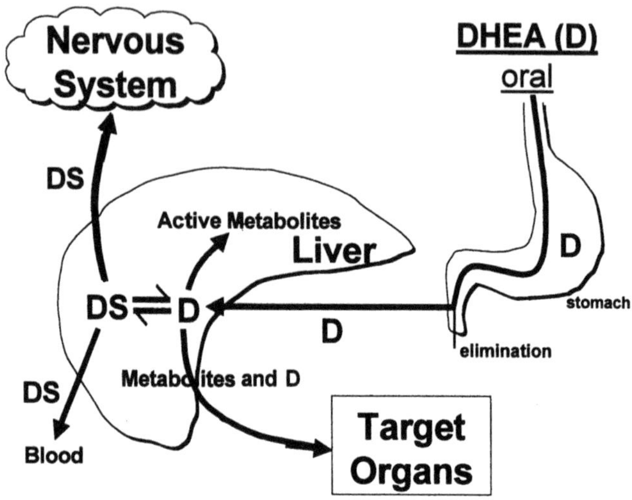

Figure 7. DHEA orally administered. Pathway and metabolism.

Table 3. DHEAge-50mg DHEA, oral. Steroid Studies: Blood Values at M0 and M12 [22].

Group	DHEAS µmol/l		Testo nmol/l		ADG nmol/l		E_2 pmol/l	
	M0	M12	M0	M12	M0	M12	M0	M12
Men < 70								
DHEA	2.9	7.22*	18.4	18.1	14.3	23.4*	71	81*
Placebo	2.65	2.66	20	18.2	15.2	16.2	73	76
Men > 70								
DHEA	2.44	8.98*	19.3	20.7	13.7	35.3*	74	81*
Placebo	2.14	2	19.3	18.6	14	15.1	74	80
Women < 70								
DHEA	2.01	5.24*	1.3	1.6	4.5	20.5*	28	37*
Placebo	2.19	2.11	1.16	1.23	3.9	4.2	27	27
Women > 70								
DHEA	1.66	7.19*	1.09	1.92*	3.3	26.4*	25	35*
Placebo	1.81	1.57	1.17	1.25	3.8	3.9	26	27

A Few Clinically Related Remarks

Aging is not a synchronous process with regard to its different characteristics. It is even more evident clinically than hormonally. The following provides a few comments that may be useful to clinicians who treat aging men.

BRAIN AND MENTAL [see 23-25]

Depression is not uncommon in aging men, associated with decrease of bioavailable testosterone [26], and androgens may have some antidepressant activity. However, there is no well-controlled study of appropriate subgroups versus age and no general recommendation is possible [25], even though DHEA administration may have interesting effects upon depressive states [27]. Slow-wave sleep and growth hormone GH decrease correlatively with age.

Alzheimer's disease is one of the more common and disabling neurodegenerative diseases of the elderly and is much less frequent in aging men than in women. Among the hypotheses formulated thus far to explain the prevalence disparity, there is the marked relative difference in circulating estradiol levels between men and women who enter menopause without hormone replacement. These women undergo a sudden decrease in circulating estrogen when compared to men, whose hormonal levels decrease with a less steep slope. The question is therefore whether estrogen derived from aromatization of circulating androgens is enough to explain this apparent protection of men with respect to women.

LIBIDO

Libido in aging men may be related to excessive decrease of testosterone, though correlation between testosterone levels and libido is weak and libido has been shown to persist for some time after castration. Elevating testosterone levels in the elderly might be required because of decreasing number and affinity of androgen receptors with increasing age, as seen in the aging rat. Due to scarce information, therefore, androgen replacement for libido preservation should be limited initially to a prudent short trial under medical supervision [28].

PROSTATE

Contrary to generally beliefs, there is no definitive evidence for deleterious effects of androgen replacement therapy on prostate [29]. Of course, men under androgen replacement therapy will be followed by repeated digital rectal examination (DRE), prostatic specific antigen measured in the blood (PSA), and transrectal ultrasonography. A specific androgen receptor modulator (SARM) such as 7α-methyl-19nor-testosterone may be of interest to avoid androgenic side effects in prostate [30,31].

BONE

It is very possible that both testosterone [32] and estradiol play a role upon bone metabolism and thus the development of osteoporosis, as suggested ([33], Figure 8). In fact in women, estrogen involvement in bone preservation has been verified by the efficacy of hormone replacement therapy. On the other hand, bone mass evolution depends very much on nutritional conditions and exercise during development. The same may be applied to muscle [34]. Frequently vitamin D deficiency is correlated to decrease of muscular strength.

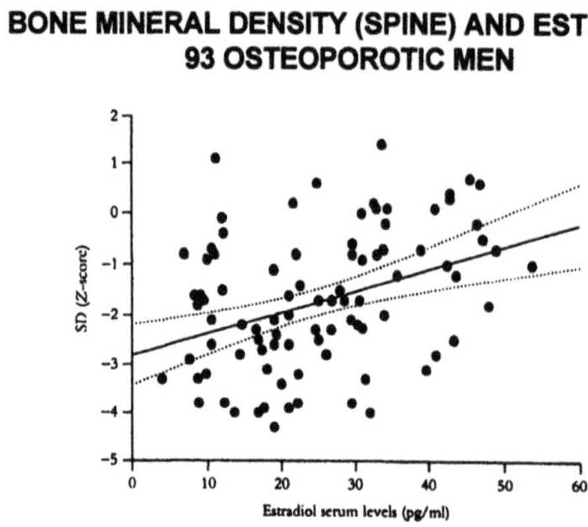

Figure 8. Bone mineral density (spine) and estradiol (93 osteoporotic men) [33].

HEART AND BLOOD VESSELS [35]

Effects of androgens upon blood lipids and the development of atheromatosis are still disputable. In spite of the higher frequency of cardiovascular events in men than in women during the reproductive years, epidemiological data show an inverse correlation between testosterone levels and atherogenic lipid profile, including a reduction in Lp(a) and an increase in insulin sensitivity. Testosterone levels, however, do not appear correlated with cardiovascular event risk. On the other hand, supraphysiological levels of androgens have been proven atherogenic and may lead to a cardiovascular pathological event. Some trials using testosterone intra-arterially have been based on studies such as that of Philipps et al. [36, Figure 9].

TREATMENT [37,38].

Uncertainties concerning the beneficial and safe use of testosterone remain [39,40]. The question is whether to prevent or to repair. However the subsequent question of what to prevent must also be asked: body composition variations, the compromising of bone status, brain degeneration and mental decline, loss of libido and impairment of sexual activity? Clearly, these targets have to be defined qualitatively and quantitatively at the clinical and biological levels, and this is globally more difficult than in women ([28], Table 4). Possible help may come from advice on better behavior, diet, and environmental conditions (psycho-social in most cases), and from the administration of hormones which is most often the least important component.

Transdermal administration of testosterone avoids the hepatic first-pass effect and may create less polycythemia than oral administration. Interestingly, patches of testosterone permit reestablishment of a nycthemeral cycle.

Orally administered DHEA has not proved to be successful when given at the dose (possibly insufficient) of 50 mg/day to healthy men of 60-80 years [41]. However higher doses should be (prudently) studied as well as the possible effects on men ≥ 80 years old A recent impressive report by Mazat et al. ([42], Table 5) showed significant correlation between mortality and low DHEAS levels in 65-70 year-old men, which opens the discussion to the potential advantage of DHEAS administration (generally at a dose in the order of 50 mg), at least in men of this age and DHEAS levels and under medical supervision (see also discussion in the PNAS commentary by S.S.C. Yen [43]).

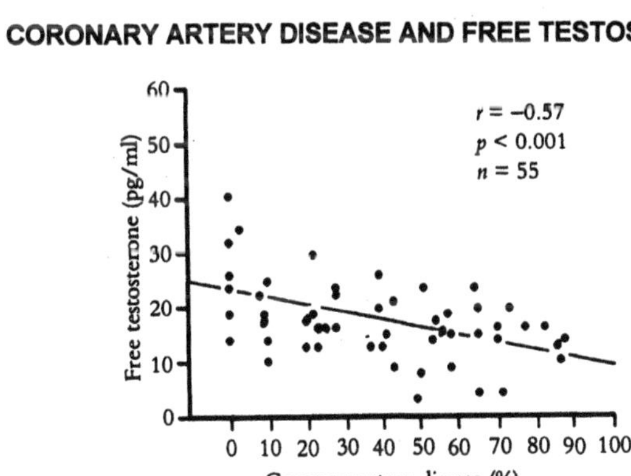

Figure 9. Coronary artery disease and free testosterone [36].

Table 4. Positive and Negative Effects of Testosterone Replacement in Older Males [28]

Postive effects	Negative effects
Enhanced libido	Increased hematocrit
Increased muscle mass	Worsening sleep apnea
Increased strength	Gynecomastia
Increased bone mineral density	Water retention
Decreased fat mass	Effects on prostate cancer
Decreased leptin	
Increased cognition	
Coronary artery vasodilatation	

Evidence-based intervention has to be positioned against anti-aging entrepreneurs who peddle DHEA, testosterone, and growth hormones at random. It remains that the disequilibrium in aging men between the unchanged level of plasma cortisol and the profound decrease of testosterone and DHEA(S) (Table 6, see also the comments on abdominal obesity of Marin and Arver, [44]) suggests that cautious studies are still indicated to try to counter this unbalanced hormonal situation effectively and safely [see also 45 and 40].

Table 5. Relative Risk of Death at Year 10 [42]

Health Parameters	Univariate analysis		
	RR	IC 95%	p
DHEAS level			
Low versus high	1.9	(1.2-2.8)	0.003
Tobacco consumption			
Smoker versus nonsmoker	2.1	(1.1-4.1)	0.03
Former smoker versus no smoker	1.7	(1.0-2.7)	0.04
Subjective health			
Poor versus good	1.5	(1.0-2.3)	0.04
Medications			
2-4 versus 0-1 medications	1.5	(0.7-3.4)	0.3
5 and more versus 0-1 medications	3.0	(1.4-6.3)	0.005

Table 6. Aging Men: Excess Cortisol, Decreased Androgen Related Symptoms

Aging Men: Excess Cortisol, Decreased Androgen Related Symptoms
Decrease musculo-skeletal skin
Increase adipose deposition
Diabetes. Insulin resistance
Impaired memory
Immuno deficit
Hypertension. Atheromatosis
Decreased facial hair growth
Decreased libido
Sexual dysfunction

References

1. Tenover JS, McLachlan RI, Dahl KD, Burger HG, de Kretser DM, Bremner WJ. Decreased serum inhibin levels in normal elderly men: Evidence for a decline in Sertoli cell function with aging. J Clin Endocrinol Metab 1988;67:455-59.
2. Vermeulen A, Deslypere JP. Testicular endocrine function in the ageing male. Maturitas 1985;7:273-79.
3. Nieschlag E, Lammers U, Freischem CW, Langer K, Wickings EJ. Reproductive functions in young fathers and grandfathers. J Clin Endocrinol Metab 1982;55:676-81.
4. Bauer J. The male climacteric: A misnomer. JAMA Dec. 2, 1944, Correspondence.
5. McKinlay JB, Longcope C, Gray A. The questionable physiologic and epidemiologic basis for a male climacteric syndrome: Preliminary results from the Massachusetts Male Aging Study. Maturitas 1989:11:103-15.
6. Werner AA. The male climacteric. JAMA 1946;132:188-94.
7. Vermeulen A, Goemaere S, Kaufman JM. Sex hormones, body composition and aging. The Aging Male 1999;2:8-15.
8. Morley JE, Kaiser FE, Perry HL III, et al. Longitudinal changes in testosterone, luteinizing hormone, and follicle-stimulating hormone in healthy older men. Metabolism 1997;46: 410-13.
9. Morley JE, Kaiser FE, Raum, WJ, et al. Potentially predictive and manipulable blood serum correlates of aging in the healthy human male: Progressive decreases in bioavailable testosterone, dehydroepiandrosterone sulfate, and the ration of insulin-like growth factor 1 to growth hormone. Proc Natl Acad Sci USA 1997;94:7537-42.
10. Veldhuis JD, Urban RJ, Lizarralde G, Johnson ML, Iranmanesh A. Attenuation of luteinizing hormone secretory burst amplitude as a proximate basis for the hypoandrogenism of healthy aging in men. J Clin Endocrinol Metab 1992;75:707-13.

11. Winters SJ, Troen P. Episodic luteinizing hormone (LH) secretion and the response of LH and follicle-stimulating hormone to LH-releasing hormone in aged men: Evidence for coexistent primary testicular insufficiency and an impairment in gonadotropin secretion. J Clin Endocrinol Metab 1982;55:560-65.
12. Bremner WJ, Vitiello MV, Prinz PN. Loss of circadian rhythmicity in blood testosterone levels with aging in normal men. J Clin Endocrinol Metab 1983;56:1278-81.
13. Seidman SN, Walsh BT. Testosterone and depression in aging men. Am J Geriatr Psychiatry 1999;7:18-33.
14. Heinemann LAJ, Zimmermann T, Vermeulen A, Thiel C, Hummel W. A new "aging males' symptoms" rating scale. The Aging Male 1999;2:105-14.
15. Mercier-Bodard C, Alfsen A, Baulieu EE. Sex steroid binding plasma protein (SBP). Acta Endocrinologica 1970;64:204-24.
16. Tremblay RR, Massé J. Usefulness and limitation of bioavailable testosterone in assessment of androgenicity during the process of aging in men. The Aging Male 1999;2: 16-21.
17. Vermeulen A, Kaufman JM, Giagulli VA. Influence of some biological indexes on sex hormone-binding globulin and androgen levels in aging or obese males. J Clin Endocrinol Metab 1996;81:1821-26.
18. Baulieu EE, Mauvais-Jarvis P. Studies on testosterone metabolism. I Conversion of testosterone-17α^3H to 5α and 5β androstane-3α, 17βdiol-17α^3H: A new "17β-hydroxyl pathway." J Biol Chem 1964;239:1569-77.
19. Krithivas K, Yurgalevitch SM, Mohr BA, et al. Evidence that the CAG repeat in the androgen receptor gene is associated with the age-related decline in serum androgen levels in men. J Endocrinol 1999;162:137-42.
20. Orentreich N, Brind JL, Rizer RL, Vogelman JH. Age changes and sex differences in serum dehydroepiandrosterone sulfate concentrations throughout adulthood. J Clin Endocrinol Metab 1984;17:1051-62.
21. Legrain S, Massien C, Lahlou N, et al. Dehydroepiandrosterone replacement administration: Pharmacokinetic and pharmacodynamic studies in healthy elderly subjects. J Clin Endocrinol Metab 2000;85:3208-17.
22. Baulieu EE, Thomas G, Legrain S, et al. Dehydroepiandrosterone (DHEA), DHEA sulfate, and aging: Contribution of the DHEAge Study to a sociobiomedical issue. Proc Natl Acad Sci USA 2000;97:4279-84.
23. Janowsky JS, Oviatt SK, Orwoll ES. Testosterone influences spatial cognition in older men. Behav Neurosci 1994;108:325-32.
24. Rubinow DR, Schmidt PJ. Androgens, brain, and behavior. Am J Psychiatry 1996;153: 974-84.
25. Sternbach H. Age-associated testosterone decline in men: Clinical issues for psychiatry. Am J Psychiatry 1998;155:1310-18.
26. Barrett-Connor E, von Mühlen DG, Kritz-Silverstein D. Bioavailable testosterone and depressed mood in older men: The Rancho Bernardo study. J Clin Endocrinol Metab 1999: 84:573-77.
27. Wolkowitz OM, Reus VI, Roberts E, et al. Dehydroepiandrosterone (DHEA) treatment of depression. Biol Psychiatry 1997;41:311-18.
28. Morley JE. Erectile dysfunction in senescence: Treatment options. In: M. Filicori, editor. Endocrine basis of reproductive function. Bologna, Italy: Monduzzi Editori, 2000; 537-50.

29. Behre HM, Nieschlag E. Testosterone treatment and the prostate. In: M. Filicori, editor. Endocrine basis of reproductive function. Bologna, Italy: Monduzzi Editori, 2000:579-86.
30. Bardin CW, Swerdloff RS, Santen RJ. Androgens: Risks and benefits. J Clin Endocrinol Metab 1991;73:4-7.
31. Cummings DE, Kumar N, Bardin CW, Sundaram K, Bremner WJ. Prostate-sparing effects in primates of the potent androgen 7α-methyl-19-nortestosterone: A potential alternative to testosterone for androgen replacement and male contraception. J Clin Endocrinol Metab 1998;83:4212-19.
32. Vanderschueren D, Vandenput L, Boonen S, Van Herck E, Swinnen JV, Bouillon R. An aged rat model of partial androgen deficiency: Prevention of both loss of bone and lean body mass by low-dose androgen replacement. Endocrinology 2000;141:1642-47.
33. Kudlacek S, Resch H, Pietschmann P, Willvonseder R. Hormones and osteoporosis in the aging male. The Aging Male 1999;2:145-50.
34. Baumgartner RN, Waters DL, Gallagher D, Morley JE, Garry PJ. Predictors of skeletal muscle mass in elderly men and women. Mechanisms of Ageing and Development 1998; 107:123-36.
35. Crook D. Androgen therapies and the risk of cardiovascular disease. In: M. Filicori, editor. Endocrine basis of reproductive function. Bologna, Italy: Monduzzi Editori, 2000;569-77.
36. Phillips GB, Pinkernell BH, Jing T-Y. The association of hypotestosteronemia with coronary artery disease in men. Arterioscler Thromb 1994;14:701-6.
37. Lunenfeld B. Hormone replacement therapy in the aging male. The Aging Male 1999;2:1-5.
38. Snyder PJ, Peachey H, Hannoush P, et al. Treatment of elderly men with testosterone. In: M. Filicori, editor. Endocrine basis of reproductive function. 2000;587-605.
39. Tenover JS. Effects of testosterone supplementation in the aging male. J Clin Endocrinol Metab 1992;75:1092-98.
40. Sih R, Morley JE, Kaiser FE, Perry HM III, Patrick P, Ross C. Testosterone replacement in older hypogonadal men: A 12-month randomized controlled trial. J Clin Endocrinol Metab 1997;82:1661-67.
41. Vermeulen, A. The future of hormone replacement therapy in the aging male. The Aging Male 2000;3:210-13.
42. Mazat L, Lafont S, Berr C, et al. Prospective measurements of dehydroepiandrosterone sulfate in a cohort of elderly subjects: Relationship to gender, subjective health, smoking habits, and 10-year mortality. Proc Natl Acad Sci USA 2001;98:8145-50.
43. Yen SCC. Dehydroepiandrosterone sulfate and longevity: New clues for an old friend. Commentary. Proc Natl Acad Sci USA 2001;98:8167-69.
44. Marin P, Arver S. Androgens and abdominal obesity. Baillières Clin Endocrinol Metab 1998;12:441-51.
45. Gooren LJG. Male reproductive health: What are the issues? In: M. Filicori, editor. Endocrine basis of reproductive function. Bologna, Italy: Monduzzi Editori, 2000;491-524.

MECHANISMS OF ESTROGEN REGULATION OF BONE TURNOVER AND BONE MASS

B. Lawrence Riggs

Introduction

Although the association of estrogen (E) deficiency with postmenopausal bone loss and osteoporosis has been appreciated for over 40 years, the mechanisms by which estrogen preserves bone mass have not been clear. However, over the last decade, there has been an enormous increase in our understanding of the mechanisms by which this occurs. E action on bone can be understood at several different levels of organization. In this paper, we will discuss E action on bone and calcium metabolism at the organ, tissue, cellular, and molecular levels.

Action of Estrogen at the Organ Level

At the organ level the principal action of E is to conserve and maintain bone mass. Indeed E and biomechanical strain are the main physiological determinants of bone mass. A deficiency of either of these determinants will lead to severe bone loss, whereas the effects of a deficiency in other calcitrophic hormones (such as parathyroid hormone, vitamin D metabolites, calcitonin, or glucocorticoids) have effects on bone that are much more modest.

Action of Estrogen at the Tissue Level

At the tissue level, E acts on the skeleton both directly and indirectly through effects on extraskeletal calcium homeostasis. See Riggs et al. [1] for details and for complete reference.

DIRECT SKELETAL EFFECTS

Direct effects are mediated through high affinity estrogen receptors (ERs) in osteoblasts and osteoclasts. Bone cells contain both the ERα and ERβ species. The overall effects of E on the skeleton are to tonically suppress bone turnover and to maintain balanced rates of bone formation and bone resorption [2]. At menopause, the withdrawal of the restraining effects of E on bone cell function, leads to a large increase in bone turnover. Bone resorption increases more than bone formation does. In a population study of 653 French women, Garnero et al. [3] found that bone formation markers increased by about 45% and bone resorption markers increased by about 90%. This large remodeling imbalance leads to a rapid phase of bone loss that gradually declines over 4 to 8 years to become asymptotic with a subsequent slow phase of bone loss that persists indefinitely [1]. Perhaps because of its greater surface-to-volume ratio, this rapid phase of bone loss is associated with an excessively high rate of cancellous bone loss whereas the parallel rate of cortical bone loss is much smaller. For example, in a two-year longitudinal study of bone loss after elective ovariectomy in perimenopausal women, Genant [4] found losses of 18% in cancellous bone by quantitative computed tomography, but only 4% in cortical bone by single photon absorptiometry. The reasons for the limited duration of this early postmenopausal, rapid loss phase are unclear. Possibly, when the amount of cancellous bone falls below some critical value, biomechanical factors act to limit the rate of further bone loss.

Indirect Skeletal Effects

These are largely responsible for the late, slow phase of bone loss in elderly women. In contrast to the rapid phase of bone loss in which a large outflow of calcium from bone enlarges the miscible pool and partially suppresses parathyroid function, the subsequent slow phase of bone loss is associated with external calcium wasting and with progressive secondary hyperparathyroidism. This is caused by the loss of effects of estrogen on extraskeletal calcium homeostasis. E acts directly on the intestine through E receptors [5] to enhance calcium absorption [6]. E also acts on the kidney to increase renal tubular calcium absorption and, thus, to maintain renal calcium homeostasis [7]. When E is deficient, the loss of these actions leads to external calcium wasting, which unless made up by large increases in calcium intake, leads to progressive secondary hyperparathyroidism and to increased bone resorption. This is associated with a decrease in bone formation, due, at least in part, to E deficiency. Thus, there is continued high bone turnover and remodeling imbalance leading to the slow bone loss that continues indefinitely. In this phase similar amounts of cortical and cancellous bone are lost.

Action of Estrogen at the Cellular Level

As originally pointed out by Frost [8], the activities of osteoclasts and osteoblasts are combined into functional assemblies called basic multicellular units (BMUs). A remodeling cycle begins with formation of a new BMU on a previously inactive surface of bone. The lining cells disappear and are replaced by multinucleated osteoclasts that construct a resorption lacunae on the endosteal surface of bone over a two-week interval. The resorption phase then is terminated, probably by osteoclast apoptosis, and, after a brief reversal phase, a team of osteoblasts is recruited that fill in the resorption cavity with new bone. In cortical bone, osteoclasts form the leading edge of a cutting cone that creates a resorption tunnel, and osteoblasts follow in their wake to convert it into a structural osteon (Haversian system). This sequence is shown schematically in the cartoon in Figure 1. (For reviews see Parfitt [9] and Manolagas [2])

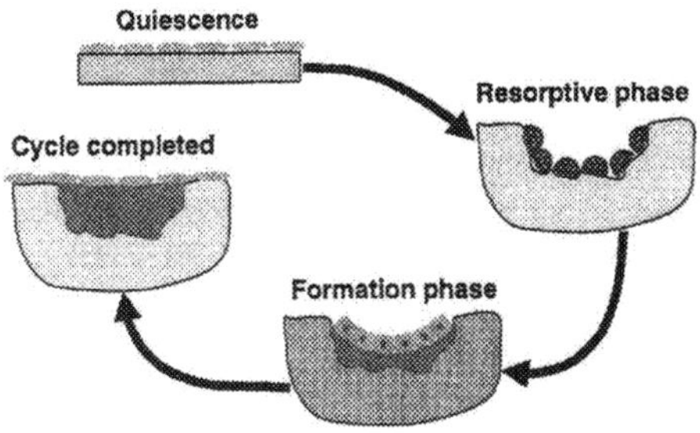

Figure 1. Cartoon demonstrating bone remodeling cycle at the level of the BMU. The resorption phase is mediated by osteoclasts that construct a resorption cavity. This is followed by a formation phase that refills the cavity with new bone. A remodeling imbalance leading to bone loss will occur if the cavity constructed by the osteoclasts is too deep, if the osteoblasts fail to refill it, or if both occur. If a remodeling imbalance exists, an increase in bone turnover (there are more BMUs) will exacerbate the rate of bone loss.

E acts to decrease osteoclast formation and activity and, by increasing apoptosis, it decreases osteoclast lifespan [10]. Controversy exists about the action of E on osteoblasts. Some evidence suggests that E increases osteoblast formation, differentiation, proliferation, and function, although results have varied among different model systems. Recently, two groups [11,2] have demonstrated that E antagonizes osteoblast apoptosis and, thus, extends osteoblast lifespan. Perhaps the strongest evidence for a direct effect of E on increasing bone formation were provided by Khastgir et al. [12] and by Tobias and Compston [13] who demonstrated large increases in cancellous bone volume and in wall thickness of trabecular packets in biopsy samples from elderly women after 6 years of percutaneous administration of high dosages of E. Whether these represent only pharmacologic effects or whether they represent an augmentation of physiologic effects of E that are insufficiently large to detect is unclear.

E deficiency affects remodeling in two ways. First, it increases the activation frequency ("birth rate") of BMUs, which leads to higher bone turnover. Second, it induces a remodeling imbalance by prolonging the resorption phase (osteoclast apoptosis is reduced [10]) and shortening the formation phase (osteoblast apoptosis is increased [2]). Also, increased osteoclast recruitment extends the progression of the BMU. As a consequence of these changes, the volume of the resorption cavity is increased beyond the capacity of the osteoblasts to refill it [9]. In cancellous bone, the extended osteoclast life span increases resorption depth leading to trabecular plate perforation and loss of trabecular connectivity [9,14]. In cortical bone, the rapid phase is associated with subendocortical cavitation and, eventually, the inner third of the cortex may assume cancellous-like characteristics [9]. When a remodeling imbalance exists, high bone turnover will exacerbate bone loss. In contrast to the osteoclast-mediated disruption of the cancellous bone microarchitecture during the rapid phase, the subsequent slow phase of bone loss is characterized by trabecular thinning in which impaired osteoblast activity plays a prominent causal role [9].

Action of Estrogen at the Molecular Level

Cytokines responsible for the paracrine regulation of bone resorption by estrogen can be grouped as being "upstream" and "downstream." Early studies focused on the role of E deficiency in increasing the production in bone of the upstream cytokines — interleukin-1 (IL-1), IL-6, tumor necrosis factor-α (TNFα), granulocyte-macrophage colony-stimulating factor, macrophage colony-stimulating factor (M-CSF), and prostaglandin-E_2 (PGE_2). These cytokines increase bone resorption, mainly by increasing the pool size of pre-osteoclasts in bone marrow. Moreover, in contrast to the downstream cytokines, ablation or overexpression of their genes do not result in the extremes of changes in bone mass — osteoporosis and osteopetrosis. Moreover, ovariectomy (OVX)-induced increases in osteoclastogenesis are attenuated or prevented by measures that impair the synthesis or response to IL-1, IL-6, TNFα or PGE_2. E also upregulates transforming growth factor-β (TGF-β), an inhibitor of bone resorption that acts directly on osteoclasts to decrease their activity and rate of apoptosis.

The downstream cytokines are the final effectors of osteoclast differentiation and function [15,16]. The long sought osteoblast-derived paracrine effector of osteoclast differentiation was identified as the receptor activator of NFκB ligand (RANKL), which is expressed by stromal-osteoblastic lineage cells. Cell-to-cell contact between these cells and osteoclast lineage cells allows RANKL to bind its membrane receptor, RANK, potently stimulating all aspects of osteoclast function; in response to RANKL signaling, osteoclast differentiation and activity increase and osteoclast apoptosis decreases. Indeed, RANKL is both necessary and sufficient for osteoclast formation, provided that permissive concentrations of M-CSF are present. The stromal-osteoblast lineage cells also secrete osteoprotegerin (OPG), a soluble decoy receptor that neutralizes RANKL. E increases OPG and decreases M-CSF and RANK. However, part of its effect on this signaling system may be indirect through E-stimulated intermediaries. Thus, IL-1 and TNFα increase RANKL, OPG, and M-CSF whereas PGE_2 increases RANKL and decreases OPG. E has not yet been shown to regulate RANKL directly. E also blocks the activity of Jun NH_2-terminal kinase (JNK) and the resulting production of c-Jun and JunD in osteoclast lineage cells [16]. Thus, it seems likely that E inhibits bone resorption by inducing small but cumulative changes in multiple E-dependent regulatory factors. These changes are shown schematically in the cartoon of Figure 2.

See Pacifici [17], Manolagas [2], Hofbauer et al. [16], and Riggs [18] for more details and for complete references.

Clinical Correlations

Loss of the actions of E outlined above can satisfactorily explain both the early and the late phases of postmenopausal bone loss in women. At menopause, the acute loss of the restraining effects of E on bone cell activity leads to an accelerated phase of loss of predominantly cancellous bone that decreases after about 4 to 8 years and disappears after about 15 to 20 years when severe depletion of cancellous bone stimulates counter-regulatory forces that limit further loss. The slow phase of bone loss, which also begins at menopause, then becomes dominant. It involves loss of both cancellous and cortical bone and continues throughout the remainder of life. It is caused by the loss of E effects on extraskeletal calcium homeostasis leading to decreased intestinal calcium absorption, increased renal calcium wasting, and, perhaps also, effects on vitamin D metabolism and loss of a direct effect on the parathyroid gland that decreases PTH secretion. These extraskeletal alterations lead to a net loss of calcium from the body that increases the level of dietary calcium intake required to prevent secondary hyperparathyroidism and increased bone turnover. These manifestations can be reversed by either E replacement (which restores extraskeletal calcium fluxes to premenopausal levels) or by large increases in dietary calcium (which offsets the net calcium losses induced by postmenopausal abnormalities in extraskeletal calcium fluxes). An age-related impairment in bone formation also contributes to the slow phase of bone loss and may be caused, at least in part, by the loss of E stimulated synthesis of bone matrix proteins by osteoblasts. However, age-related factors may also contribute to the decrease in bone formation.

See Riggs et al. [1] for details and more complete references. The interaction of these mechanisms is shown in the cartoon in Figure 3.

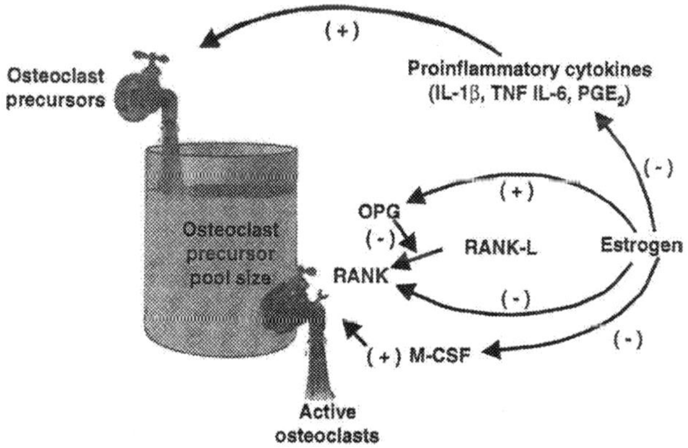

Figure 2. Cartoon illustration of the relationship among various factors regulating osteoclastogenesis. The "upstream" pro-inflammatory cytokines (IL-1β, TNF, IL-6, and PGE_2) act mainly to increase the pool size of osteoclast precursors and this action is inhibited by E. The "downstream" cytokines act to regulate the differentiation to active osteoclasts. This is facilitated by RANK-L and M-CSF. RANK-L acts through its receptor, RANK, on preosteoclasts and this action is inhibited by OPG. E decreases RANK and increases OPG. Thus, the overall action of E is to suppress osteoclast differentiation. Also, but not shown in the cartoon, E decreases osteoclast activity and decreases osteoclast life span by increasing osteoclast apoptosis.

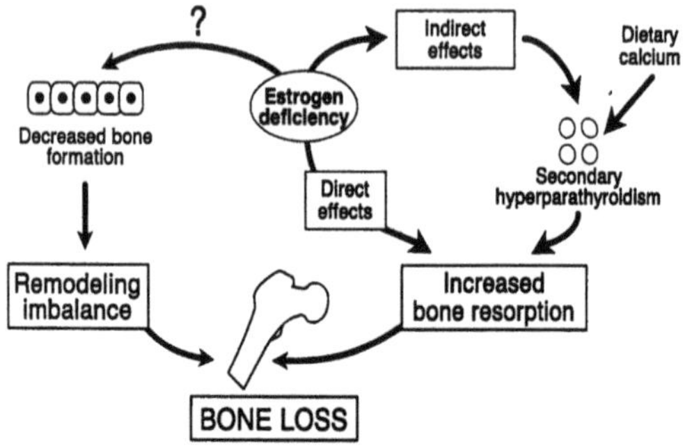

Figure 3. Schematic representation of the mechanisms by which E deficiency leads to bone loss. See text for details. With permssion, J Bone Miner Res 13:763-773, 1998.

Summary and Conclusions

E conserves bone mass by restraining bone turnover and maintaining the balance between bone resorption and bone formation. E acts on the skeleton both directly through high affinity ER in osteoblasts and osteoclasts and indirectly by enhancing intestinal calcium absorption and renal calcium conservation. E enhances bone formation by increasing osteoblast function and decreasing apoptosis. E decreases bone resorption by restraining osteoclastogenesis and osteoclast action and by increasing osteoclast apoptosis. These actions are both direct and indirect. Paracrine effects of a number of cytokines elaborated by bone marrow cells mediate the indirect actions. The surprising complexity of E action on bone can be explained by its linkage to reproductive mechanisms that are critical to fetal and neonatal survival.

References

1. Riggs BL, Khosla S, Melton LJ III. A unitary model for involutional osteoporosis: Estrogen deficiency causes both type I and type II osteoporosis in postmenopausal women and contributes to bone loss in aging men. J Bone Miner Res 1998;13:763-73.
2. Manolagas SC. Birth and death of bone cells: Basic regulatory mechanisms and implications for the pathogenesis and treatment of osteoporosis. Endocr Rev 2000;21:115-37.
3. Garnero P, Sornay-Rendu E, Choppy M, Delmas PD. Increased bone turnover in late postmenopausal women is a major determinant of osteoporosis. J Bone Miner Res 1996; 11:337-49.
4. Genant HK, Cann CE, Ettinger B, Gordan GS. Quantitative computed tomography of vertebral spongiosa: A sensitive method for detecting early bone loss after oophorectomy. Ann Intern Med 1982;97:699-705.
5. Arjmandi BH, Salih MA, Herbert DC, Sims SH, Kalu DN. Evidence for estrogen receptor-linked caclium transport in the intestine. Bone Miner 1993;21:63-74.

6. Gennari C, Agnusdei D, Nardi P, Civitelli R. Estrogen preserves a normal intestinal responsiveness to 1,25-dihydroxyvitamin D_3 in oophorectomized women. J Clin Endocrinol Metab 1990;71:1288-93.
7. McKane WR, Khosla S, Burritt MF, et al. Mechanism of renal calcium conservation with estrogen replacement therapy in women in early postmenopause - a clinical research center study. J Clin Endocrinol Metab 1995;80:3458-64.
8. Frost HM. Bone dynamics in metabolic bone disease. J Bone Joint Surg 1966;48:1192-1203.
9. Parfitt AM. Skeletal heterogeneity and the purposes of bone remodeling implications for the understanding of osteoporosis. In: Marcus R, Feldman D, Kelsey J, editors. Osteoporosis. 2nd Edition. San Diego: Academic Press, in press.
10. Hughes DE, Dai A, Tiffee JC, Li HH, Mundy GR, Boyce BF. Estrogen promotes apoptosis of murine osteoclasts mediated by TGF-β. Nat Med 1996;2:1132-36.
11. Gohel A, McCarthy M-B, Gronowicz G. Estrogen prevents glucocorticoid-induced apoptosis in osteoblasts in vivo and in vitro. Endocrinology 1999;140:5339-47.
12. Khastgir G, Studd J, Holland N, Alaghband-Zadah J, Fox S, Chow J. Anabolic effect of estrogen replacement on bone in postmenopausal women with osteoporosis: Histomorphometric evidence in a longitudinal study. J Clin Endocrinol Metab 2001;86: 289-95.
13. Tobias JH, Compston JE. Does estrogen stimulate osteoblast function in postmenopausal women? Bone 1999;24:121-24.
14. Eriksen EF, Landgahl B, Vesterby A, Rungby J, Kassem M. Hormone replacement therapy prevents osteoclastic hyperactivity: A histomorphometric study in early postmenopausal women. J Bone Miner Res 1999;14:1217-21.
15. Suda T, Takahashi N, Udagawa N, Jimi E, Gillespie MT, Martin TJ. Modulation of osteoclast differentiation and function by the new members of the tumor necrosis factor receptor and ligand families. Endocr Rev 1999;20:345-57.
16. Hofbauer LC, Khosla S, Dunstan CR, Lacey DL, Boyle WJ, Riggs BL. The roles of osteoprotegerin and osteoprotegerin ligand in the paracrine regulation of bone resorption. J Bone Miner Res 2000;15:2-12.
17. Pacifici R. Estrogen, Cytokines, and pathogenesis of postmenopausal osteoporosis. J Bone Miner Res 1996;11:1043-51.
18. Riggs BL. The mechanisms of estrogen regulation of bone resorption. J Clin Invest 2000; 106:1203-4.

GENETICS OF OSTEOPOROSIS

Luigi Gennari, Lucia Becherini, Alberto Falchetti, Laura Masi, and Maria Luisa Brandi.

Introduction

Osteoporosis (OP) is the most prevalent metabolic bone disease among developed countries and it is defined as a systemic skeletal disease characterized by low bone mass and microarchitectural deterioration of bone tissue with a consequent increase in bone fragility and susceptibility to nontraumatic fracture [1]. OP recognizes a complex multifactorial pathogenesis. Although there are several environmental influences on bone mineral density (BMD), such as diet (calcium intake, alcohol consumption) and lifestyle factors (smoking and physical exercise), a genetic contribution to the pathogenesis of OP, accounting from 50% to 80% of the inter-individual variability in bone mass, has been recognized [2]. In rare instances, OP could be inherited in a simple Mendelian manner. Examples of this include familial osteoporotic syndromes due to mutations in the aromatase gene and estrogen receptor alpha (ERα) gene [3,4]. Families have also been described in which high bone mass is inherited as an autosomal dominant trait, consistent with the effect of a single gene located on chromosome 11 [5]. However, except for these rare conditions, OP has to be considered a multifactorial disease in which genetic determinants are modulated by hormonal, environmental, and nutritional factors. Most multifactorial diseases showing a clear genetic component, including OP, are often called "polygenic" diseases, to emphasise their determination by multiple genetic factors. Given the complex biology of the skeleton it is likely that bone mass is under the control of a large number of genes, many of which exert relatively small effects on BMD (minor genes) whereas a few contribute substantially to variation in this trait (major genes). It is also likely that complex gene-environment interactions exist. There are many candidate genes implicated in the determination of BMD and in the pathogenesis of OP, ranging from those encoding for cytokines to those encoding for calciotropic hormones, for their receptors, and for matrix bone proteins. A list of possible candidate genes for OP is reported in Table 1. Possibly the same osteoporotic phenotype could be the result of different genetic and/or environmental interaction. It is also possible that some individuals having one or more predisposing alleles and thus genetically at risk for OP, never became osteoporotic (incomplete penetrance), or, conversely, that individuals with no predisposing alleles may develop OP with age, due to nongenetic factors (phenocopy).

Table 1. Potential Candidate Genes for Osteoporosis

Candidate Genes for Osteoporosis
Adhesions molecules and ligands (i.e. integrins)
Bone matrix proteins
- Collagenic
- Non-collagenic
Calciotropic Hormones and Their Receptors
- Calcitonin and Calcitonin Receptor
- Vitamin D and Vitamin D Receptor
- PTH and PTH Receptors
- Calcium Sensing Receptor
Cytokines, Growth Factors, and Their Receptors (IL-6, IL-1, IGF-I, etc.)
Enzymatic Metabolic Pathways (Aromatase, Metalloproteinases, etc.)
Sex Hormones and Their Receptors
- Androgen and Androgen Receptor
- Estrogen and Estrogen receptors

In the past years, several epidemiological and clinical observations have underlined the importance of genetics in the pathogenesis of OP. First of all, there is the existence of racial differences in bone mineral density and bone turnover: black women shows higher mean BMD values at different skeletal sites with respect of white women with the same age and similar weight, height, calcium intake, and physical activity level [6-8]. Such a difference in bone mass is associated with a higher prevalence of OP in white than in black women. Similarly, different BMD values have been observed between Polynesian and European populations [9]. These variations in the incidence of OP between ethnic and racial groups may relate to environmental factors, but may also reflect inherited differences in susceptibility. Family studies also confirmed the existence of a genetic contribution in OP, showing a correlation in BMD values between mothers and daughters, particularly at the lumbar spine [10,11]. If compared to age-matched women, daughters of women with OP have a reduced bone mineral content and an higher risk of fracture after menopause [10]. Moreover, several epidemiological studies confirmed the importance of a positive family history of OP as a risk factor for the development of osteoporotic fractures [11-15]. Finally twin pairs have been successfully used in human quantitative genetics of several diseases including OP. The comparative analysis of intra-pair differences between monozygote and dizygote twins (in terms of concordance and discordance) might be useful in evaluating the genetic and environmental contribution on bone mass, with the possibility of measuring how much phenotypic variance is caused by the environment. While in dizygote twins (who share 50% of genes) intra-pair BMD differences may be due both to genetic and environmental factors, in monozygote twins (who share 100% of genes) intra-pair BMD differences are exclusively due to environmental factors. Twin data are usually expressed in terms of concordance. In practice the demonstration of a genetic component for a given disease, through twin pairs analysis, is based on the following criteria: 1) if a trait (or a disease) is "totally due to genetic factors" then 100% monozygote twin pairs will be concordant for this trait or they will both lack it, while 50% dizygote twin pairs (sharing 50% of genes) will be concordant for this trait; 2) if a trait is "not genetically determined" the concordance between monozygote and dyzigote twin pairs will be similar and significantly lower than 100%; and 3) if a trait is "multifactorial", with an important genetic component, monozygote twin pairs will be concordant more than dyzygote twin pair, even though for less than 100%. Recently results from several twin studies demonstrated a higher concordance in bone mass and serum osteocalcin levels in monozygote twin pairs with respect to dizygotes, underlying a relevant genetic influence on bone metabolism [2]. Other twin studies showed similar high degree of heritability for other bone parameters such as quantitative ultrasound and bone geometry [16-18]. Since the monozygotic twin pair concordance in BMD values is lower than 100%, it appears that the interaction of genetic and environmental factors causes OP. Such a model of disease is called "threshold model" and presumes a continuously distributed and genetically determined susceptibility for the disease. Just a part of the individuals above a given "threshold" will became osteoporotic, expecially if exposed to appropriate environmental influences. Possibly, these promoting environmental factors might have a particularly increased effect in those individuals genetically predisposed for the disease. The genetic effect on bone may also be site-specific, with different genes regulating bone density at different skeletal sites. Moreover, the possibility that a significant part of the heritability of bone mass is related to shared genetic contributions to skeletal size and body composition, cannot be excluded.

The main strategies commonly employed for identification and characterization of genes that are involved in the pathogenesis of complex disorders like OP are linkage analysis in multigeneration pedigrees, allele sharing methods in sib-pairs, association studies in unrelated affected and not affected subjects, and experimental crosses in animals [19]. In practice, all of these approaches search for evidence of an association between a phenotypic disease characteristic and a series of polymorphic genetic markers. With regard to OP, the two main phenotypic characteristics are low BMD and fracture. While the former is a quantitative continuous trait, the latter is a qualitative categorical variable. Recently few genetic linkage studies and a consistent number of candidate-gene association studies have identified several loci and genes that appear to be involved in the regulation of bone mass and the pathogenesis of osteoporotic fractures [20-22].

Candidate Genes Association Studies

To date, most efforts toward understanding the genetic determinants of BMD and osteoporotic risk have largely relied on population-based case-control association studies of genes known to be involved in bone metabolism. By this approach positive and negative associations have been reported for several candidate genes but the individual contribution of these genes to the pathogenesis of OP is still controversial [20-22]. Conflicting results may relate to major pitfalls of association studies in late onset disorders like OP, mainly due to inappropriate choice of the control group, to population admixture, and to competing risk leading to selection bias [23]. Moreover, a positive association can arise for 3 reasons: 1) a given allele is effectively a cause of the disease; 2) a given allele does no cause the trait but is in linkage disequilibrium with the actual cause; and 3) the results are artifacts of population admixture.

VITAMIN D RECEPTOR GENE STUDIES

Among the several candidate genes, the gene encoding for the vitamin D receptor (VDR) was the first to be proposed as a major locus for the genetic effect on bone mass. The VDR gene possess several polymorphic sites, whose the one detected by the restriction endonuclease *Bsm I* in intron 8 was associated with BMD in the Australian population [24]. After this original report, conflicting data have been published on the association of the diallelic *Bsm I* RFLP in the VDR gene and BMD both in premenopausal and postmenopausal women [20-22]. Similarly, studies examining the relationship of this polymorphism with skeletal growth, bone turnover markers, rates of bone loss, intestinal calcium absorption, and osteoporotic fractures yielded conflicting results. A meta-analytical approach, incorporating the results from 16 studies revealed a weak contribution of the allelic variant at the 3' end of the gene on the variation of BMD values [25], while a more recent meta-analysis concluded that BMD associates to VDR polymorphisms at high confidence levels and both genetic and nongenetic factors can interfere with the unmasking of the effects of VDR gene variants on bone phenotype [26]. There may be several explanations for the discrepancy among these studies. First, interactions of environmental factors such as dietary calcium intake appeared to represent an important confounding factor in VDR polymorphism analysis [20,27-29]. Moreover, linkage disequilibrium with other bone metabolism-related genes on chromosome 12 (i.e. collagen type 1 and retinoic acid receptor genes) cannot be excluded. Finally, the limited size of samples, differences in genotype distribution among different ethnic groups and interactions with other genes, all have to be considered as potential confounders. Other polymorphic genes, such as the one encoding for ERα, have been shown to modulate VDR gene effect in the determination of BMD, confirming the existence of gene-gene interaction [30]. All together, these findings may contribute to explaining contradictory data among published studies, suggesting the possibility of modifying the genetically determined BMD through appropriate lifestyle changes. However, polymorphisms at the 3'end of VDR gene are anonymous polymorphisms, as they do not code for different aminoacids in the VDR protein. Therefore, a major question is how these allelic differences may be related to functional differences in VDR activity. An alternative hypothesis is that these 3'-end polymorphisms affect VDR gene transcription and/or mRNA stability, as suggested by Morrison et al., in their minigene reporter constructs analysis [24]. Moreover, preliminary data revealed an interesting linkage between the VDR 3'-end allelic variants and the differences in the length of a microsatellite poly(A) repeat at the 3'-end untranslated region of the VDR gene, approximately 1kb upstream of the poly(A) tail, a region which is important for mRNA stability [31,32]. Alleles *a*, *b*, and *T* are highly associated with a long length of poly(A) repeats, while alleles *A*, *B*, and *t* are linked to a short poly(A) length. Although it is still not established whether this repeat microsatellite is the functional relevant locus, it has been speculated that by analogy to tandem repeats in other genes, the length of poly(A) may affect mRNA stability. Possibly VDR alleles associated to decreased BMD values and to an higher risk of osteoporosis could be responsible of a decreased number of VDRs due to a reduction in the cellular VDR mRNA levels. To date, however, quantitative PCR analysis on pheripheral blood leucocytes as well as in fibroblasts did not support a firm evidence of significative differences in VDR amounts among VDR 3'-end genotypes [33-35]. A further complicating factor in interpreting the role of the VDR 3'-end allelic variants is that their degree of linkage disequilibrium with the poly(A) repeats is imperfect and vary among different populations, such that some ethnic group exhibit a very tight linkage, while in others the presence of *Bsm I* and *Apa I* sites or the absence of *Taq I* site is not a good predictor of a long poly(A) repeat length [32].

Recently, a new diallelic (ATG/ACG) polymorphic VDR variant has been described in exon 2 of the gene, detectable with the restriction endonuclease FokI [36]. This polymorphism is responsible of a 3 aminoacid difference in VDR length between FF and ff individuals and the short form of the VDR gene (FF) gave approximately 1.7-fold greater increase in transcription activation in transfected HeLa cells [37]. Mexican-American postmenopausal women with ff genotype showed lower lumbar BMD than those with FF genotype [36]. This relationship confirmed in Japanese [37], North-American [38], and Italian [39] populations was not evidenced in French [40] and Swiss [41] women, even though a significant association of this genotype with differences in urinary type I collagen cross-linked n-telopeptide was observed in the French population [40]. Of particular interest a novel region in the VDR N-terminal segment required for functional interaction with transcription factor II B (TFIIB) has been recently detected [42], confirming that VDR similar to ER and GR possess an activation function 1-like domain N-terminal of the zinc fingers. It has also been demonstrated that as a direct result of differential interaction of the two *Fok I* receptor isoforms with TFIIB at this N-terminal region, the "F" hVDR possesses more potent transcriptional activity, providing the mechanistic basis for the enhanced BMD associated with FF versus ff genotypes [42].

ESTROGEN RECEPTOR GENE STUDIES

The importance of the ERs genes in the determination of BMD is supported by several observations : 1) osteoblasts, osteoclasts, and bone marrow stromal cells bear ERs and are modulated by estrogen [43] ; 2) homozygote inactivating mutation of the ERα gene caused OP in a male patient [3] ; and 3) KO mice for ERα gene exhibit a low BMD [44]. It is possible that common allelic variants of the ERα, may cause milder estrogen resistance, which becomes evident by aging and/or by menopausal hypogonadism, leading to clinical disorders such as OP. Both intronic polymorphisms (recognized by the restriction endonuclease PvuII and XbaI) and polymorphic variable number of (TA)n repeats upstream the ERα, have been associated with BMD in the Japanese population [45,46]. Similar studies in other populations yielded conflicting results [20-22]. Recently, we investigated the role of these polymorphisms at the ERα gene locus in a large sample of postmenopausal Italian women [47]. We found a strong linkage disequilibrium between intron 1 (Pvu II and Xba I) polymorphic sites and also between these sites and the microsatellite (TA)n dinucleotide repeat polymorphism, with a high degree of coincidence of the short TA alleles and the presence of Pvu II and Xba I restriction sites. Interestingly, a statistically significant correlation between the (TA)n repeat allelic variants and OP was observed, with subjects with a low number of repeats (TA < 15) showing the lowest BMD values and the highest vertebral fracture risk. Two studies in American and Danish populations recently confirmed this observation [48,49]; however, one performed in a Scottish population, observed no overall association between the TA repeat number and BMD [50]. All the positive studies are concordant and demonstrate a significant association between reduced BMD values and the presence of a low number of TA repeats. The molecular mechanism underlying how bone mineralization is affected by the variation in the number of dinucleotide repeats is still unclear. However, because of its position, in between promoter A and B of the ERα gene and next to a regulatory region, it is possible to speculate that allelic variation due to different (TA)n dinucleotide repeats length might have physiological relevance by affecting promoter usage and/or mRNA transcription.

Collagen Gene Studies

Collagen type I is the major constituent of bone matrix proteins and, therefore, collagen type I genes (COLIA1 and COLA2) have been proposed as candidate genes in the determination of bone mass. Indeed, the osteoporotic phenotype of Osteogenesis Imperfecta is due to mutations that affect the coding regions of collagen type I genes [51]. Recently, Grant et al. showed that a G/T polymorphism in the first intron of COLIA1 gene strongly segregated with BMD and osteoporotic fractures [52]. Additional data in larger samples of different populations support these findings [53-55]. A recent cross-section large-scale study indicates that the unfavorable COLIA1 allele (the T variant, arbitrary termed "s" allele) acts as a marker for accelerated age-related bone loss rather than a marker for lower peak bone mass [56]. However, a small study in a Finnish population [57] showed no significant association between the COLIA1 Sp1 polymorphism and bone mass or fracture, nor did another study in US twins [58]. A recent meta-analysis confirmed the significant associations between COLIA1 alleles and BMD, BMI, and osteoporotic fractures [59]. The association with fracture was stronger than expected on the basis of the observed differences in BMD and BMI, suggesting an additional effect on bone strength. Moreover, functional *in vitro* analyses supported evidence of allele-specific differences in binding of the Sp1 protein to the polymorphic recognition site, in collagen protein production and in bone strength in samples derived from patients with different COLIA1 genotypes [59].

OTHER CANDIDATE GENE STUDIES

Polymorphisms at others candidate genes such as interleukin 6 gene [60], TGF beta gene [61], apolipoprotein E gene [62], calcitonin receptor gene [63], androgen receptor gene

[48], osteocalcin gene [48], and aromatase gene [64] have been related to BMD in some isolated studies. These observations have not yet been confirmed by other independent studies and certainly other genes, with great or even greater effects both on BMD and bone metabolism, are still awaiting for their mapping and identification.

Linkage Analysis

Interestingly, three different bone-related phenotypes, OP pseudoglioma-syndrome, familial high bone mass, and autosomal recessive osteopetrosis have been now linked to the same locus on chromosome 11q12-13, suggesting this region plays an important role in regulating skeletal homeostasis [65-67]. The same quantitative trait loci (QTL) has been also supposed to correlate to BMD variation in the normal female population [70]. In the past few years, both linkage and sib-pairs analysis defined multiple additional QTL supposed to regulate bone mass, but results are again conflicting and the responsible genes remain to be defined [21,22]. In part this could be due to the fact that linkage analysis is ideal for looking for loci that are necessary, even if not sufficient, for disease expression, but may be much less powerful for finding loci that are neither necessary nor sufficient for disease expression, so-called susceptibility loci. In the latter case, different approaches, such as nonparametric allele-sharing methods (i.e. affected sib-pair analysis, linkage disequilibrium and transmission/disequilibrium test) have far greater power [19,69]. Recruitment of a large sib-pairs number should become necessary for performing linkage studies by haplotype sharing or transmission/disequilibrium test in humans [70]. Affected relatives should show excess allele sharing even in the presence of incomplete penetrance, phenocopy, genetic heterogeneity, and high frequency disease alleles [19]. Nonparametric linkage approaches testing multiple candidate genes in large pedigrees could result interesting, as well. Preliminary data from such a study demonstrated a suggestive linkage of the parathyroid hormone receptor type 1 to OP [71]. A limiting factor to linkage analysis of multiple candidate gene is actually represented by the lack of accurate statistical software to clearly define the threshold of significance.

Animal Studies

Linkage studies in experimental animals provide an additional strategy for identifying the genes involved in the regulation of bone mass. Comparative genetics could add useful information on potential interesting genes in humans once quantitative trait loci in animal models (i.e. rodents, primates) will be identified [72]. Genes identified in murine analyses can usually be mapped to particular human chromosomal regions because of the high degree of synteny that exists between the mouse and human genomes. Recent studies of various genetically homogeneous inbred mouse strains, with significant differences in skeletal phenotypes, revealed several QTLs involved in the regulation of bone mass [21,73]. Further studies are required to identify the responsible genes and to determine if these genes are also involved in regulating bone mass in humans.

Conclusions

OP affects hundreds of millions of patients throughout the world, causing pain and disability with great impact on individuals and on society as whole. Evidence has been given that this disorder recognize a complex genetic component. The identification of involved genetic pathways is certainly difficult and represent a great challenge in the next future. As in other multifactorial diseases (i.e. hypertension and diabetes) the disease initiation, progression and severity may be influenced by multiple environmental factors with multiple genes in a given individual. Several large-scale investigations involving thousands of patients and genome-wide screening now underway may make possible identification of multiple gene variations associated with an increased risk for OP. However, the importance of genetic heterogeneity, including ethnicity, as well as environmental, hormonal, and constitutional confounders (i.e. skeletal and body size) will need to be taken into serious account in the future genetic studies. Gene-gene and gene-environment as well as pharmacogenomic interactions in human and animal models will be critical targets for future research. Further developments in molecular genetic, such as microarray chips, will allow simultaneous large-scale differential identification of thousands of genes' polymorphisms segregating with the disease. All these efforts will certainly improve our knowledge of the pathogenesis of these debilitating disorders, allowing earlier preventive strategies as well as the development of more appropriate and effective treatment options.

References

1. Consensus Development Conference. Diagnosis, prophylaxis and treatment of osteoporosis. Am J Med 1993;94:646-50.
2. Smith DM, Nance WE, Kang KW, Christian JC, Johnston CC. Genetic factors in determining bone mass. J Clin Invest 1973;52:2800-8.
3. Smith EP, Boyod J, Frank GR, Talahashi H Cohen RM, Specker B, Williams TC, Lubahn DB, Korach KS. Estrogen resistance caused by a mutation in the estrogen-receptor gene in a man, N Engl J Med 1994;331:1056-61.
4. Morishima A, Grumbach MM, Simpson ER, FisherC, Qin K. Aromatase deficiency in male and female sibilings caused by a novel mutation and the physiological role of estrogens. J Clin Endocrinol Metab 1995;80:3689-98.
5. Johnson ML, Gong G, Kimberling W, Recker SM, Kimmel DB, Recker RB. Linkage of a gene causing high bone mass to human chromosome 11 (11q12-13). Am J Hum Genet 1997;60:1326-32.
6. Luckey MM, Meier DL, Mandeli IP, Da Costa MC, Hubbard ML, Goldsmith SI.. Radial and vertebral bone density in white and black women: Evidence for racial differences in premenopausal bone homeostasis. J Clin Endocrinol Metab 1989;69:762-70.
7. Daniels LD, Pettifor JM, Schnitzler CM, Russell SW, Patel DN. Ethnic differences in bone density in female South African nurses. J Bone Miner Res 1995;10:359-67.
8. Schnitzler CM, Pettifor JM, Mesquita JM, Bird MDT, Schnaid E, Smyth AE. Histomorphometry of iliac crest bone in 346 normal black and white South African adults. Bone Miner 1990;10:183-99.

9. Cundy T, Cornish J, Evans MC, Gamble G, Stapleton J, Reid IR. Sources of interracial variation in bone mineral density. J Bone Miner Res 1995;10:368-73.
10. Seeman E, Hopper JL, Bach LA, et al. Reduced bone mass in daughters of women with osteoporosis. N Engl J Med 1989;320:554-58.
11. Hansen MA, Hassager C, Jensen SB, Christiansen C. Is heritability a risk factor for postmenopausal osteoporosis? J Bone Miner Res 1992;7(9):1037-43.
12. Lonzer MD, Imrie R, Rogers D, Worley D, Licata A, Secic M. Effects of heredity, age, weight, puberty, activity, and calcium intake on bone mineral density in children. Clin Pediatr 1996;35:185-89.
13. Evans RA, Marel GM, Lancaster EK, Kos S, Evans M, Wong SY. Bone mass is low in relatives of osteoporotic patients. Ann Intern Med 1988;109:870-73.
14. Soroko SB, Barrett-Connor E, Edelstein SL, Kritz-Silverstain D. Family history of osteoporosis and bone mineral density at the axial skeleton: The Rancho Bernardo Study. J Bone Miner Res 1994;9:761-69.
15. Diaz MN, O'Neill TW, Silman AJ. The influence of family history of hip fracture on the risk of vertebral deformity in men and women: The European Vertebral Osteoporosis Study. Bone 1997;20:145-49.
16. Arden NK, Baker J, Hogg C, Baan K, Spector TD. The heritability of bone mineral density, ultrasound of the calcaneous and hip axis length: A study of postmenopausal twins. J Bone Miner Res 1996;11:530-34.
17. Flicker L, Faulkner KG, Hopper JL,et al. Determinants of hip axis length in women aged 10-89 years: A twin study. Bone 1996;8:41-45.
18. Howard GM, Nguyen TV, Harris M, Kelly PJ, Eisman JA. Genetic and environmental contributions to the association between quantitative ultrasound and bone mineral density measurements: A twin study. J Bone Miner Res 1998;13:1318-27.
19. Lander ES, Schork NJ. Genetic dissection of complex traits. Science 1994;265:2037-48.
20. Eisman JA. Genetics of osteoporosis. Endocr Rev 1999;20:788-804.
21. Stewart TL, Ralston SH. Role of genetic factors in the pathogenesis of osteoporosis. J Endocrinol 2000;166:235-45.
22. Brandi ML, Gennari L, Matucci Cerinic M, et al Genetic markers of osteoarticular disorders: facts and hopes. Arthritis Research 2001;45: in press.
23. Econs MJ, Speer MC. Genetic studies of complex diseases: Let the reader beware. J Bone Miner Res 1996;11:1835-40.
24. Morrison NA, Cheng JQI, Akifumi T, et al. Prediction of bone density from vitamin D receptor alleles. Nature 1994;367:284-87.
25. Cooper GS, Umbach DM. Are vitamin D receptor polymorphisms associated with bone mineral density? A meta-analysis. J Bone Miner Res 1996;11:1841-49.
26. Gong G, Stern HS, Cheng SC, et al. The association of bone mineral density with vitamin D receptor gene polymorphisms. Osteoporos Int 1999;9:55-64.
27. Ferrari SL, Rizzoli R, Slosman DO, Bonjour JP. Do dietary calcium and age explain the controversy surrounding the relationship between bone mineral density and vitamin D receptor gene polymorphisms? J Bone Miner Res 1998;13:363-70.
28. Kiel DP, Myers RH, Cupples LA, et al. The BsmI vitamin D receptor restriction fragment length polymorphism (bb) influences the effect of calcium intake on bone mineral density. J Bone Miner Res 1997;12:1049-57.
29. Dawson-Hughes B, Harris SS, Finneran S. Calcium absorption on high and low calcium intake in relation to vitamin D receptor genotype. J Clin Endocrinol Metab 1995;80:3657-

61.
30. Gennari L, Becherini L, Masi L, et al. Vitamin D and estrogen receptor allelic variants in postmenopausal women: Evidence of multiple gene contribution on bone mineral density. J Clin Endocrinol Metab 1998;83:939-44.
31. Haussler MR, Whitfield GK, Haussler CA, et al. The nuclear vitamin D receptor: Biological and molecular regulatory properties revealed. J Bone Miner Res 1998;13:325-49.
32. Ingles SA, Haile RW, Henderson BE, et al. Strength of linkage disequilibrium between two vitamin D receptor markers in five ethnic groups: Implications for association studies. Cancer Epidemiol Biomarkers Prev 1997;6:93-98.
33. Mocharla H, Butch AW, Pappas AA, et al. Quantification of vitamin D receptor m RNA by competitive polymerase chain reaction in PBMC: Lack of correspondence with common allelic variants. J Bone Miner Res 1997;12:726-33.
34. Gross C, Musiol IM, Eccleshall TR, Mallory PJ, Feldman D. Vitamin D receptor gene polymorphism: Analysis of ligand binding and hormone responsiveness in cultured fibroblasts. Biochem Biophys Res Commun 1998;242:467-73.
35. Durrin LK, Haile RW, Ingles SA, Coetzee GA. Vitamin D receptor 3'-untranslated region polymorphisms: Lack of effect on mRNA stability. Biochim Biophys Acta 1999;1453:311-20.
36. Gross C, Eccleshall TR, Malloy PJ, Villa ML, Marcus R, Feldman D. The presence of a polymorphism at the translation initiation site of the vitamin D receptor gene is associated with low bone mineral density in postmenopausal Mexican-American women. J Bone Miner Res 1996;11:1850-55.
37. Arai H, Myamoto K, Taketani Y, et al. A vitamin D receptor gene polymorphism in the translation initiation codon: Effect on protein activity and relation to bone mineral density in Japanese women. J Bone Miner Res 1997;12:915-21.
38. Harris SS, Eccleshall TR, Gross C, Dawson-Hughes B, Feldman D. The vitamin D receptor start codon polymorphism (Fok I) and bone mineral density in premenopausal American black and white women. J Bone Miner Res 1997;12:1043-48.
39. Gennari L, Becherini L, Mansani R, et al. Fok I polymorphism at translation initiation site of the vitamin D receptor gene predicts bone mineral density and vertebral fractures in postmenopausal Italian women. J Bone Miner Res 1999;14:1379-86.
40. Eccleshall TR, Garnero P, Gross C, Delmas PD, Feldman D. Lack of correlation between start codon polymorphism of the vitamin D receptor gene and bone mineral density in premenopausal French women : The OFELY study. J Bone Miner Res 1998;13:31-35.
41. Ferrari SL, Rizzoli R, Manen D, Slosman D, Bonjour JP. Vitamin D receptor gene start codon polymorphisms (Fok I) and bone mineral density: Interaction with age, dietary calcium, and 3'-end region polymorphisms. J Bone Miner Res 1998;13:925-30.
42. Jurutka PW, Remus LS, Whitfield GK, et al. The polymorphic N terminus in human vitamin D receptor isoforms influences transcriptional activity by modulating interaction with transcription factor IIB. Mol Endocrinol 2000;14:401-20.
43. Eriksen EF, Colvard DS, Berg NJ, et al. Evidence of estrogen receptors in normal human osteoblast-like cells. Science 1988;241:84-86.
44. Korach KS. Insights from the study of animals lacking functional estrogen receptor. Science 1994;266:1524-27.
45. Kobayashi S, Inoue S, Hosoi T, Ouchi Y, Shiraki M, Orimo H. Association of bone mineral density with polymorphism of estrogen receptor gene. J Bone Miner Res 1996;11:

306-11.
46. Han KO, Moon IG, Kang YS, Chung HY, Min HK, Han IK. Non association of estrogen receptor genotypes with bone mineral density and estrogen responsiveness to hormone replacement therapy in Korean postmenopausal women. J Clin Endocrinol Metab 1997;82: 991-95.
47. Becherini L, Gennari L, Masi L, et al. Evidence of a linkage disequilibrium between polymorphisms in the human estrogen receptor alpha gene and their relationship to bone mass variation in postmenopausal Italian women. Hum Mol Genet 2000;12;9:2043-50.
48. Sowers M, Willing M, Burns T, et al. Genetic markers, bone mineral density and serum osteocalcin levels. J Bone Miner Res 1999;14:1411-19.
49. Langdahl BL, Lokke E, Carstens M, Stenkjaer LL, Eriksen EF. A TA repeat polymorphism in the estrogen receptor gene is associated with osteoporotic fractures but polymorphisms in the first exon and intron are not. J Bone Mineral Res 2000;15:2222-30.
50. Albagha OM, McGuigan FE, Reid DM, Ralston SH. Estrogen receptor alpha gene polymorphisms and bone mineral density: Haplotype analysis in women from the United Kingdom. J Bone Mineral Res 2001;16:128-34.
51. Sykes B. Bone disease cracks genetics. Nature 1990;348:18-20.
52. Grant SFA, Reid DM, Blake G, Herd R, Fogelman I, Ralston SH Reduced bone density and osteoporosis associated with polymorphic SP1 site in the collagen type I alpha 1 gene. Nat Genet 1996;14:203-5.
53. Uitterlinden AG, Burger H, Huang Q, et al. Relation of alleles of the collagen type Iα1 gene to bone density and the risk of osteoporotic fractures in postmenopausal women. N Engl J Med 1998;338:1016-21.
54. Garnero P, Borel O, Grant SFA, Ralston SH, Delmas PD. Collagen Iα1 Sp1 polymorphism, bone mass, and bone turnover in healthy French postmenopausal women: The OFELY study. J Bone Miner Res 1998;13:813-17.
55. Langdahl BL, Ralston SH, Grant SFA, Eriksen EF. An Sp1 binding site polymorphism in the COLIA1 gene predicts osteoporotic fractures in men and women. J Bone Miner Res 1998;13:1384-89.
56. Keen RW, Woodford-Richens KL, Grant SFA, Ralston SH, Lanchbury JS, Spector TD. Polymorphism at the type I collagen (COLIA1) locus is associated with reduced bone mineral density, increased collagen turnover. Arthritis Rheum 1996;42:285-90.
57. Liden M, Wilen B, Ljunghall S, Melhus H. Polymorphism at the Sp1 binding site in the collagen type I alpha gene does not predict bone mineral density in postmenopausal women in Sweden. Calcif Tissue Int 1998;63:293-95.
58. Hustmyer FG, Lui G, Johnston CC, Christian J, Peacock M. Polymorphism at the Sp1 binding site of COLIA1 and bone mineral density in pre-menopausal female twins and elderly fracture patients. Osteoporosis Inter 1999;9:346-50.
59. Mann V, Hobson EE, Li B, et al. A COL1A1 Sp1 binding site polymorphism predisposes to osteoporotic fracture by affecting bone density and quality. J Clin Invest 2001:107:899-907.
60. Murray RE, McGuian F, Grant SFA, Reid DM, Ralston SH. Polymorphisms of the interleukin-6 gene are associated with bone mineral density. Bone 1997;21:89-92
61. Langdahl BL, Knudsen JY, Jensen HK, Gregersen N, Eriksen EF. A sequence variation : 713-delC in the transforming growth factor-β1 gene has higher prevalence in osteoporotic women than in normal women and is associated with very low bone mass in osteoporotic women and increased bone turnover in both osteoporotic and normal women. Bone 1997;

20:289-94.

62. Shiraki M, Shiraki Y, Aoki C, Inoue S, Kaneki M, Ouchi Y. Association of bone mineral density with apolipoprotein E phenotype. J Bone Miner Res 1997;12:1438-45.
63. Masi L, Becherini L, Colli E, et al. Polymorphisms of the calcitonin receptor gene are associated with bone mineral density in postmenopausal Italian women. Biochem Biophys Res Commun 1998;248:190-95.
64. Masi L, Becherini L, Gennari L, et al. Polymorphism of the aromatase gene in postmenopausal Italian women: Distribution and correlation with bone mass and fracture risk. J Clin Endocrinol Metab 2001;86:2263-69.
65. Gong Y, Vikkula M, Boon L, et al. Osteoporosis-pseudoglioma syndrome, a disorder affecting skeletal strength and vision, is assigned to chromosome region 11q12-13. Am J Hum Genet 1996;59:146-51.
66. Johnson ML, Gong G, Kimberling W, Recker SM, Kimmel DB, Recker RB. Linkage of a gene causing high bone mass to human chromosome 11 (11q12-13). Am J Hum Genet 1997;60:1326-32.
67. Heaney C, Shalev H, Elbedour K, et al. Human autosomal recessive osteopetrosis maps to 11q13, a position predicted by comparative mapping of the murine osteosclerosis (oc) mutation. Hum Mol Genet 1998;7:1407-10.
68. Koller DL, Rodriguez LA, Christian JC, et al. Linkage of a QTL contributing to normal variation in bone mineral density to chromosome 11q12-13. J Bone Miner Res 1998;13:1903-8.
69. Risch N, Merikangas K. The future of genetic studies of complex human diseases. Science 1996;273:1516-17.
70. Spielman SR, McGinnis RE, Ewens WJ. Transmission test for linkage disequilibrium: The insulin gene region and insulin-dependent diabetes mellitus (IDMM). Am J Hum Genet 1993;52:506-16.
71. Duncan EN, Brown MA, Sinsheimer J, et al. Suggestive linkage of the parathyroid receptor type 1 to osteoporosis. J Bone Miner Res 1999;14:1993-99.
72. VandeBerg JL, Williams-Blangero S. Advantages and limitations of non human primates as animal models in genetic research on complex disease. J Med Primatol 1997; 26(3):113-19.
73. Klein RF, Mitchell SR, Phillips TJ, Belknap JK, Orwoll ER. Quantitative trait loci affecting peak bone mineral density in mice. J Bone Miner Res 1998;13:1648-56.

The Intrauterine Programming of Osteoporosis

Cyrus Cooper, Muhammad K. Javaid, Karen Walker-Bone, Elaine M. Dennison, and Nigel K Arden

Introduction

Osteoporosis is a skeletal disorder characterized by low bone mass and microarchitectural deterioration of bone tissue with a consequent increase in the risk of fracture. These fractures typically occur at the hip, spine, and distal forearm; the annual cost attributable to them in England and Wales is £1.7 billion, with over 90% of this figure ascribed to hip fracture [1]. Figure 1 shows the history of advances in the field of osteoporosis over the previous three millennia. The recognition that fractures might be a consequence of bone fragility was initiated in the writings of Hippocrates; palaeopathological studies of bone specimens removed from burial sites dating as early at the 8th century AD confirm that osteoporotic vertebral collapse has occurred among elderly individuals throughout the ages. Our recent enhanced understanding of the disorder, however, stems from the work of orthopedic surgeons such as Sir Astley Cooper in 1825, who documented the descriptive characteristics of age-related fractures, and the observations of histopathologists in France and Germany at around the same time, who first coined the time "osteoporosis" to denote the rarification of trabecular architecture observed in the central part of vertebral bodies from patients who were elderly, when compared with those who had died at younger ages. The modern era of osteoporosis research originated in the research of Dr. Albright in the United States, who first documented osteoporotic vertebral deformity as a consequence of estrogen deficiency in postmenopausal women. These astute clinical observations heralded a period in which we developed techniques for the noninvasive assessment of bone mineral density; validated several pharmacological approaches to the prevention and treatment of age-related bone loss; defined osteoporosis densitometrically; and developed high risk and population-based strategies to combat the disorder.

The bone mass of an individual in later adult life depends upon the peak attained during skeletal growth, and the subsequent rate of bone loss. Preventive strategies against osteoporosis may be aimed at either increasing the peak bone mass attained, or reducing the rates of bone loss. There is evidence to suggest that peak bone mass is inherited, but current genetic markers are only able to explain a small proportion of the variation in individual bone mass or fracture risk [2]. It is likely that environmental influences during early life interact with the genome in establishing the functional level of a variety of metabolic processes involved in skeletal growth. This editorial will address the role played by such environmental influences during intrauterine, or very early postnatal life. It will review the conceptual basis of the fetal origins hypothesis; epidemiological studies pointing to the fetal programming of later osteoporosis risk and animal evidence relating to the programming of skeletal growth and metabolism.

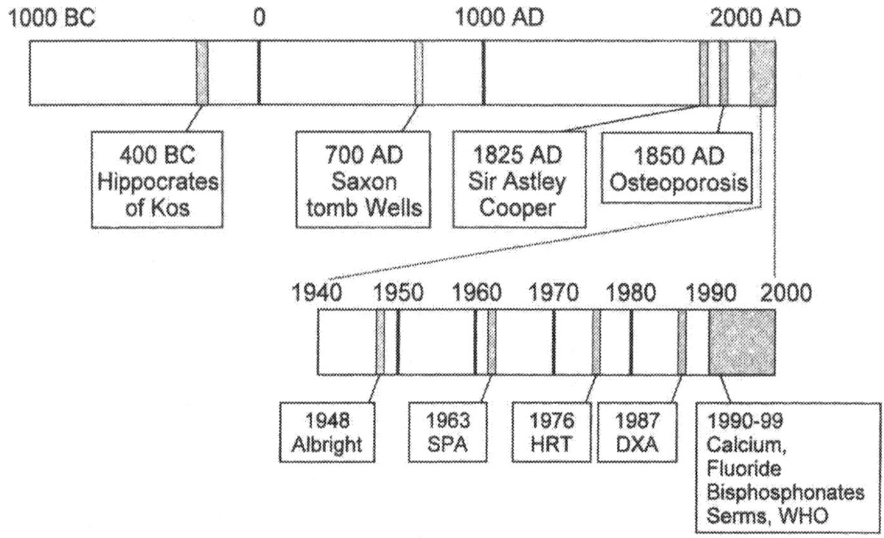

Figure 1. Historical development of research into osteoporosis over three millennia.

Epidemiological studies of coronary heart disease performed over a decade ago demonstrated strong geographic associations between death rate from the disorder in 1968-1978, and infant mortality in 1901-1910 [3]. Subsequent research, based on individuals whose birth records had been preserved for seven decades, revealed that men and women who were undernourished during intrauterine life, and therefore had low birthweight or were thin at birth, had an increased risk for coronary heart disease, hypertension, noninsulin dependent diabetes, and hypercholesterolemia [4]. These associations are explained by a phenomenon known as programming [5]; this term describes persisting changes in structure and function caused by environmental stimuli acting at critical periods during early development. During embryonic life, the basic form of the human baby is laid down in miniature. However, the body does not increase greatly in size until the fetal period when a rapid growth phase commences, which continues until after birth [6]. The main feature of fetal growth is cell division. Different tissues of the body grow during periods of rapid cell division, so called "critical" periods [7]. Their timing differs for different tissues; for example, the kidney has one in the weeks immediately before birth, while the long bones accelerate their rate of growth during the second trimester of gestation. The main adaptive response to a lack of nutrients and oxygen during this period of growth is to slow the rate of cell division, especially in tissues which are undergoing critical periods at the time. This reduction in cell division is either direct, or mediated through altered concentrations of growth factors or hormones (in particular insulin, growth hormone and cortisol).

It is not in question that the human skeleton can be programmed by undernutrition. Rickets has served as a long-standing example of undernutrition at a critical stage of early life, leading to persisting changes in structure. What is new is the realization that some of the body's "memories" of early undernutrition become translated into pathology and thereby determine disease in later life. Evidence has now accumulated that such intrauterine programming contributes to the risk of osteoporosis in later life.

Programming of Osteoporosis

Evidence that the risk of osteoporosis might be modified by environmental influences during early life stems from four groups of studies:

(a) bone mineral measurements undertaken in cohorts of adults whose detailed birth and/or childhood records have been preserved;

(b) detailed physiological studies exploring the relationship between candidate endocrine systems which might be programmed (GH/IGF-1; hypothalamic-pituitary adrenal, gonadal steroid) and age-related bone loss;

(c) studies characterizing the nutrition, body build, and lifestyle of pregnant women and relating these to the bone mass of their newborn offspring; and

(d) studies relating childhood growth rates to the later risk of hip fracture.

The first epidemiological evidence that osteoporosis risk might be programmed came from a study of 153 women born in Bath during 1968-69 who were traced and studied at age 21 years [8]. Data on childhood growth were obtained from linked birth and school health records. There were statistically significant ($p < 0.05$) associations between weight at one year and bone mineral content (BMC), but not density, at the lumbar spine and femoral neck; these relationships were independent of adult weight and body mass index. The data suggested a discordance between the processes which govern skeletal growth, and those which influence mineralization. They also provide direct evidence that the trajectory of bone growth might be programmed, an assertion previously only supported by inference from measurements of body height. The association between weight in infancy and adult bone mass was replicated in a second cohort study of 238 men and 201 women aged 60-75 years, who were born and still lived in Hertfordshire [9]. In this study, there were highly significant relationships between weight at one year and adult bone area at the spine and hip ($p < 0.005$); the relationships with BMC at these two sites were weaker but remained statistically significant ($p < 0.02$). They also remained after adjustment for known genetic markers of osteoporosis risk, such as polymorphisms in the gene for the vitamin D receptor [10], and for collagen IA1, and after adjustment for lifestyle characteristics in adulthood which might have influenced bone mass (physical activity, dietary calcium intake, cigarette smoking, and alcohol consumption). More recently, we have demonstrated that birthweight is a significant predictor of BMC at the lumbar spine, femoral neck, and whole body among 143 men and women aged 70-75 years. In this study, birthweight was a predictor not only of bone area and bone mineral content, but also of bone mineral density and volumetric bone mineral density at the lumbar spine, femoral neck, and whole body, among women (Figure 2). This study confirms that genetic and/or environmental influences during intrauterine life, rather than early postnatal life, explain the previously observed associations between weight at one year and adult bone mass.

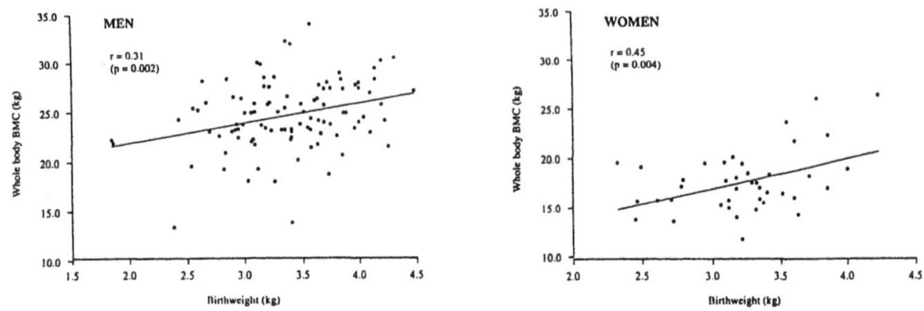

Figure 2. Relationship between birthweight and whole body bone mineral content assessed by dual energy X-ray absorptiometry among 143 men and women aged 70-75 years [derived from ref. 11].

To explore further the potential role of hypothalamic-pituitary function and its relevance to the pathogenesis of osteoporosis, profiles of circulating GH and cortisol were compared with bone density among groups of men and women whose birth records had been preserved. These studies revealed that birthweight and weight in infancy were predictors of basal levels of GH and cortisol during late adult life [12-14]. The levels of these two skeletally active hormones were also found to be determinants of prospectively determined bone loss rate. The data are compatible with the hypothesis that environmental stressors during intrauterine or early postnatal life alter the sensitivity of the growth plate to GH and cortisol. The consequence of such endocrine programming would be to reduce peak skeletal size, perhaps also to reduce mineralization, and to predispose to an accelerated rate of bone loss during later life [12-14].

The third piece of epidemiological evidence that osteoporosis might be programmed stems from investigation of a series of mothers through pregnancy; anthropometric and lifestyle maternal characteristics were related to the bone mineral of their newborn offspring [15,16]. After adjusting for sex and gestational age, neonatal bone mass was strongly, positively associated with birthweight, birth length, and placental weight. Other determinants included maternal and paternal birthweight, and maternal triceps skinfold thickness at 28 weeks (Figure 3). Maternal smoking, and maternal energy intake at 18 weeks gestation, were negatively associated with neonatal BMC at both the spine and whole body. The independent effects of maternal and paternal birthweight on fetal skeletal development support the notion that paternal influences, for example through the imprinting of growth promoting genes such as IGF-2, contribute strongly to the establishment of the early skeletal growth trajectory, while maternal nutrition and body build modify fetal nutrient supply and subsequent bone accretion, predominantly through influences on placentation.

Most evidence relating the intrauterine environment to later osteoporosis stems from studies utilizing noninvasive assessment of bone mineral. The clinically important consequence of reduced bone mass is fracture, and data are now available which directly link growth rates in childhood with the risk of later hip fracture [17]. Studies of a unique Finnish cohort in whom birth and childhood growth data were linked to later hospital discharge records for hip fracture, have permitted follow-up of around 7,000 men and women who were born in Helsinki University Central Hospital during 1924-1933. Body size at birth was recorded and an average of 10 measurements were obtained of height and weight throughout childhood. Hip fracture incidence was assessed in this cohort using the Finnish hospital discharge registration system. After adjustment for age and sex, there were two major determinants of hip fracture risk: tall maternal height ($p < 0.001$), and low rate of childhood growth (height, $p = 0.006$; weight, $p = 0.01$). The effects of maternal height and childhood growth rate were statistically independent of each other, and remained after adjusting for socioeconomic status. The data are compatible with endocrine programming influencing the risk of hip fracture. In addition, the observation that fracture subjects were shorter at birth, but of average height by age 7 years, suggests that hip fracture risk might be particularly elevated among children in whom growth of the skeletal envelope is forced ahead of the capacity to mineralize, a phenomenon which is accelerated during pubertal growth.

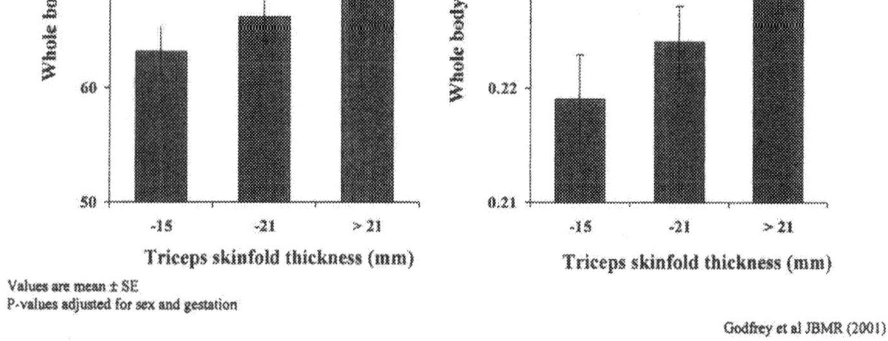

Figure 3. Maternal fat stores (assessed by triceps skinfold thickness at 28 weeks of gestation) and whole body bone mineral content in the neonate [derived from ref. 16].

Numerous animal experiments have shown that hormones, undernutrition, and other influences that affect development during sensitive periods of early life permanently program the structure and physiology of the body's tissues and systems. A remarkable example is the effect of temperature on the sex of reptiles [18]. If the eggs of an American alligator are incubated at 30° C, all the offspring are female. If incubated at 33° C, all the offspring are male. At temperatures between 30° and 33° C, there are varying proportions of females and males. It is believed that the fundamental sex is female, and a transcription factor is required to divert growth along a male pathway. Instead of the transcription factor being controlled genetically by a sex chromosome, it depends on the environment, specifically temperature.

Organ systems in the body are most susceptible to programming during periods when they are growing rapidly. During the first two months of life, the embryonic period, there is extensive differentiation of progenitor cells, without rapid cell replication. Thereafter, in the fetal period, the highest growth rates are observed. Growth slows in late gestation and continues to slow in childhood. The high growth rates of the fetus compared with the child are mostly the result of cell replication; the proportion of cells which are dividing becomes progressively less as the fetus becomes older. Slowing of growth is a major adaptation to undernutrition. Experiments on rats, mice, sheep, and pigs have demonstrated that protein or calorie restriction of the mother during pregnancy and lactation is associated with smaller offspring [18,19-21]. In general, the earlier in life that undernutrition occurs, the more likely it is to have permanent effects on body size [22]. Early in embryonic life, growth is regulated by the supply of nutrients and oxygen. At some point shortly after birth, growth begins to track. In humans, tracking is demonstrated by the way in which infants grow along centile curves. Once tracking is established, it is no longer possible to make animals grow faster by offering them unlimited food. The rate of growth has become set, homeostatically controlled by feedback systems. After a period of undernutrition, they will regain their expected size. This contrasts with the effects of undernutrition during intrauterine life, in which skeletal development is slowed and the peak skeletal proportions attained following the completion of linear growth are reduced.

There are three cellular mechanisms for the induction of programming. First, the nutrient environment may permanently alter gene expression; one example of this is permanent change in the activity of metabolic enzymes such as HMG-CoA reductase [23]. Second, early nutrition may permanently reduce cell numbers. The small, but normally proportioned rat produced by undernutrition before weaning, has been shown to have fewer cells in its organs and tissues [24]. Growth retarded human babies have reduced numbers of cells in their pancreas which may limit insulin secretion [25], and reduced size of their airways which may limit respiratory function [26]. Third, certain clones of cells may be altered by environmental adversity during development; for example, an altered balance of the TH-1 and TH-2 lymphocyte subtypes might predispose to atopic disease in later life [27]. Evidence from the human studies outlined above suggests that skeletal development might be programmed as a consequence of the first two of these mechanisms.

Conclusions

Undernutrition and other adverse influences arising in fetal life or immediately after birth have a permanent effect on body structure, physiology, and metabolism. The specific effects of undernutrition depend on the time and development at which it occurs; rapidly growing fetuses and neonates are more vulnerable. Its effects include altered gene expression, reduced cell numbers, imbalance between cell types, altered organ structure, and changes in the pattern of hormonal release and tissue sensitivity to these hormones. Evidence is now accumulating from human studies that programming of bone growth might be an important contributor to the later risk of osteoporotic fracture. Body weight in infancy is a determinant of adult bone mineral content, as well as of the basal levels of activity of the GH/IGF-1 and HPA axes. Epidemiological studies have suggested that maternal smoking and nutrition during pregnancy influence intrauterine skeletal mineralization. Finally, childhood growth rates have been directly linked to the risk of hip fracture many decades later. Further studies of this phenomenon are required in order that effective preventive strategies against osteoporosis throughout the life course may be delineated and more effectively applied.

References

1. Royal College of Physicians. Osteoporosis: Clinical guidelines for prevention and treatment. The Royal College of Physicians of London, 1999.
2. Ralston S. Do genetic markers aid in risk assessment? Osteoporosis Int 1998;8(Suppl.1): S37-S42.
3. Barker DJP. Fetal origins of coronary heart disease. BMJ 1995;311:171-74.
4. Barker DJP. The fetal origins of adult disease. Proceedings of the Royal Society of London (B) 1995;262:37-43.
5. Lucas A. Programming by early nutrition in man. In: Bock GR, Whelan J, editors. The childhood environment and adult disease. New York: John Wiley, 1991: 38-55.
6. Walpert L. The triumph of the embryo. Oxford: Oxford University Press, 1991.
7. Widdowson EM, McCance RA. The determinants of growth and form. Proceedings of the Royal Society of London 1974;185: 1-17.
8. Cooper C, Cawley MID, Bhalla A, et al. Childhood growth, physical activity and peak bone mass in women. J Bone Min Res 1995;10:940-47.
9. Cooper C, Fall C, Egger P, Hobbs R, Eastell R, Barker D. Growth in infancy and bone mass in later life. Ann Rheum Dis 1997;56:17-21.
10. Keen R, Egger P, Fall C, et al. Polymorphisms of the vitamin D receptor, infant growth and adult bone mass. Calcif Tiss Int 1997;60:233-35.
11. Gale CR, Martyn CN, Kellingray S, Eastell R, Cooper C. Intrauterine programming of adult body composition. J Clin Endocrinol Metab 2001;86:267-72.
12. Fall C, Hindmarsh P, Dennison E, Kellingray S, Barker D, Cooper C. Programming of growth hormone secretion and bone mineral density in elderly men; an hypothesis. J Clin Endocrinol Metab 1998;83:135-39.
13. Dennison E, Hindmarsh P, Fall C, et al. Profiles of endogenous circulating cortisol and bone mineral density in healthy elderly men. J Clin Endocrinol Metab 1999;84:3058-63.

14. Phillips DIW, Barker DJP, Fall CHD, et al. Elevated plasma cortisol concentrations: A link between low birthweight and the insulin resistance syndrome? J Clin Endocrinol Metab 1998;83:757-60.
15. Dennison E, Godfrey K, Wheeler T, Taylor S, Kellingray S, Cooper C. Determinants of neonatal bone mass. Bone 1997;20:26S (abstract).
16. Godfrey K, Walker-Bone K, Robinson S, et al. Neonatal bone mass: Influence of parental birthweight, maternal smoking, body composition, and activity during pregnancy. J Bone Min Res 2001;16:1-10.
17. Cooper C, Eriksson JF, Forsen T, Osmond C, Tuomilehto J, Barker DJP. Childhood growth trajectory as a strong determinant of later risk of hip fracture: A prospective study. Calcif Tissue Int 1999;64(Suppl.1):S38.
18. Barker DJP. Programming the baby. In: Barker DJP, editor. Mothers, babies and health in later life. London: Churchill Livingstone, 1998:13-41.
19. McCance RA, Widdowson EM. The determinants of growth and form. Proceedings of the Royal Society of London (B) 1974;185:1-17.
20. Smart JL, Massey RF, Nash SC, Tonkiss J. Effects of early life undernutrition in artificially reared rats: Subsequent body and organ growth. Br J Nutr 1987;58:245-55.
21. Chow BF, Lee CJ. Effect of dietary restriction of pregnant rats on body weight gain of the offspring. J Nutr 1964;82:10-18.
22. McCance RA, Widdowson EM. Nutrition and growth. Proceedings of the Royal Society of London (B) 1962;156:326-37.
23. Brown SA, Rogers LK, Dunn JK, Gotto AM, Patsch W. Development of cholesterol homeostatic memory in the rat is influenced by maternal diets. Metabolism 1990;39:468-73.
24. McLeod KI, Goldrick RB, Whyte HM. The effect of maternal malnutrition on the progeny in the rat: Studies on growth, body composition and organ cellularity in first and second generation progeny. Australian J Exp Biol Med Sci 1972;50:435-46.
25. Snoeck A, Remacle C, Reusens B, Hoet JJ. Effect of a low protein diet during pregnancy on the fetal rat endocrine pancreas. Biol Neonate 1990;57:107-18.
26. Matsui R, Thurlbeck WM, Fujita Y, Yu SY, Kida K. Connective tissue, mechanical, and morphometric changes in the lungs of weanling rats fed a low protein diet. Pediatr Pulmonol 1989; 7:159-66.
27. Godfrey KM, Barker DJP, Osmond C. Disproportionate fetal growth and raised IGE concentration in adult life. Clin Exp Allergy 1994;24:641-48.

THE ROLE OF MENOPAUSE IN BONE AND JOINT HEALTH: IMPLICATIONS FOR OSTEOARTHRITIS AND OSTEOPOROSIS

MaryFran Sowers

Introduction

The health of joint tissue is a reflection of the health of bone and cartilage and the tissues that make up these organs including the contributing Type I and Type II collagens. These tissues may respond not only to ovarian and growth hormone stimulation, they also may be linked to other biological responses including reaction to oxidation and cytokine release. It is still an open question as to whether the menopausal transition impacts joint health. It is the purpose of this presentation to identify the potential for a menopause relationship to influence bones and other tissues of the joint and consider how this is related to osteoporosis and osteoarthritis.

Osteoporosis is defined as a loss of bone accompanied by micro-fracture [1]. The concept of osteoporosis has been operationally defined in a concept paper published under the auspices of the World Health Organization whereby osteoporosis is a bone mineral density value < 2.5 SD below a young adult normal value [2]. Apart from fractures, particularly of the spine, femoral head, and wrist, osteoporosis is associated with back pain, loss of height associated with microfracture of vertebral bodies, dowager's hump, and in instances where compromise of the spinal column is substantial, limitations in breathing as the rib cage increasingly rests on the pelvis.

Osteoarthritis, by definition, reflects the degeneration of articular cartilage together with changes in subchondral bone and intra-articular inflammation. This failure of the tissue in joints is manifest as softening of tissue, fibrillation, ulcerations, and loss of articular cartilage, the formation of osteophytes (bony protrusions), bony cysts, and ultimately exposure of the subchondral bone. Apart from total compromise of the joint requiring replacement, osteoarthritis is associated with joint pain, tenderness, limitations in movement, crepitus (the crackling sound arising from bone rubbing against bone), effusion (the accumulation of fluid into the joint space), and localized inflammation.

Relationship of Osteoporosis and Osteoarthritis

It has been recognized for some time that osteoporosis and osteoarthritis are linked. An example of that is shown in Table 1 where the data are shown that initiated the understanding that those with osteoporosis are much less likely to have osteoarthritis. Foss and Byers showed that men and women below the 10th percentile of cortical bone density had virtually no osteoarthritis [3]. In contrast, men and women with cortical bone density above the 90th percentile included virtually no men or women with osteoporosis, but did include more than half of men and women with osteoarthritis. We have observed a similar relationship in pre- and perimenopausal women [4].

Table 1. Bone Density (2nd Metacarpal Cortical Area) in 140 Cases of Femoral Neck Fracture and 100 Cases of Osteoarthritis

	Osteoarthritis		Osteoporosis	
	Male	Female	Male	Female
Number	32	68	19	121
Above 90th	(47%)	(53%)	(0%)	(2%)
Below 10th	(3%0	(0%)	(63%)	(42%)

Relationship of Osteoporosis and Osteoarthritis to the Menopause Transition

EPIDEMIOLOGICAL STUDIES

There are very few studies that allow the investigation of both osteoporosis and osteoporosis in relation to the menopause [5]. The Southeast Michigan cohort is uniquely positioned to do so [6]. The Southeast Michigan cohort is an amalgamation of two independent studies that have been organized to have common protocols with respect to studies of bone, characteristics of osteoarthritis, and ovarian hormones. The Michigan Bone Health Study is a population-based study located at Tecumseh, Michigan that includes data from 602 Caucasian women who are currently aged 34 to 54 years and for whom osteoarthritis studies, including x-rays of hands and knees, were taken in 1992, 1996, 1998, and 2000. The other component of the Southeast Michigan cohort includes Study of Women's Health Across the Nation (SWAN), a population-based study located in the Detroit area that encompasses data from 319 African-American and 227 Caucasian women, aged 46-56 years, for whom osteoarthritis studies have been completed in 1996,1998, and 2000 [6].

One approach to determining if there is a menopausal association with osteoporosis and osteoarthritis is to examine the association of follicle stimulating hormone (FSH) with the frequency of osteoarthritis and bone mineral density as an indicator of osteoporosis risk. FSH is the communication link that rises as the feedback between pituitary and ovary become increasingly deranged during the perimenopausal period. As shown in Figure 1, FSH concentrations rise in the Southeast Michigan population with age, an age that is coincident with the time of the transition. As shown in Figure 2, as FSH concentrations rise, the bone mineral densities become lower.

FSH concentrations are linked to osteoarthritis. As shown in Table 2, there is little osteoarthritis prior to age 40 years in the Southeast Michigan population; however, after that age, the prevalence is greater than 11% in the knees and greater than 16% in the hands. Further, there is an association osteoarthritis with FSH concentrations apart from the associations of BMI and age, well-known risk factors for osteoarthritis. There is a greater risk of OA with higher FSH concentrations, shown in Table 3.

Cellular and Molecular Studies

From the cellular/molecular viewpoint, it is useful to ask whether the materials of the joint are responsive to the presence or absence of ovarian products associated with the menopausal transition. The bone of osteoporosis involves bone matrix: type I collagen and bone turnover cells, osteoclasts and osteoblasts. Osteoarthritis involves the articular cartilage. This cartilage is primarily type II collagen fibers and accompanying proteoglycans, as well as Types IX and XI collagen, and water, chondrocytes. Further there is also involvement of the bone matrix type I collagen and the bone turnover cells. Figure 3 shows that Type I and Type II collagen differ only by one of the three chains of the triple helical construction.

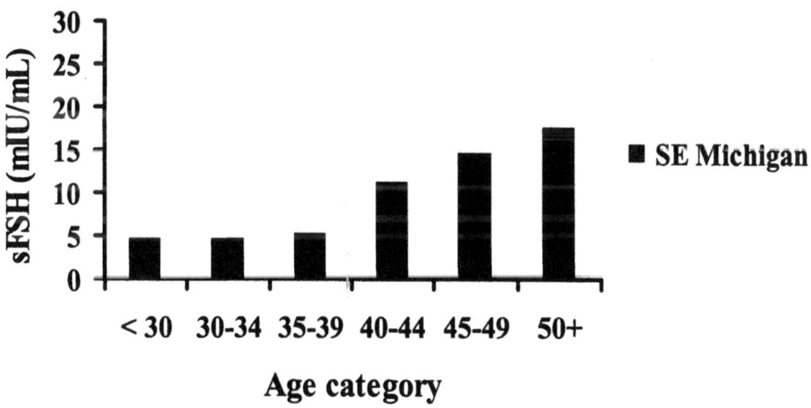

Figure 1. sFollicle stimulating hormone (FSH) concentration (baseline) by age group.

Figure 4 shows the mechanisms by which hormones and cytokines may influence cellular and molecular activities of both bone and cartilage. Estradiol and cytokines such as IL-1 interact to act on the synthesis of procollagens. In turn, the globulin molecules are lysed from these molecules to form the Type I or Type II collagen triple helix. Ultimately, degradation is associated with cytokine activity. These activities have been described with respect to both bone and cartilage material [5].

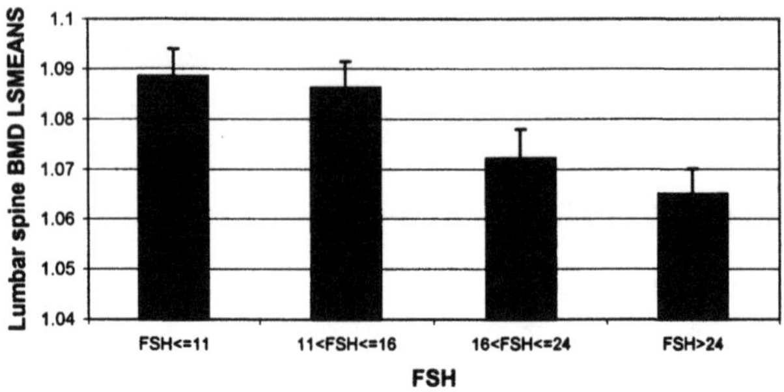

Figure 2. Bone mineral density* in Swan according to quartiles of FSH concentration.
* after adjusting for ethnicity, BMI, and physical activity

Tissue	Chains	Collagen Genes	Chromosome	Procollagen Molecule	
I	2-α1 (I)	COL1A1	17	$\alpha 1(I)_2\alpha 2(I)$	Bone
	1-α2 (I)	COL1A2	7		
II	3-α1 (II)	COL2A1	12	$\alpha 1(II)_3$	Cartilage
III	3-α1(III)	COL3A1	2	$\alpha 1(III)_3$	Skin

Figure 3. The three major types of collagen.

Table 2. The Prevalence/100 of Osteoarthritis of the Hand and Knee in the Southeast Michigan Cohort of Women

N	Age	Knee OA		Hand OA	
		Prevalence (P)		Prevalence (P)	
		P	(95% CI)	P	(95% CI)
1053	27-55	11.5	(9.6, 13.4)	16.4	(14.2, 18.5)
73	27-34	1.4	(-1.3, 4.0)	0.0	—
149	35-39	1.3	(-0.5,3.2)	1.3	(-0.5, 3.2)
400	40-44	15.0	(11.5, 18.5)	13.5	(10.2, 16.7)
375	45-49	13.3	(9.89, 16.77)	25.1	(20.7, 29.5)
56	50-55	14.4	(5.1, 23.4)	23.2	(12.2, 34.1)

Table 3. The Odds of Osteoarthritis of the Knee: Follicle Stimulating Hormone and Obesity (BMI)

	Osteoarthritis (95% CI)	p-value
OA of the Knee		
1996 point prevalence		0.0001
FSH < 11, BMI < 30	reference	
FSH > 11, BMI < 30	2.0 (0.8-5.5)	
FSH ≤ 11, BMI > 30	8.6 (3.5-21.3)	
FSH > 11, BMI > 30	10.3 (4.3-24.2)	
1996-1998 incidence		0.0003
FSH < 11, BMI < 30	reference	
FSH > 11, BMI < 30	1.28 (0.56-2.91)	
FSH ≤ 11, BMI > 30	3.76 (1.72-8.26)	
FSH > 11, BMI > 30	2.93 (1.39-6.18)	

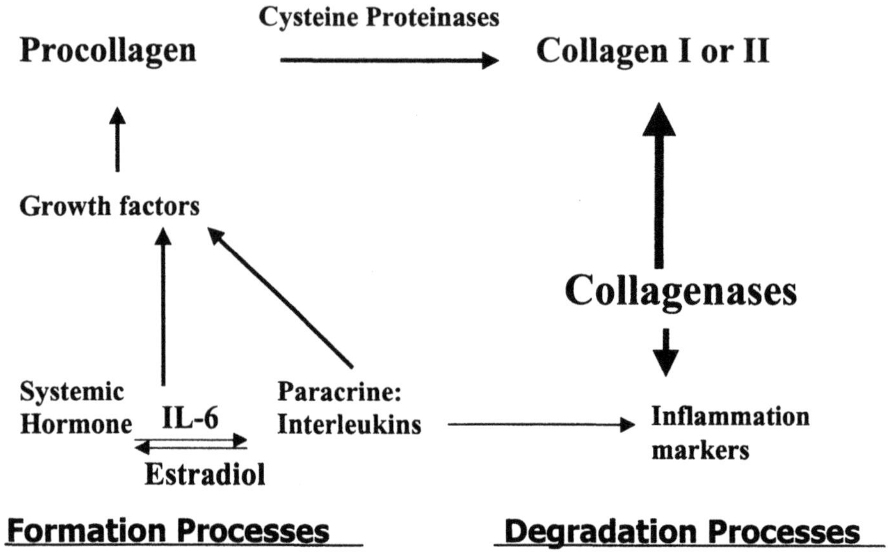

Figure 4. Hormones, cytokines, and the cellular/molecular activities related to bone and cartilage.

Estradiol or its absence may affect bone by several mechanisms including synthesis or suppression of the collagen matrix in which calcium hydroxyapatite is deposited and by modulating the excess expression of cytokines. In tissue culture systems, estrogen is reported to stimulate collagen synthesis in rat uteri and femur [7]. In aortic smooth muscle cells, estrogen was associated with a shift of Type 1 to Type III procollagen fractions in cattle [8]. Estrogens may have an indirect role in bone through their influence on cytokine expression, when controlled cytokine action plays a role in normal tissue turnover and repair. Cytokines that have been extensively studied the interleukins (IL-1, IL-6) and transforming growth factor β, and tumor necrosis factor-α. Estradiol was associated with an increase in the synthesis and release of IL-1 in macrophages [9]. Estradiol (as well as testosterone) has also been shown to modulate the IL-6 release induced by IL-1.

There are several approaches whereby estrogen in the menopause could affect osteoarthritis. There may be an indirect role of estrogens via the maintenance of bone, a direct role of estrogens in collagen synthesis or suppression, or an indirect role for estrogen in modulating the excess expression of cytokines. There is evidence of the availability of estrogen receptors to undertake these roles. Tsai and Lui [10] have reported the presence of estrogen receptors in the cartilage of rabbit femoral condyle. It has been suggested that the up-regulation of estrogen receptors represent the effort to repair arthritic changes in cartilage [11]. Sheridan and others have reported that cells important to arthritic processes may have estrogen receptors [11-13] in some cells from dogs, rabbit and baboon but not all studies demonstrate this [14].

There have been hypothesized relationships between osteoarthritis and ovarian hormone levels, usually estrogen, but the hypotheses that have emerged are bidirectional. A protective effect for estrogen was first suggested by observations of increased risk of osteoarthritis during the menopausal transition. Studies, both *in vivo* and *in vitro*, suggest that estrogen may be chondrodestructive but bone protective, potentially though the up-regulation of estrogen receptors. Likewise, hormone replacement therapy has been evaluated with the understanding that a factor that is causal of disease can be identified when that factor is replaced in a system where it is absent. The results of studies that address these issues are relatively consistent in bone, but are frequently contradictory in studies of osteoarthritis [5].

There are several reasons that studies to date may be so contradictory. Consistently defining osteoarthritis has been difficult and there are important substantial interspecies differences affecting the interpretation of studies in animal models. Studies in humans frequently have insufficient sample sizes to sort out whether the response is related to the initiation, progression or severity of the disease(s). There are also difficulties in characterizing the exposures to hormones. In studies of hormone replacement therapies, responses have varied according to the dose and type of formulation, as well as the timing in the disease course. Studies have also tended to address issues related to estrogen, but failed to consider other important hormones such as androgen levels. In light of these limitations, well-defined and well-executed studies in this area are critical. A more complete understanding can have an important impact in populations and could provide an opportunity for needed therapeutic interventions [5].

References

1. Consensus Development Conference Statement. Prophylaxis and treatment of osteoporosis. J Am Med Assoc 1991;90:107-10.
2. NIH Consensus development conference statement. Proceedings of the Osteoporosis Prevention, Diagnosis and Therapy Conference 2000;Mar 27-29.
3. Foss MVL, Byers PD. Bone density, osteoarthritis of the hip, and fractures of the upper end of the femur. Ann Rheum Dis 1972;13:259-64.
4. Sowers MF, Lachance L, Jamadar D, Hochberg M, Crutchfield M, Jannausch ML. The associations of bone mineral density and bone turnover markers with osteoarthritis of the hand and knee in pre- and peri-menopausal women. Arth Rheum 1999;42:483-89.
5. Sowers MF. Estrogens and osteoarthritis; hormone replacement, menopause, and aging. In: Lobo RA, Kelsey J, Marcus R, editors. Menopause: Biology and pathobiology San Diego, CA: Academic Press, 2000: 535-43.
6. Sowers MF, Lachance L, Hochberg M, Jamadar D. Prevalence of radiographically defined osteoarthritis of the hand and knee in a population of pre- and perimenopausal women. Osteoarthritis Cartilage 2000;8:69-77.
7. Smith QT, Allison DJ. Changes of collagen content in skin, femur and uterus of 17β-estradiol benzoate-treated rats. Endocrinology 1966;79:486-92.
8. Beldekas JC, Smith B, Gerstenfeld LC, Sonenshein GE, Franzblau C.Effects of 17β-estradiol on the biosynthesis of collagen in cultured bovine aortic smooth muscle cells.

Biochemistry 1981;20:2162-67.
9. Hu SK, Mitcho YL, Rath NC. Effect of estradiol on interleukin 1 synthesis by macrophages. Int J Immunopharmacol 1988;10:247-52.
10. Tsai CL, Liu TK. Osteoarthritis in women: Its relationship to estrogen and current trends. Life Sci 1992;50:1737-44
11. Sheridan PJ, Aufdemorte TB, Holt GR, Gates GA. Cartilage of the baboon contains estrogen receptors. Rheumatol Int 1985;5:279-81.
12. Young PCM, Stack MT. Estrogen and glucocorticoid receptors in adult canine articular cartilage. Arthrit Rheum 1982;25:568-73.
13. Rosner IA, Manni A, Malemud CJ, Boja B, and Moskowitz KW. Estrogen receptors in articular chondrocytes. Biochem Biophys Res Commun 1982;10:1378-82.
14. Kan KW, Cruess RL, Posner BI, Guyda HJ, Solomon S. Hormone receptors in the epiphysial cartilage J Endocrinol 1984;103:125-31.

NOVEL COMPOUNDS ACTING THROUGH RECEPTORS AND ENZYME MEDIATORS

Trevor M. Penning

Introduction

This article will introduce novel steroids that have an optimal profile for the prevention of postmenopausal osteoporosis. These agents have a duality of function: they can activate the estrogen receptor (ER) but they also regulate the amount of ligand available for the ER via enzyme inhibition in a tissue-specific manner. These agents have the same clinical profile as selective estrogen receptor modulators (SERMS) but a different mode of action. This article will develop these mechanistic concepts.

Steroid Hormone Action and SERMS

Steroid hormones, such as estrogens, dissociate from sex-steroid binding globulins, enter target cells and bind to their nuclear receptors [1]. In the case of estrogens these receptors are ERα and Erβ [2]. The receptor-ligand complex dissociates from its chaperone proteins, dimerizes and binds to estrogen response elements (EREs) on the promoter regions of structural genes to cause new gene transcription, a process known as trans-activation [3] (Figure 1).

This now appears to be an oversimplification of steroid hormone action. Binding of the dimerized receptor to a hormone response element, will lead only to a partial response and gene transcription may increase only 5-fold over basal levels. Ligands that give this response are referred to as partial agonists/antagonists. To obtain a maximal response the receptor-ligand complex recruits co-activators, e.g. SRC-1, so that gene transcription can increase by up to 30-fold over basal levels [4,5] (Figure 2). Ligands that give this response are complete agonists. The receptor-ligand complex may also recruit co-repressors, e.g. NcoR-1, so that gene transcription is abrogated leading to no gene transcription over basal levels. Ligands that cause this response are complete antagonists. Thus a graded response is achieved where co-activators and co-repressors act as the rheostat. The recruitment of these co-regulators is dependent upon the conformation elicited in the receptor by the ligand [6]. Ligands can generate tissue specific responses because the expression of the co-regulators is tissue selective. Ligands that induce tissue specific responses by this mechanism are known as selective steroid receptor modulators.

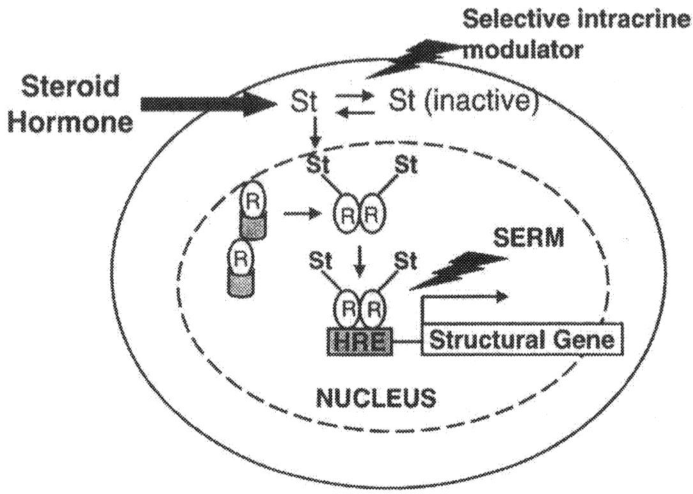

Figure 1. Mechanism of action of steroid hormones in target tissues. St = steroid hormone; R = receptor; HRE = hormone response element; and SERM = selective estrogen receptor modulator.

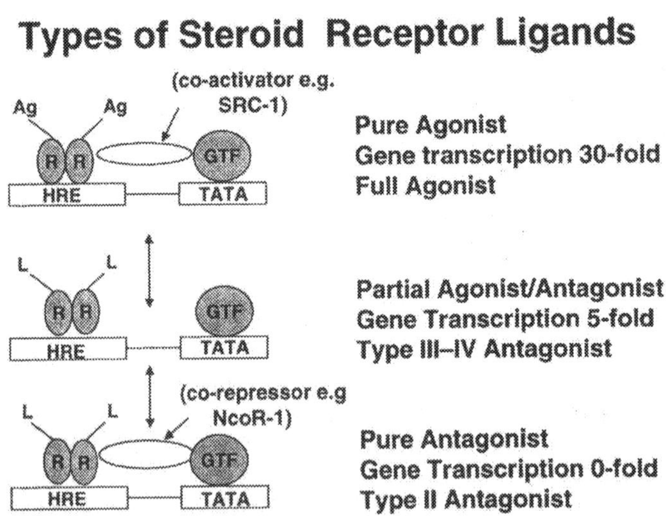

Figure 2. Types of steroid receptor ligands. R = steroid receptor; Ag = agonist; L = ligand; HRE = hormone response element; GTF = general transcription factors; and TATA = TATA box

SERMS compete with 17β-estradiol for the ER, the receptor-ligand complex induces gene transcription in a tissue specific manner by the recruitment of co-regulators. The first agent of this class is tamoxifen, Figure 3. It is an estrogen in the bone, cardiovascular system, and uterus but it is an anti-estrogen in the breast and CNS [7]. If its estrogenic properties in the uterus were eliminated it would have a more desirable profile for the prevention and treatment of postmenopausal symptoms, i.e. it would be one step closer to a designer estrogen. The second agent of this class is raloxifene. It is an estrogen in the bone and cardiovascular system, but an anti-estrogen in the uterus, breast, and CNS [8]. It thus has a more desirable profile for the treatment of postmenopausal osteoporosis. Its anti-estrogenic effects in the CNS would, however, still promote the incidence of vasomotor flashes. These agents should be contrasted with ICI 164,382 and ICI 187,720 which act as complete anti-estrogens (full antagonists) in all tissues [9]. They are primarily used for the hormonal ablative therapy of breast cancer when tamoxifen fails, thus increasing estrogenicity is seen across ligands: tamoxifen > raloxifene > ICI 164,384, and ICI 187,720.

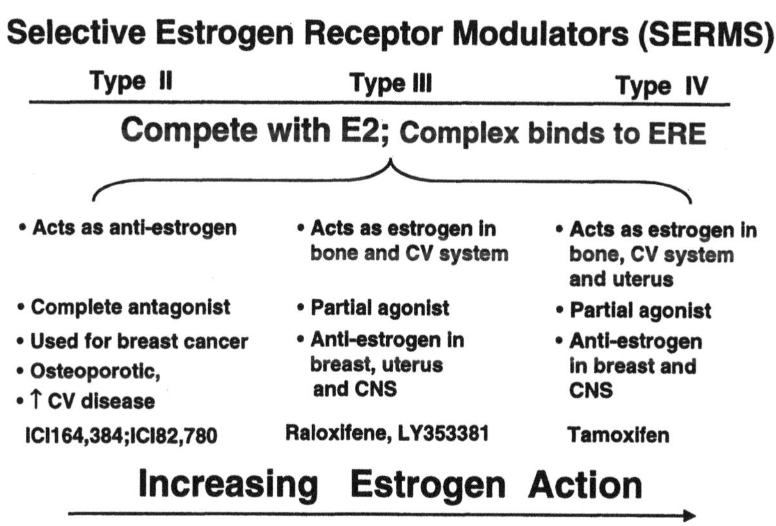

Figure 3. Increasing estrogenicity of SERMs.

Enzymes Involved in the Intracrine Formation of Steroid Hormones

SERMs are not the only agents that can give a tissue specific hormone response. There is evidence that similar effects may be achieved by enzyme inhibition. Steroid target tissues have their own profile of enzymes that can synthesize and eliminate active hormones (intracrine regulation) [10]. This phenomenon may be even more important when gonadal steroids are no longer produced as is the case at menopause.

A number of well-characterized steroidogenic reactions occur in target tissues, and in many instances these reactions have been targeted with enzyme inhibitors with therapeutic benefit. For example, in male prostate testosterone acts as a pro-hormone and is converted to 5α-dihydrotestosterone (5α-DHT) by type 2 5α-reductase [11]. 5α-DHT is essential for the normal and abnormal growth of the prostate, and inhibitors of type 2 5α-reductase, e.g. finasteride, can be used for the hormonal ablative therapy of benign prostatic hyperplasia and prostate cancer [11]. In the breast, peripheral aromatase activity (CYParom) will catalyze the conversion of Δ^4-androstenedione and testosterone to estrone and 17β-estradiol, respectively. Both steroidal (4-hydroxy-androstenedione) and nonsteroidal (Arimidex) CYParom inhibitors have now been developed for the hormonal ablative therapy of breast cancer [12]. A third example, involves the intracrine formation of progesterone from pregnenolone in the endometrium and placenta. This reaction is catalyzed by the type 1 3β-hydroxysteroid dehydrogenase and can be blocked by epostane. Epostane will deprive the endometrium of progesterone and can be used as abortifacient and postcoital contraceptive [13]. It thus has the same clinical outcome as RU486 but a different mode of action. RU486 is a progesterone receptor antagonist while epostane blocks the enzymatic formation of progesterone locally. It is thus apparent that drugs already exist to block the intracrine formation of androgens, estrogens and progestins in a tissue discrete manner.

This suggests that pre-receptor regulation of steroid hormone action can occur via enzymes that control ligand availability. Other enzymes that can regulate ligand access are the: steroid 5α/5β-reductases; the steroid sulfatases and steroid sulfotransferases, which respectively, liberate active hormone from their sulfate esters or eliminate active hormone by sulfate conjugation; and the hydroxysteroid dehydrogenases (HSDs), which convert potent steroid hormones into their cognate inactive metabolites. Target tissues contain their own specific profile of these enzymes, so that enzyme inhibitors can regulate the amount of active hormone present in a tissue specific manner. This has lead to the concept of "selective intracrine modulators." These agents will inhibit tissue specific enzymes that regulate the amount of ligand available for a steroid receptor, they will have the same effect as SERMs but a different mode of action.

HSDs are well-characterized targets for selective intracrine modulation. For each sex hormone there are a pair of HSDs which by acting as reductases or oxidases will either convert active hormone into their cognate inactive metabolite or vice-versa. They can thus regulate ligand occupancy for ER, AR (androgen receptor), and PR (progesterone receptor) [14].

For the ER the estrogenic type 1 17β-HSD acts exclusively as a reductase and will convert E1 (a weak estrogen) to E2 (a potent estrogen) and acts as the "on-switch" for the receptor [15] (Figure 4). By contrast the type 2 17β-HSD acts exclusively as an oxidase and will convert E2 to E1 and is the "off-switch" for the receptor [15]. The type 1 17β-HSD is expressed in the breast and the type 2 17β-HSD is distributed ubiquitously. For the AR, the type 2 3α-HSD acts as a reductase and will convert 5α-DHT (a potent androgen) to 3α-androstanediol (a weak androgen) and acts as the "off switch" for the receptor. By contrast, the type 3 3α-HSD acts as an oxidase and will convert 3α-androstanediol to 5α-DHT and is the "on switch" for the receptor [16]. Both isoforms are found in the prostate. For the PR, 20α-HSD by acting as a reductase will convert progesterone (active hormone) to 20α-hydroxyprogesterone (inactive progestin) and acts as the "off switch" for the receptor. 20α-HSD will also act as an oxidase and will convert 20α-OHP to P and turn on the PR.

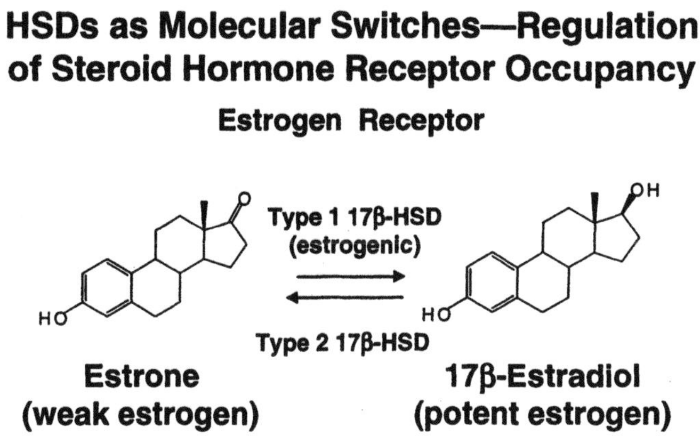

Figure 4. Pre-receptor regulation of steroid hormone action and type 1 17β-HSD.

Persuasive evidence exists to demonstrate that the type 1 17β-HSD is a target for selective intracrine modulation. The transient expression of its cDNA shows that it acts exclusively as reductase and will only convert E1 to E2 [10] a property that is also observed in cultured cells [17]. It is co-expressed in human breast epithelial cells with ERα and ERβ [18]. Thus its pattern of expression suggests that it regulates trans-activation of the ER. Its level of expression is elevated 20-fold in epithelial and stromal cells of human breast tumors indicating a role in the E2 dependent growth of the breast [19]. It is also co-expressed with aromatase in invasive lobular carcinoma [20]. Thus 17β-HSD is expressed in the same tissue as aromatase which makes its substrate estrone. Therefore inhibition of type 1 17β-HSD type is desirable to prevent E2 action in the breast.

Selective Intracrine Modulators in the Clinic

Are there selective intracrine modulators in the clinic, i.e. compounds that will inhibit tissue specific enzymes that regulate the amount of ligand available for a steroid receptor? A prototypic agent is tibolone [(7α,17α)-17-hydroxy-7-methyl-19-norpregn-5(10)-en-20-yn-3-one (Org OD 14)], Figure 5.

Tibolone exerts its effects by selective steroid (estrogen) receptor activation. This is achieved by a duality of function involving tissue specific modulation of enzymes that control ligand access to the ER (intracrine regulation) and by activation of the ER *per se* by its 3-hydroxy- metabolites. Tibolone is activated by metabolism to 3α and 3β-hydroxymetabolites . These metabolites will inhibit breast sulfatase with IC_{50} values of 0.08 μM and prevent the liberation of active estrogens from the sulfated pool [21]. These same metabolites also inhibit type 1 17β-HSD and prevent the conversion of E1 to E2 in the breast [22]. The combined effect is to deprive the breast ER of its estrogen. However, these same metabolites have no effect on bone sulfatase so that the ER in the bone has access to its ligands [23]. Thus the 3α- and 3β-hydroxymetabolites allow estrogenic effects in the bone but not the breast. In addition the 3α- and 3β-hydroxymetabolites can lead to ER activation in the bone [24].

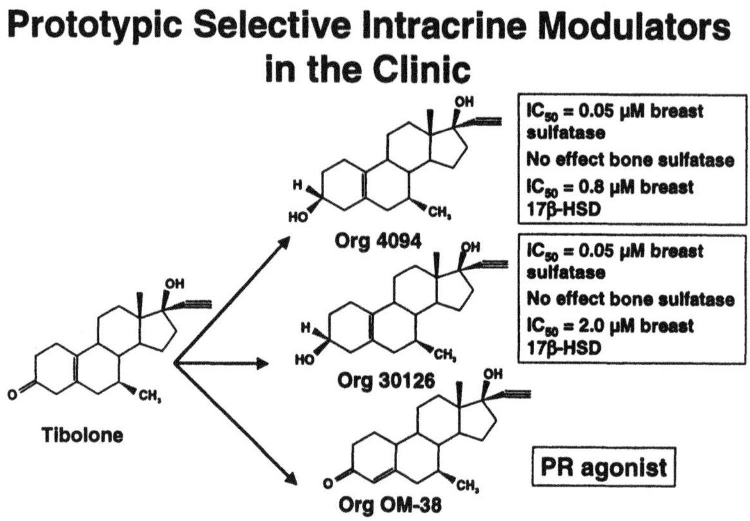

Figure 5. Prototypic selective intracrine modulators in the clinic.

A further beneficial effect of tibolone is that its Δ^4-ene metabolite, produced in the endometrium by type 1 3β-hydroxysteroid dehydrogenase, acts as PR agonist thus preventing estrogen stimulation of this tissue [25]. Thus by working through its metabolites tibolone can act as a tissue selective intracrine modulator and activator of the ER and PR. Because of its tissue specific effects in the bone it has an optimal profile for the treatment of postmenopausal osteoporosis. Clinical data also indicates that it reduces the incidence of hot flashes due to its estrogenic effects in the CNS [26], Figure 6.

Summary

In conclusion, SERMS work at the level of the ER and can produce a graded transcriptional response. By contrast selective intracrine modulators alter the activity of enzymes that convert potent steroid hormones into their cognate inactive metabolites and regulate ligand access to the ER in a tissue-specific manner. Tibolone exerts its effects via its metabolites working by both mechanisms.

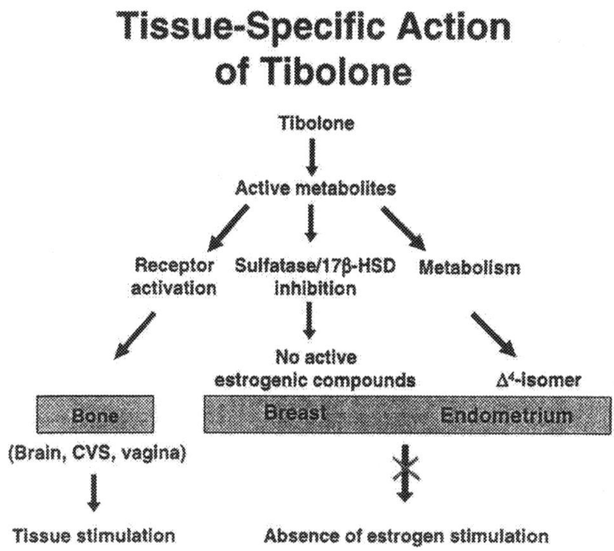

Figure 6. Tissue specific action of tibolone.

References

1. Carcon-Jurica MA, Schrader WT, O'Malley BW. Steroid receptor family: structure and functions. Endocrine Rev 1990;11:201-20.
2. Kuiper GGJM, Nilson S, Gustaffsson J-A. Characteristics and function of the novel estrogen receptor β. In: O'Malley BW, editor. Hormones and signaling. New York: Academic Press, 1998: 90-112.
3. Truss M, Beato, M. Steroid hormone receptors: interaction with deoxyribonucleic acid and transcription factors. Endocrine Rev 1993;14:459-79.
4. Wijayartane AL, Nagcl SC, Paige LA, et al. Comparative analysis of mechanistic differences among antiestrogens. Endocrinology 1990;140:5828-40.
5. Klinge C. Estrogen receptor interaction with co-activators and co-repressors. Steroids 2000;65:227-51.
6. Brzozwoski AM, Pike AC, Dauter Z, et al. Molecular basis of agonism and antagonism in the estrogen receptor. Nature 1997;389:753-58.
7. O'Regan RM, Jordan VC. Tamoxifen to raloxifene and beyond. Semin Oncol 2001;28: 260-73.
8. Jordan VC, Morrow M. Tamoxifen, raloxifene, and the prevention of breast cancer. Endocrine Rev 1999;20:253-78.
9. Nicholson RI, Francis AB, McClelland RA, Manning DL, Gee JMW. Pure anti-oestrogens (ICI 164,384 and ICI 182,780) and breast cancer: is the attainment of complete oestrogen withdrawal worthwhile? Endocrine Related Cancer 1994;4:5-19.

10. Labrie F, Luu-The V, Lin S-X, et al. Intracrinology: Role of the family of 17β-hydroxysteroid dehydrogenases in human pathology and disease. J Mol Endocrinol 2000; 25:1-16.
11. Jin Y, Penning, TM. Steroid 5α-reductases and 3α-hydroxysteroid dehydrogenases: Key enzymes in androgen metabolism. In: Seckl, JR, Walker, BR editors. Disorders of steroid metabolism. Holly, JMP, series editor. Best Practice & Research: Clinical Endocrinology and Metabolism. London: Bailliare Tindall 2000;15:79-94.
12. Miller WR Aromatase inhibitors. Endocrine Related Cancer 1996;3:65-79.
13. Crooji MJ, de Nooyer CC, Rao BR, Berends GT, Gooren LJ, Janssens, J. Termination of early pregnancy by the 3β-hydroxysteroid dehydrogenase inhibitor epostane. N Engl J Med 1988;319:813-17.
14. Penning TM. Molecular endocrinology of hydroxysteroid dehydrogenases. Endocrine Rev 1997;18:281-305.
15. Peltoketo H, Luu-The V, Simard J, Adamski J. 17β-hydroxysteroid dehydrogenase (HSD) 17-ketosteroid (KSR) family; nomenclature and main characteristics of the 17-HSD/KSR enzymes. J Mol Endocrinol 1999;23:1-11.
16. Penning TM, Burczynski ME, Jez JM, et al. Human 3α-hydroxysteroid dehydrogenase isoforms (AKR1C1-AK1C4) of the aldo-keto reductase superfamily: functional plasticity and tissue distribution reveals roles in the inactivation and formation of male and female sex hormones. Biochem J 2000;351:67-77.
17. Miettinen MM, Mustonen MV, Poutanen MH, Isomaa VV, Vihko, RK. Human 17β-hydroxysteroid dehydrogenase type 1 and type 2 isoenzymes have opposite activities in cultured cells and characteristic cell- and tissue-specific expression. Biochem J 1966;314: 839-45.
18. Jarvinen TAH, Pelto-Huikko M, Holli K, Isola J. Estrogen receptor β is co-expressed with ERα and PR and associated with nodal stats, grade and proliferation rate in breast cancer. Amer J Pathol 2000;156:29-35.
19. Spiers V, Green, AR, Atkin, SL. Activity and gene expression of 17β-hydroxysteroid dehydrogenase type 1 in primary cultures of epithelial and stromal cells derived from normal and tumorous human breast tissue: The role of IL-8 . J Steroid Biochem & Mol Biol 1998;67:267-74.
20. Sasano H, Frost AR, Saitoh R, et al. Aromatase and 17β-hydroxysteroid dehydrogenase type 1 in human breast carcinoma. J Clin Endcorinol 1996;81:4042-46.
21. Chetrite G, Kloosterboer HJ, Pasqualini JR. Effect of tibolone (Org OD14) and its metabolites on estrone sulphatase activity in MCF-7 and T-47D mammary cancer cells. Anti-cancer Res 1997;17:135-40.
22. Chetrite G, Kloosterboer HJ, Phillipe J-C, Pasqualini, JR. Effects of Org OD14 (Livial) and its metabolites on 17β-hydroxysteroid dehydrogenase activity in hormone-dependent MCF-7 and T-47D breast cancer cells. Anti-cancer Res 1999;19:261-68.
23. Kloosterboer HJ, de Gooyer ME. Tibolone inhibits sulfatase activity in breast but not in the bone. Proceedings 9th International Menopause Symposium 1999 Oct 17-21; Yokohama, Japan P349.
24. Kloosterboer HJ. Tibolone a steroid with a tissue-specific mode of action. J Steroid Biochem & Mol Biol 2001;76:231-38.
25. Tang B, Markiewicz L, Kloosterboer HJ, Gurpride E. Human endometrial 3β-hydroxysteroid dehydrogenase/isomerase can locally reduce intrinsic estrogenic/

progestagenic activity ratios of a steroidal drug (Org OD14). J Steroid Biochem & Mol Biol 1993;45:345-51.

26. Al-azzawi F, Wahab M, Habiba M, Akkad A, Mason T. Continuous combined hormone replacement therapy compared with tibolone. Obstet Gynecol 1999;93:258-64.

TIBOLONE IS EFFECTIVE IN PREVENTING POSTMENOPAUSAL BONE LOSS

J.C. Gallagher

Introduction

Tibolone is a synthetic compound, which binds to estrogen, progesterone, and androgen receptors. Previous studies have shown favorable effects on bone, the vagina, the cardiovascular system, climacteric symptoms, mood, and libido without detrimental estrogen-like stimulation of the breast and endometrium [1-4]. Studies have indicated that tibolone increases bone mineral density (BMD) relative to baseline or placebo over periods ranging from 6 months to 3 years [3]. Two large, multicenter, randomized, double-blind, placebo-controlled, dose-finding studies were performed in North America. These studies were intended to evaluate the efficacy of different doses of tibolone in the prevention of bone loss in early postmenopausal women, and to determine the minimum effective dose of tibolone.

Methods

DESIGN AND PARTICIPANTS

Seven hundred seventy participants were randomized to 5 treatment groups: 0.3, 0.625, 1.25, or 2.5 mg tibolone or placebo daily for 2 years. In addition, all participants received supplemental calcium carbonate (500 mg/day). The patients were healthy postmenopausal women within 4 years of menopause, without clinical or radiologic evidence of osteoporosis. Two multicenter studies were carried out, depending on whether the center used Lunar or Hologic DEXA machines.

The mean age of the participants was 52.4 (± 3.3) years. They averaged 2.5 (± 1.6) years postmenopause. Participants' mean body mass index (BMI) was 25.1 (± 3.7) kg/m^2. The dropout rate ranged from 28% to 36%. Twelve percent of the participants withdrew for nondrug-related reasons and 11% discontinued treatment due to adverse effects. The intent-to-treat group included 656 women.

EFFICACY MEASURES

The primary outcome measures included the assessment of BMD of the lumbar spine, total hip, and femoral neck, while secondary measures included assessments of two bone biochemical markers, serum osteocalcin and urine cross-linked N-telopeptides of bone collagen (NTX). BMD was measured by DEXA using either Hologic or Lunar densitometers. Serum osteocalcin was measured in the Mayo Clinic assay system; urinary NTX assays were measured with a commercially available system (Osteomark, Mochida Pharmaceutical Co., Japan).

STATISTICAL ANALYSIS

Statistical analysis was based on an intent-to-treat population. Treatment groups were compared by analysis of variance (ANOVA). The BMD and bone marker results presented here consist of pooled data from both DEXA studies. All results are expressed as percentages of change from baseline.

Results

LUMBAR SPINE BMD

Figure 1 shows the dose-dependent increase in lumbar spine BMD by tibolone. Spine BMD was significantly different from placebo for all doses of tibolone at 24 months ($p = 0.0001$). Furthermore, the difference in BMD relative to placebo was significant from 6 months onward ($p < 0.05$). The 3 higher doses of tibolone increased spine BMD, with increases of more than 2% for the 2.5 mg dose. The percent change in BMD between the highest dose of tibolone (2.5 mg) and placebo after 24 months was nearly 5%.

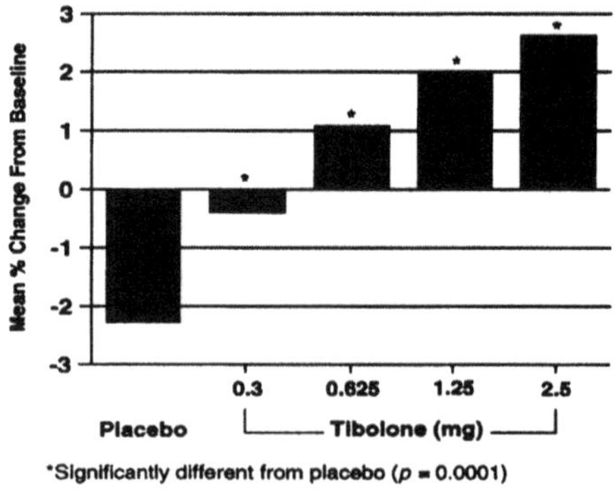

Figure 1. Mean percent change from baseline in BMD of lumbar spine for each treatment group at 24 months

TOTAL HIP BMD

Tibolone dose-dependently increased total hip BMD (Figure 2). The 3 higher tibolone doses increased total hip BMD by 24 months (p = 0.0001), with increases of up to approximately 2% for the highest dose of tibolone (2.5 mg). The percent change in BMD between the 2.5 mg dose of tibolone and placebo after 24 months was approximately 4%.

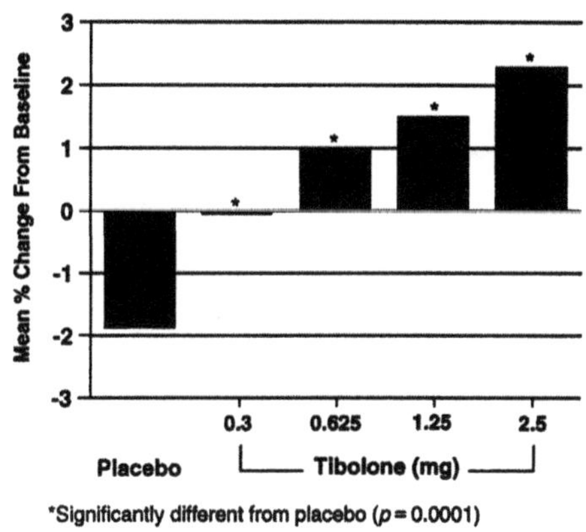

Figure 2. Mean percent change from baseline in BMD of total hip for each treatment group at 24 months

FEMORAL NECK BMD

All doses of tibolone produced a significant difference in femoral neck BMD after 24 months (p = 0.0001) compared to placebo (Figure 3). Treatment with the 1.25 and 2.5 mg doses resulted in greater BMD relative to placebo at all time points subsequent to the 6-month mark ($p \leq 0.001$).

BONE BIOCHEMICAL MARKERS

The highest dose of tibolone (2.5 mg) significantly (p = 0.0001) reduced serum osteocalcin by approximately 20% relative to placebo after 24 months of treatment (Figure 4). The effect of the intermediate doses of tibolone (0.625 mg and 1.25 mg) were less pronounced, but were still statistically significant ($p \leq 0.001$).

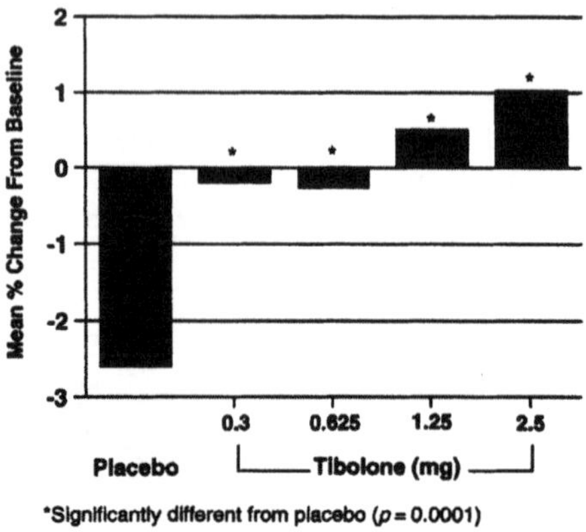

Figure 3. Mean percent change from baseline in BMD of femoral neck for each treatment group at 24 months

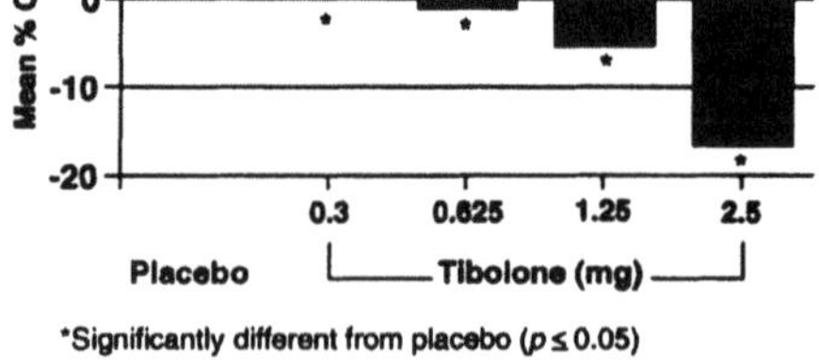

Figure 4. Mean percent change from baseline in serum osteocalcin for each treatment group at 24 months

Figure 5 illustrates changes in urinary NTX levels with tibolone treatment (because the distribution was not normal, medians rather than median are plotted). The 2 lower doses of tibolone (0.3 and 0.625 mg) reduced median NTX levels by more than 20% from baseline and the 2 higher doses (1.25 and 2.5 mg) reduced median NTX levels by more than 40%. With the exception of the lowest dose (0.3 mg) at 6 months, all doses of tibolone reduced NTX levels, relative to placebo, from the 6-month mark onward ($p \leq 0.001$).

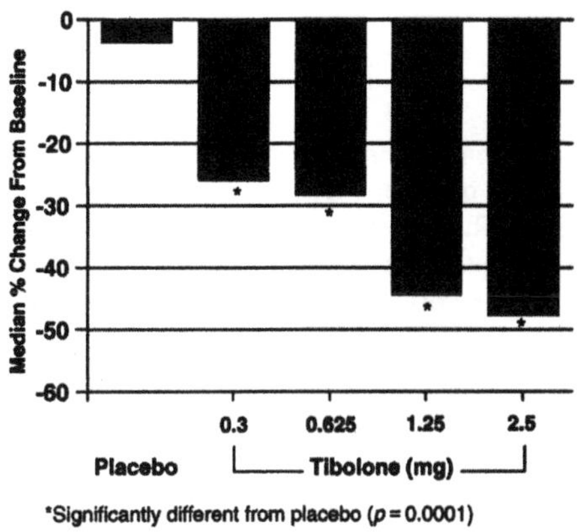

Figure 5. Median percent change from baseline in urinary cross-linked N-telopeptides for each treatment group at 24 months

Discussion

Previous studies have shown that tibolone, a tissue-specific compound, has potent effects on BMD, similar to those of estrogen [3,5]. In the studies presented here, daily doses of 0.625 mg or higher of tibolone progressively increased BMD in lumbar spine and total hip over a 2-year span in early postmenopausal women. With regard to femoral neck density, there was an increase in BMD only on the 1.25 mg and 2.5 mg doses. At all skeletal sites, placebo-treated participants consistently lost bone density over the 2-year time period despite calcium supplementation. The substantial decreases in serum osteocalcin and urinary NTX levels observed with the higher doses of tibolone are consistent with a significant dose-dependent decrease in bone turnover and inhibition of bone resorption.

The present investigation has indicated that, while all four doses of tibolone revealed significant positive effects on bone density, the 1.25 mg/day dose appears to be the optimum dose for the prevention of bone loss at the femoral neck as well as the spine. As with estrogens, the increase in BMD was greater in the spine than the femoral neck. In comparison to other therapeutic agents, tibolone 1.25 mg per day has an effect on spine and total hip BMD similar to that of other antiresportive agents, such as bisphosphonates and estrogens [6,7]. In summary, tibolone is a tissue-specific compound that is effective for preventing osteoporosis in postmenopausal women.

Acknowledgments

This work described above was made possible by many investigators who worked on tibolone in the USA.

References

1. Kloosterboer HJ. Tibolone and its metabolites: Pharmacology, tissue specificity and effects in animal models of tumors. Gynecol Endocrinol 2001;11(Suppl.1):63-68.
2. Kloosterboer HJ, Sands R. Intracrinology: The secret of the tissue-specificity of tibolone. Journal of British Menopause Society 2000;Supplement S2:23-27.
3. Moore RA. Livial: A review of clinical studies. Br J Obstet Gynaecol 1999;106(Suppl.19): 1-21.
4. Tang B, Markiewicz L, Kloosterboer HJ, Gurpide E. Human endometrial 3 beta-hydroxysteroid dehydrogenase/isomerase can locally reduce intrinsic estrogenic/ progestagenic activity ratios of a steroidal drug (Org OD 14). J Steroid Biochem Molec Biol 1993;45(5):345-51.
5. Ederveen AG, Kloosterboer HJ. Tibolone exerts its protective effect on trabecular bone loss through the estrogen receptor. J Bone Miner Res 2001;16:in press.
6. Black DM, Cummings SR, Karpf DB, et al. Randomised trial of effect of alendronate on risk of fracture in women with existing vertebral fractures. Lancet 1996;348:1535-41.
7. Ravn, P., Bidstrup, M., Wasnich, R.D., et al. Alendronate and estrogen-progestin in the long-term prevention of bone loss: Four-year results from the early postmenopausal intervention cohort study. A randomized, controlled trial. Ann Intern Med 1999;131(12); 935-42.

Sex Hormones and the Immune System: Implications for Menopause and Autoimmunity

Gil Mor

Introduction

It has long been suspected that there is a strong interaction between sex hormones and the immune system. Several observations support this concept such as the dimorphic nature of the two genders, alterations in the immune response after gonadectomy or sex steroid hormone treatment, modification of the immune response during pregnancy, and the identification of steroid hormone receptors in cells of the immune system support this concept. Numerous *in vitro* and *in vivo* experiments have demonstrated that sex hormones affect and modify the actions of cells of the immune system. In addition, considerable evidence has accumulated suggesting that the interaction between estrogen and cells of the immune system can have non-immune regulatory effects. Thus, the role of estrogen in prevention of bone loss is mediated by mechanisms involving the inhibition of proinflammatory cytokines by bone marrow cells [1-3].Moreover, disorders frequently affecting women after menopause, such as cardiovascular disease, osteoporosis, or neurodegenerative disorders, can be ascribed to the loss of sex hormone-dependent regulation of physiological functions, as well as to a modification of the non-immune functions of resident immune cells [4].

In this review we will outline the complex relationships between the menopause, sex hormones, target immune cells, and cytokines, stressing the implications of these phenomena on immune and non-immune regulation and autoimmunity during different stages of a woman's life. Particular emphasis is given to the time following menopause.

The Classical Immune System

The immune system eliminates foreign material in two ways: natural/innate immunity and adaptive immunity. Natural immunity produces a relatively unsophisticated response that prevents access of pathogens to the body. This is a primitive evolutionary response that occurs without the need of prior exposure to similar pathogens. For example, macrophages and granulocytes engulf invading microorganisms at the site of entry. These macrophages are estrogen-sensitive.

Adaptive immunity is an additional, more sophisticated response found in higher forms such as humans. Cells of the innate immune system process phagocytose foreign material and present its antigens to cells of the adaptive immunity for possible reactions. This immune response is highly specific and normally is potentiated by repeated antigenic encounters. It is also hormonally sensitive. Adaptive immunity consists of two types of immune responses: humoral immunity in which antibodies are produced and cellular immunity which involves cell lysis by specialized lymphocytes (cytolytic T cells). The adaptive immunity is characterized by an anamnestic response, that enables the immune cells to "remember" the foreign antigenic encounter and react to further exposures to the same antigen faster and more vigorously; and by the use of cytokines for communication and regulation of the innate immune response.

Immune cells mediate their effects by releasing cytokines and thus establishing particular microenvironments. T helper lymphocytes (Th) that originate from the thymus play a major role in creating a specific microenvironment for a particular organ or tissue. Following an immune challenge immune cells produce cytokine, the type of which determines their differentiation into T helper-1 (Th-1) or T-helper 2 (Th-2) lymphocytes. For example, Th-1 lymphocytes secrete interleukin-2 (IL-2) and interferon-γ (INF- γ) setting the basis for a pro-inflammatory environment. Conversely, the Th-2 lymphocytes secrete cytokines such as IL-4 and IL-10 which are predominately involved in antibody production following an antigenic challenge. The actions of the two types of lymphocytes are closely intertwined, both acting in concert and responding to counter regulatory effects of their cytokines. For example Th1 cytokines produce pro-inflamatory cytokine that while acting to reinforce the cytolitic immune response, also down-regulate the production of Th2 type cytokines (for review see 5-7). Thus, women during the reproductive years are more likely to develop a Th-1 response after challenge with an infectious agent or antigen, except during pregnancy when a Th-2 environment prevails (see below and 8).

NON-IMMUNE REGULATORY FUNCTIONS OF LEUKOCYTES AND THEIR PRODUCTS

Migratory immune cells, especially macrophages, not only provide protection against foreign antigens but also, through the production of cytokines and hormones, have an active role in the regulation of cell growth and function of almost all the tissues in the body. Similarly, leukocytes express receptors for hormones and neurotransmitters, which make them targets for the action of hormones in the local microenvironment. We have named the immune cells as the "migratory or portable endocrine system" [4].

This non-immune regulation is extremely active in reproductive tissues and sensitive to sex steroids . In general we can characterize this relationship as one in which the balance between cytolitic and humoral immunity is dependent on gonadal function-hormone availability. Examples of the interaction between sex hormones and the immune system can be summarized as follows:

Sex differences in the immune response and the effect of menopause. Physiologic, experimental, and clinical data confirm differences in immune responses between the two sexes [9]. During reproductive years females tend to have a more vigorous immune response: higher immunoglobulin concentrations, stronger primary and secondary responses, increased resistance to the induction of immunological tolerance and a greater ability to reject tumors and homografts [10]. A recent report has shown changes in allergy sensitivity between males and females at about the age of 15 (when male testosterone and in females estrogen levels increase) [11].

During the climateric the function of the immune system becomes more similar to that in men. This alteration is both functional and in the cellular composition. We have shown that the number of circulating macrophage precursors (monocytes) increases during menopause. This estrogen-regulated function could be due to increase of bone marrow precursor or a decrease of cell migration into tissues. Hormone replacement therapy decreases the monocyte number to levels found in premenopausal women [12]. Moreover, in animal studies, ovariectomy upregulates myeloid cell differentiation into the monocyte-macrophage lineage and increases thymic weight while estrogen replacement decreases the number of thymocytes and the size of the thymus [13].

Further evidences of a role for estrogen as an immunomodulator is provided by the observation that the incidence of a great variety of autoimmune diseases which are by far and large over-represented in reproductive-age women [14], dramatically decrease following the menopause [15,16].

Sexual hormones and autoimmunity; implications for menopause. The predominance of autoimmune disease among women suggests that sex hormones may modulate immune-susceptibly. This covers a broad range of autoimmune disorders, ranging from organ-specific (such as Graves' disease) to generalized, such as systemic lupus erythematosis (SLE). Although, multiple sclerosis (MS), SLE, and rheumatoid arthritis (RA) are different diseases and probably differ in etiology, the common link is the prevalence of these diseases in women [17]. The reasons for the sex bias in autoimmune diseases are unclear but may include such factors as sex-related differences in immune responsiveness, response to infection, sex steroid effects, and sex-linked genetic factors. Women may have greater susceptibility to autoimmune diseases, in part because of more robust immune responses, yet have a better prognosis, perhaps as a result of heightened recovery mechanisms [18]. Elucidation of the precise cellular and molecular mechanisms by which sex hormones alter immune function as well as the signal transduction pathways involved is vital to understanding gender differences in autoimmunity.

Most attention has been directed toward the sex steroids, estrogens and progesterone, which are produced in the ovary. The findings that estrogen has a biphasic effects on normal immune responses [19,20] and in autoimmune diseases has helped to explain many contradictory results from *in vitro* as well as *in vivo* studies using different doses of estrogen or progesterone. There are natural fluctuations in the levels of sex hormones during the menstrual cycle and pregnancy. These changes can also be induced by oral contraceptives and by estrogen replacement therapy after menopause. In addition, the recent identification of a second estrogen receptor has prompted new areas of investigation.

Alterations in the course of autoimmune diseases during pregnancy underscore the presence of sex-hormone modulation of the immune microenvironment. During pregnancy as well as pre- and post-partum there are differences between the diseases. In MS and RA there is a decrease in disease severity during the 9 months of gestation, with a return to pre-pregnancy levels after birth. This is in contrast to SLE where some studies show that the disease worsens during pregnancy, whereas others show no change. Elevations of serum estradiol are often found in female patients with SLE, and often can be linked to active disease [21,22]. For example, one study has shown that peripheral blood cells from patients with SLE respond to estrogen treatment with a reduction of TNF-α [23]. Because this cytokine regulates apoptosis, the failure to maintain its production during pregnancy may disturb programmed cell death of activated immunocompetent cells in SLE and thereby enhances autoimmunity. Conversely, estrogens prevent apoptosis in synovial macrophages [24] and reduce apoptosis in human peripheral blood cells [25].In women, the onset of symptoms in MS appears to be earlier than in men, but men tend to exhibit a rapid progression and more severe disease course. In SLE women first show disease symptoms during childbearing years, whereas men tend to show disease later in life [14]. Although the differences remains unexplained, they are real. It has been proposed that the differences in the rate of disease progression and presentation are due to sex-linked genetic factors and to the effects of sex hormones on injury and repair mechanisms [26].

Gender differences in the course of autoimmune disease have clinical implications. For example, should therapy be initiated differently in men and women? The possible role of hormone replacement therapy should be considered in cases of autoimmune disease.

Regulation of reproductive functions by immune cells and their products (cytokines): implications for the menopause. Recent data has provided evidence of a feed-back loop between reproductive hormones, mainly estrogen, and the expression, distribution, and activity of cytokines [27]. *In vitro* studies using mice cell cultures showed that while androgens decreased the production of IFN-γ, IL-4, and IL-5 [28], estrogen enhanced IFN-γ production by murine lymphoid cells [29]. Moreover, estrogen treatment of macrophages from male mice increased IL-1 secretion [30]. In CD4+ T cell clones from MS patients, both IL-10 and IFN-γ production were increased in the presence of estradiol [31].Likewise, cytokines can regulate endocrine and reproductive functions. In human pituitary cells *in vitro*, IL-1β induces the release of the gonadotrophins, LH and FSH. IL-6 has also been shown to promote the release of FSH and LH in amounts similar to the released in response to gonadotrophin-releasing hormone (GnRH). As an example, in women with acute or chronic severe illness, delays in ovulation and even chronic anovulation can commonly develop, and IL-1β is thought to play a major role in suppressing LH release. IL-1β acts to inhibit the estrogen-induced surge in LH release, there by supporting the hypothesis that cytokines are involved in causing the anovulation observed in women with severe illness [32,33]. Other cytokines of gonadal origin such as activin and inhibin (members of the TGF-β family) modulate the release of FSH from the pituitary.

A growing body of evidence indicates that IL-6 and other cytokines modulate the rate of formation of steroid hormones in the gonads and adrenal cortex as well as in extraglandular tissues. Hence, IL-6 inhibits formation of progesterone in granulosa cells and TGF-β acts in a number of steroid-producing endocrine cells to inhibit steroidogenesis, in part by a mechanism of inhibition of gene transcription [34].

Cytokines are also important for reproduction, TGF-β acts in the stromal endometrial cells to counteract the action of progesterone by way of a progesterone receptor-independent process in a gene-specific manner affecting the function of endometrial cells. The expression of TGF-β in the endometrium seems to be related to blatocyst implantation [34]. It has been shown that during implantation there is a wave-like propagation of the TGF-β immunoreactivity in the endometrium that begins at the site of implantation and proceeds outward to involve the entire endometrium in a decidual response [35].

Using an animal model for SLE, we showed that tamoxifen, or a specific antibody against estradiol had beneficial effects on the clinical manifestations of the SLE-model mice by restoring the level of cytokines to the normal levels observed in the control mice. These findings suggest that cytokine modulation could be the basis to explain the effect of estrogen on the immune system and the therapeutic use of selected estrogen receptor modulators (SERMS) on autoimmune disease [36].

These results indicate a strong interaction between the endocrine and immune systems and support our definition of the immune cells as "migratory endocrine cells." These cells have the potential for *in situ* modulation of reproductive functions, such as ovulation, and serve as targets for steroid hormones, participating in multiple autocrine and paracrine circuits.

An integrated hypothesis of sex steroids hormones, cytokines and autoimmune diseases during the transition to menopause. As we pointed out above, it is now generally agreed that the immune responses may polarize into cytokine environments characteristic of Th1 and Th2 cells. In general, the normal reproductive women has a strong tendency to respond to foreign antigens by developing a Th1-type 1 (type 1) immune response (cell mediated) and by expressing high levels of pro-inflammatory cytokines [16,37]. However, during pregnancy, there is a decrease in cellular immunity and enhancement of humoral immunity, characterized by higher levels of anti-inflammatory cytokines [38]. Both human and murine pregnancies, particularly at the maternal fetal interface, have been shown to exhibit a strong shift in cytokine balance from type 1 to type 2.

Although no autoimmune disease can be considered exclusively type 1- or type 2 cytokine-driven, it is generally agreed that the clinical manifestations of MS and RA primarily reflect a nonspecific response by excessive number of macrophages present plus a specific cell-mediated type-1 immune response. In contrast, SLE is considered to be antibody-mediated disease dependent on type 2 cytokines. Hence, the particular hormone environment during pregnancy favors a Th-2 response, which halts the progression of the Th-1 immune response associated with MS and RA while further enhancing the ongoing Th-2-antibody-promoting response associated with SLE [15,16]. Studies of peripheral blood cells from pregnant women confirm the down-regulation of proinflammatory cytokines and enhancement of anti-inflammatory cytokines production [23,39].

Menopause represents a low estrogen state and possibly a type 1 immune environment. This would be consistent with changes in other tissues studied such as bone.

Estrogen receptors and immune cells. Estrogen modulates its effect by binding to estrogen receptors (ER) present in the immune target cells. The ER is a nuclear transcription factor that regulates gene expression [40]. Some of the genes regulated by estrogens are pS2, progesterone receptor, bcl2 apoptosis inhibitor, Fas Ligand and other growth-related genes responsible for estrogen's effects on cell death and proliferation. Others and we have shown ER in human peripheral blood mononuclear cells, thymocytes, spleen cells. Rat peritoneal macrophages and human leukemic cells and the monocytic leukemia cell line J111 [41-45]. The recent discovery of a second estrogen receptor, ERβ [46,47], presents new possibilities for control of immune targets by different selective estrogen receptor modulators.

One of the main immune cells targets for the action of estrogen is the monocytes/macrophages. We characterized the expression of ERs in human peripheral monocytes as well as in tissue macrophages including brain macrophages or macroglia [42,48].

Changes in the Immune System During Menopause

A relationship between sex hormones and the immune system during the menopause is clear. We have demonstrated that in postmenopausal women the number of peripheral blood monocytes is increased and the percentage of estrogen receptor positive monocytes is relatively decreased [12]. Further more, estrogen replacement therapy for a period of three months led to a decline in the numbers of monocytes to the values observed in young women and to an increase in percentage of ER positive monocytes. Interestingly, no change was observed in the total leukocytes among all study participants [12]. Similarly, it was demonstrated that in ovariectomized rats there is an upregulation of myeloid cell differentiation into the monocyte-macrophage lineage [13]. Another study [49] showed that short-term estradiol replacement in healthy postmenopausal women induced a significant reduction in Natural Killer cell (NK) activity but left antibody-dependent cytotoxicity unaffected. Although the NK cell activity dropped significantly after 3 weeks of estradiol treatment, it did not reach levels of untreated premenopausal women, further underscoring the important role of estrogen in autoimmune diseases [50,51].

Conclusion

This review has presented a limited view on selected topics in the broad interaction between the immune system sex steroids and the menopause. Based on these studies, it is clear that sex hormones, and estrogen in particular, modulate the activation of immune cells in immune and non-immune functions. Although gender differences in autoimmune diseases are well recognized, sexual dimorphism in the immune response and the importance of sex hormones in promoting differences between men and women need further study.

During the menopause, deficiency of estrogen results in a failure of estrogen's regulation of the immune system, and this may in turn play an important role in the development of climacteric symptomatology and disease. We believe that understanding of the tight bond between the immune system and sex hormones will open up for further study in this regard, and promote the understanding and development of potential preventive and therapeutic possibilities for the menopausal woman.

References

1. Jilka R, Hangok G, Girasole G, et al. Increased osteoclast development after estrogen loss: Mediation by interleukin-6. Science 1992;257:88-91.
2. Kitazawa R, Kimble RB, Vannice JL, Kung VT, Pacifici R. Interleukin-1 receptor antagonist and tumor necrosis factor binding protein decrease osteoclast formation and bone resorption in ovariectomized mice. J Clin Invest 1994;94:2397-406.
3. Kimble RB, Kitazawa R, Vannice JL, Pacifici R. Persistent bone-sparing effect of interleukin-1 receptor antagonist: A hypothesis on the role of IL-1 in ovariectomy-induced bone loss. Calcif Tissue Int 1994;55:260-65.
4. Mor G, Naftolin F. Oestrogen, menopause and the immune system. JBMS 1998;4:4-8.
5. van der Meer JW, Vogels MT, Netea MG, Kullberg BJ. Proinflammatory cytokines and treatment of disease. Ann N Y Acad Sci 1998;856:243-51.
6. van Deuren M, Dofferhoff AS, van der Meer JW. Cytokines and the response to infection. J Pathol 1992;168:349-56.
7. Mor G, Klinman D, Shapiro S, et al. Complexity of the cytokine and antibody response elicited by immunizing mice with Plasmodium yoelii circumsporozoite protein plasmid DNA. J Immunol 1995;155:2039-46.
8. Weetman AP. The immunology of pregnancy. Thyroid 1999;9:643-46.
9. Ahmed S, Penhale W, Talal N., Sex hormones, immune response and autoimmune disease. Am J Path 1985;121:531-51.
10. Schuurs A, Verheul H. Effects of gender and sex steroids on the immune response. J Steroid Biochem 1990;35:157-72.
11. Verheul H, Tittes E, Kelder J, Schuurs A. Effects of steroids with different endocrine profiles on the development, morphology and function of the bursa of Fabricious in chickens. J Steroid Bioch 1986;25: 665-75.
12. Ben-Hur H, Mor G, Insler V, et al. Menopause is associated with a significant increase in blood monocyte number and a relative decrease in the expression of estrogen receptors in human peripheral monocytes. AJRI 1995;34:363-69.
13. Erben RG, Raith S, Eberle J, Stangassinger M. Ovariectomy augments B lymphopoiesis and generation of monocyte-macrophage precursors in rat bone marrow. Am J Physiol 1998;274:E476-83.
14. Talal N. Autoimmunity and sex revisited.Clin Immunol Immunopathol 1989;53:355-57.
15. Cutolo M, Sulli A, Seriolo B, Accardo S, Masi AT. Estrogens, the immune response and autoimmunity. Clin Exp Rheumatol 1995;13:217-26.
16. Wilder RL. Hormones, pregnancy, and autoimmune diseases. Ann NY Acad Sci 1998;840: 45-50.
17. Whitacre CC, Reingold SC, O'Looney PA. A gender gap in autoimmunity. Science 1999; 283:1277-78.
18. Olsen N, Kovacs W. Gonadal steroids and immunity. Endocrine Rev 1996;17:369-84.

19. Polan M, Daniele A, Kuo A. Gonodal steroids modulate human monocyte interleukin-1 (IL-1) activity. Fert Steril 1988;49:964-68.
20. Polan ML, Loukides J, Nelson P, et al. Progesterone and estradiol modulate interleukin-1-beta messenger ribonucleic acid levels in cultured human peripheral monocytes. J Clin Endoc Metab 1989;69:1200-6.
21. Lahita RG, Bradlow HL. Klinefelter's syndrome: Hormone metabolism in hypogonadal males with systemic lupus erythematosus. J Rheumatol 1987;14(Suppl.13):154-57.
22. Lahita RG, Bradlow HL, Ginzler E, Pang S, New M. Low plasma androgens in women with systemic lupus erythematosus. Arthritis Rheum 1987;30:241-48.
23. Wilder RL, Elenkov IJ. Hormonal regulation of tumor necrosis factor-alpha, interleukin-12 and interleukin-10 production by activated macrophages. A disease-modifying mechanism in rheumatoid arthritis and systemic lupus erythematosus? Ann NY Acad Sci 1999;876:14-31.
24. Evans MJ, MacLaughlin S, Marvin RD, Abdou NI. Estrogen decreases in vitro apoptosis of peripheral blood mononuclear cells from women with normal menstrual cycles and decreases TNF-alpha production in SLE but not in normal cultures. Clin Immunol Immunopathol 1997;82:258-62.
25. Vegeto E, Pollio G, Pellicciari C, Maggi A. Estrogen and progesterone induction of survival of monoblastoid cells undergoing TNF-alpha-induced apoptosis. FASEB J 1999; 13:793-803.
26. Poser S, Kurtzke JF, Poser W, Schlaf G. Survival in multiple sclerosis. J Clin Epidemiol 1989;42:159-68.
27. Adashi E. The potential relevance of cytokines to ovarian physiology:The emerging role of resident ovarian cells of the white blood cell series. End Rev 1990;11:454-63.
28. Araneo BA, Dowell T, Diegel M, Daynes RA. Dihydrotestosterone exerts a depressive influence on the production of interleukin-4 (IL-4), IL-5, and gamma-interferon, but not IL-2 by activated murine T cells. Blood 1991;78:688-99.
29. Fox HS, Bond BL, Parslow TG. Estrogen regulates the IFN-gamma promoter. J Immunol 1991;146:4362-67.
30. Hu S-K, Mitcho Y, Rath N. Effect of estradiol on Interleukin 1 synthesis by macrophages. Int J Immunopharmac 1988;10:247-52.
31. Gilmore W, Weiner LP, Correale J. Effect of estradiol on cytokine secretion by proteolipid protein- specific T cell clones isolated from multiple sclerosis patients and normal control subjects. J Immunol 1997;158:446-51.
32. Jasper M, Norman RJ. Immunoactive interleukin-1 beta and tumour necrosis factor-alpha in thecal, stromal and granulosa cell cultures from normal and polycystic ovaries. Hum Reprod 1995;10:1352-54.
33. Bonello N, McKie K, Jasper M, et al. Inhibition of nitric oxide: Effects on interleukin-1 beta-enhanced ovulation rate, steroid hormones, and ovarian leukocyte distribution at ovulation in the rat. Biol Reprod 1996;54:436-45.
34. Kruessel JS, Huang HY, Wen Y, Kloodt AR, Bielfeld P, Polan ML. Different pattern of interleukin-1 beta-(IL-1 beta), interleukin-1 receptor antagonist- (IL-1ra) and interleukin-1 receptor type I- (IL-1R tI) mRNA-expression in single preimplantation mouse embryos at various developmental stages. J Reprod Immunol 1997;34:103-20.
35. Tabibzadeh S. Human endometrium: An active site of cytokine production and action. End Rev 1991;12:272-90.
36. Dayan M, Zinger H, Kalush F, et al. The beneficial effects of treatment with tamoxifen and

anti-oestradiol antibody on experimental systemic lupus erythematosus are associated with cytokine modulations. Immunol 1997;90:101-8.
37. Elenkov IJ, Hoffman J, Wilder RL. Does differential neuroendocrine control of cytokine production govern the expression of autoimmune diseases in pregnancy and the postpartum period? Mol Med Today 1997;3:379-83.
38. Chaouat G, Cayol V, Mairovitz V, Dubanchet S. Localization of the Th2 cytokines IL-3, IL-4, IL-10 at the fetomaternal interface during human and murine pregnancy and lack of requirement for Fas/Fas ligand interaction for a successful allogeneic pregnancy. Am J Reprod Immunol 1999;42:1-13.
39. Ostensen M. Sex hormones and pregnancy in rheumatoid arthritis and systemic lupus erythematosus. Ann NY Acad Sci 1999;876:131-43; discussion 144.
40. Evans R. The steroid and thyroid hormone receptor superfamily. Science 1988;240:889-95.
41. Carbone A, Piantelli M, Musiani P, et al. Estrogen binding sites in peripheral blood monuclear cells and thymocytes from 2 myasthenia bravis patients. J Clin Lab Immunol 1986;21:87-91.
42. Mor G, Zaltsman Y, Barnard G, Ben-Hur H,Kohen F. Evidence for the presence of estrogen receptor in monocytes. Endoc J 1993;1:387-95.
43. Cohen J, Danel L, Gordier G, Saez S, Revillard J. Sex steroid receptors in peripheral T cells; abscence of androgen receptors and restriction of estrogen receptors to OKT 8 positive cells. J Immun 1983;131:2767-71.
44. Zaltsman Y, Mor G, Globerson A, Thole H, Kohen F. Expression of estrogen receptors in thymocytes. Endoc J 1993;1:211-17.
45. Gulshan S, McCruden A, Stimson W. Oestrogen receptors in macrophages. Scand J Immunol 1990;31:691-97.
46. Kuiper GGJM, Enmark E, Pelto-Huikko M, Nilsson S, Gustafsson J-A. Cloning of a novel estrogen receptor expressed in rat prostate and ovary. Proc Natl Acad Sci USA 1996;93: 5925-30.
47. Kuiper GGJM, Gustafsson J-A. The novel estrogen receptor-β subtype: Potential role in the cell- and promoter-specific actions of estrogens and anti-estrogens. FEBS Letters 1996; 410:87-90.
48. Mor G, Nilsen J, Horvath T, et al. Estrogen and microglia: A regulatory system that affects the brain. J Neurobio 1999;40:484-96.
49. Albrecht AE, Hartmann BW, Scholten C, Huber JC, Kalinowska W, Zielinski CC. Effect of estrogen replacement therapy on natural killer cell activity in postmenopausal women. Maturitas 1996;25:217-22.
50. Lahita RG. Emerging concepts for sexual predilection in the disease systemic lupus erythematosus. Ann NY Acad Sci 1999;876:64-69; discussion 69-70.
51. Lahita RG. The role of sex hormones in systemic lupus erythematosus. Curr Opin Rheumatol 1999;11:352-56.

Routes of HRT Administration. When to Use Oral Or Transdermal Administration

Göran Samsioe

Introduction

As with most pharmacologic agents, estrogens and progestogens can be administered by several modes of administration. Indeed such steroids could be given as eye drops, intranasal spray, tablets, transdermal patches, transdermal cream, implants, depo injections, intrauterine devices, vaginal pessaries, or suppositories.

Apart from a finer adjustment of dose there seem to be small, if any, clinical differences between the various modes of administration of the progestogen. This report will therefore focus on estrogens, but it goes without saying that from a practical (more than theoretical) point of view it is preferable to use the same route of administration for both the estrogen and the progestogen components in combined HRT regimens.

The three most common routes of estrogen adminstration are tablets, patches, and skin cream. These modes will be discussed more in detail while other application forms will be mentioned more briefly.

The most common and widespread mode is the oral tablet. Tablets consist of an estrogen sometimes esterified to valerate or sulphate as the active ingredient. Other esters as well as side chains exist but prior to absorption estrogen molecules are freed from these in the gut by enzyme activity. The oral administration is dependent on the function of the gastrointestinal (GI) tract, as well as on other oral items which may influence GI function and interfere with steroid resorption. In essence, oral estrogens are mainly absorbed by the intestines and enter the liver and portal circulation. Dependent on the velocity of liver blood flow and hepatic enzyme activity, some estrogen will be metabolized in a first pass effect. In addition some is excreted into the bile and as conjugates (mainly glucoronides and sulphates) and further emptied into the intestine again. In the colon bacterial enzyme activity deconjugates the molecules once more and estrogen is partly reabsorbed and hence subject to enterohepatic circulation, the degree of which may vary greatly among individuals. Estrogens are mainly excreted via feces but some water soluble metabolites may undergo renal excretion.

Estrogen Metabolism

Estradiol and its metabolites are endogenously produced hormones and therefore metabolized more specifically than other substances of exogenous or synthetic origin commonly used in drugs. In essence, estradiol is metabolized to estrone and further breakdown occurs through several metabolic pathways.

The two dominating pathways go either via 16- hydroxylation of the D–ring resulting in metabolites with decreasing estrogen activity with estriol being the most abundant end product. Estriol in turn still possesses (weak) estrogenic activity and is mainly excreted via urine either as conjugates but some also as the free steroid molecule. The other major pathways are via 2- or 4-hydroxylation of the A-ring. These pathways give rise to a number of metabolites often referred to as cathecol-estrogens with almost no estrogenic activity.

Smoking stimulates the 2 and 4 pathways. This fact has been brought forward as one reason why smokers have less estrogenic influence than nonsmokers, as illustrated by the fact that smokers have an earlier menopause and lower bone mass than their nonsmoking counterparts [1]. Also hyperthyroidism and weight reduction stimulate this pathway. Drugs such as cimetidine promote the 16OH pathway and endometrial proliferation. Additionally vaginal bleeds are not infrequent in cimetidine users. The pathway is further enhanced by hypothyroidism, liver cirrhosis, and obesity (hyperinsulinism) [2].

Estradiol also undergoes eneterohepatic circulation. In essence estradiol, estrone, and most metabolites are conjugated in the liver and then excreted into the bile. At low estrogen concentrations glucoronides dominate but with increasing estrogen amounts, as during pregnancy, the percentage of sulphate conjugates increases. Once in the gut a deconjugation process takes place. This is alomost entirely dependent on hydrolases present in bacteria of the intestinal flora. Once deconjugated some 80% re-enters the intestinal veins which empty into the portal vein and hence the estrogens reach the liver once more. For this reason estrogen concentrations in the portal vein and in the liver are always higher than in the peripheral circulation. But so is also the ratio between various estrogen components, a possibility which could explain differences between various oral preparations although ratios in peripheral circulation might be very similar.

In recent years it has become evident that (hepatic) clearance of estrogen declines substantially with with age. Hence a woman of 65 or more may require only half the dose as compared to a woman of 50. It is not difficult to understand that events interfering with the enterohepatic circulation will also disturb estrogen metabolism.

Apart from liver diseases, impaired intestinal function will also decrease the bioavailability of estrogens. Malabsorption and diarrhea are obvoius causes. But estrogens also adsorb to fibers and fiber-rich diets such as those commonly used by vegetarians. Use of bulk laxatives also decreases estrogen re-uptake as more estrogens are subject to fecal excretion adsorbed to these laxatives.

Estrogen pharmacology is also dependent on the influence of food, as food in general induces cholecystokinin which in turn enhances hepatic blood flow leading to reduced hepatic breakdown and metabolism Fewer side effects due to oral therapy are theoretically achieved when estrogen tablets are ingested with a meal. If a meal contains fat so that chylomicrons are formed by the intestine, then some estrogen might dissolve in these chylomicrons and then enter the circulation via the lymph system and the thoracic duct which in turn empties into the jugular vein [3].

From this abbreviated description of estrogen metabolism it is evident that oral administration is highly dependent on GI function and hepatic activity. Hence it is easily explicable why after oral administration there is such a tremendous variation in the amount of estrogen reaching the peripheral circulation, not only among individuals, but also intra-individually.

Pharmacology of Exogenously Administered Estrogens

In general oral administration follows a so-called first order pharmacokinetics. This means that there is an absorption phase during which plasma concentrations rise rapidly. This is followed by a distribution phase in which the drug is distributed to target tissues. It is during this phase that plasma concentration reaches its maximum and starts to decline. The third phase is the elimination phase during which the drug leaves the body mainly via excretion or metabolism. Ideally the drug should eliminated in 24 hours to avoid accumulation or return of symptoms. Unfortunately this is not always the case as a large variability exists between individuals. This variability is dependent on the rate of absorption as influenced by GI tract function. The volume of distribution is also highly variable and for lipophilic agents such as steroids which are mainly dependent on the amount of body fat. Hepatic and renal functions are the main determinants of the elimination phase, both of which may be variable and as a rule of thumb decrease with age.

Thus it is easy to understand that plasma concentrations will vary immensely among individuals but generally reaching a peak some 1-2 hours after tablet ingestion and than followed by a decrease. As estrogens are lipophilic they may accumulate in LDL and VLDL particles at peak plasma concentrations. This may be of importance for the antoxidative effect by estrogens.

It should also be remembered that tablet ingestion includes the administration of vehicles such as lactose which may cause problems in subjects with lactose intolerance. Some tablets also contain dyes to which allergic reactions may occur.

Factors that enhance target tissue concentrations after oral administration:

- Alcohol
- Grapefruit juice
- Tagamet (cimitidine)
- Certain tranqulizers,sleeping pills
- Liver malfunction

Factors that diminish target tissue concentrations:

- Smoking

- GI-malfunction (sprue,MB Chron Colitis)
- Use of broadspectrum antibiotics

Factors that enhance liver metabolism:

- Certain enzyme inductors of the cytochrome P450 enzyme systems.

Understanding estrogen metabolism is a prerequisite for the choice of the best mode of administration of estrogen. .From a pharmacologic standpoint three different groups could be distinguished:

1. Those that display a first order pharmacokinetics with extensive enterohepatic circulation and metabolism: tablets;
2. Those displaying a first order pharmacokinetics with little enterohepatic metabolism: gel, cream, and nasal spray; and
3. Those displaying in essence a zero order pharmacokinetics with little enterohepatic metabolism: implants, patches, and depo injections.

The zero order pharmacokinetics is characterized by a constant rate of drug delivery. After a short phase (for establishing equilibrium) the amount of drug eliminated per time unit equates that of drug delivered and hence plasma concentrations remain fairly stable. For estrogens this means that the ratio of concentration between portal and peripheral circulation is lower with a zero order than with a first order pharmacokinetics. Hence the ratio E2/E1 could be close to 1 using a patch or a cream. But as the patch has a constant delivery of E2, the ratio is highest when systems such as patches, depo injections, or implants are being used.

Clinical Implications

At first glance it would seem prudent to avoid tablets. But we have a long standing experience that tablets work in most cases and that they are by far the cheapest mode of administration. Therefore oral administration is the first line choice for most women. As was mentioned before estradiol is initially converted to estrone. After oral administration of estradiol the E2/E1 ratio is 0.7 indicating that some 70% of ingested estradiol is converted to estrone. After ingesting estrone as contained in conjugated equine estrogens, some estradiol is also formed. From a clinical standpoint there is little or no differences if one chooses estrone or estradiol in tablets. Some biochemical differences can be shown but the clinical importance of these, if any remains obscure in the average woman.

Thus the question may be asked: When should other modes be employed? Other modes should be used firstly in women with any hepatic disorder as one cannot guarantee that she would have the same quantitative as well as qualitative response by oral estrogens. It should also be considered in women with a long lasting disturbance of the enterohepatic circulation such as in sprue, constant use of bulk laxatives, short bowel syndrome, etc. Also in heavy smokers or users of medication that might interact with hepatic metabolism, nonoral routes are preferred.

For women, in whom a constant estrogenic influence is desirable, patches could be used. Other conditions include diabetes and pre-stages of type II diabetes, hypertriglyceridemia, and migraine.

For gel and especially patches, the dose can be individualized by trimming the patch to a smaller size. This is very useful when it is difficult to titrate a suitable dose by oral therapy as the steps between two tablets may be too crude. The same also holds true for nasal sprays whereas dose release from implants cannot be changed at this time. Also the brand names of tablets gels and patches are of importance as one study compared several patches marked 50 ug and found serum concentrations varying from 35-75 pg/ml depending on the brand name.

Typical signs of estrogen overdose include breast tenderness, weight gain, bloating, and nausea. These are also common nuisance side effects in the beginning of treatment prior to the new metabolic "steady state" being established. There is also a large inter-individual variation. The reasons for this are largely unknown. The discovery of more than one estrogen receptor is an intriguing possibility and most organs contain both alpha and beta receptors but the distribution of these receptors may vary from one individual to another. In addition there seem to additional estrogen binding sites as well as totally nongenomic effects which further add to the complexity. Use of information in clinical practice remains to be clarified.

Interactions with drugs which induce increased activity of the cytochrome P450 enzyme systems in the liver may also enhance estrogen breakdown. Hence concomitant medication with barbiturates and phenantoin may cause spotting or break-through bleeds.

The biologic effects of estrogen are largely dependent on the nonprotein-bound substances. Estrogen is transported in plasma bound to either sex hormone binding globulin (SHBG) or albumin.SHBG, which is mainly synthesized in the liver and is stimulated by estrogens. After oral administration the amount of SHBG is higher than after transdermal patches. Hence the biologic activity of sex steroids at a given plasma concentration is higher with transdermal administration than after tablets.

Given the various types doses and modes of administration that exist today one can hardly say that there are any absolute contraindications for estrogen therapy. Nonetheless caution is worthwhile in patients with a recent history of breast cancer or venous thromboembolism. Unfortunately we have scarce information on the impact by different modes of administration on these two important events. I t would seem intriguing to use nonoral administration in women at an increased risk of thrombosis as most coagulant factors are produced by the liver. But this holds true also for several anticoagulant factors as well as factors of the fibrinolytical system. Alcohol also retards hepatic metbolism of estrogens and estrogen tablet intake together with alcohol should best be avoided.

Vaginal administration is particularly used when treatment of urogenital problems in the elderly is the major indication. By vaginal administration of low daily doses such as 5-10 ug estradiol per day, it is possible to target the estrogen sensitive urogenital organs without obtaining endometrial proliferation.

Summary and Conclusions

Apart from the financial aspects, oral therapy is preferred when a more pronounced liver effect is desirable. Conditions that benefit from that are hypercholesterolemia, low HDL levels, and high levels of homocystein and Lp(a). Oral therapy is best avoided in conditions with GI and hepatic malfunction, alcohol abuse, risk of gallstone formation, as well as lactose intolerance.

Transdermal therapy is to be preferred when SHBG should not be increased as in relative testosterone deficiency, hypertriglycerdemia, diabetes, features of the metabolic syndrome such as hypertension and hyperinsulinemia, heavy smoking, or migraine. Transdermal therapy is best avoided in subjects with skin diseases and allergic reactions to the components of patches or creams. It should be emphasized that there are no huge data bases to suggest any major clinical differences between transdermal and oral administration of HRT. Additionally both therapies appear to be equally safe.

References

1. Lobo RA. Clinical aspects of hormonal replacement. In: Lobo RA, Editor. Treatment of the postmenopausal woman: Basic and clinical aspects. Second edition. Philadelphia: Lippincott Williams & Wilkins, 1999:125-139.
2. Barnes RB,Levrant SG. Pharmacology of estrogens. In: Lobo RA. Editor. Treatment of the postmenopausal woman: Basic and clinical aspects. Second edition. Philadelphia: Lippincott Williams & Wilkins, 1999: 95-104.
3. Dahlgren E, Crona N, Janson PO, Samsioe G. Oral replacement with estradiol-cycloctyl acetate: A new estradiol analogue. Effects on serum lipids, proteins, gonadotrophins, estrogens and uterine endometrial morphology. Gynecol Obstet Invest 1985;20(2):84-90.

THE ROLE OF ANTIANDROGENS IN PERI- AND POSTMENOPAUSAL HRT

H.P.G. Schneider

Introduction

Progesterone is the only natural progestogen with significant biological function. However, it is not well absorbed unless administered in a micronized form, which has been unavailable until recent years. Addition of a hydroxyl group at C_{17} of progesterone results in a loss of progestational activity. Acetylation of the 17-hydroxyl group gives rise to 17-hydroxy-progesterone acetate, which has some progestational activity. This compound offers an important starting point in the development of a number of synthetic progestogens. Elongation of the carboxyl side chain at C_{17} of 17-hydroxyprogesterone acetate gives rise to long-acting progestogens, when used parenterally; one such example is 17-hydroxyprogesterone caproate. Various manipulations of the 17-hydroxyprogesterone acetate molecule, primarily at C_6, have produced potent oral as well as parenteral progestogens (Figure 1). The addition of a methyl group at C_6 of 17-hydroxyprogesterone acetate gives rise to medroxyprogesterone acetate. Formation of a double-bond between C_6 and C_7 of this compound yields megestrol acetate. If to the latter molecule a methyl group is substituted at C_6 with a chloral group and attachment of a methylene group so that it is shared jointly by C_1 and C_2 gives rise to cyproterone acetate (CPA).

Alteration of the testosterone molecule by ethinylation at C_{17} causes the steroid to lose androgenicity substantially and to acquire both progestational properties and oral activity. 17α-ethinyl testosterone or ethisterone was first synthesized in 1939 in Berlin. Removal of the methyl group at C_{10} of ethisterone further increases the progestogenic activity of the molecule and virtually eliminates its androgenicity. The resulting product is norethindrone (also called norethisterone). The addition of a methyl group on C_{18} of norethindrone gives rise to a norgestrel, which consists of a racemic mixture of levonorgestrel and dextronorgestrel. Levonorgestrel is the biologically active form of norgestrel and is one of the most potent orally active progestogens. A number of other 19-nortestosterone derivatives have been synthesized from norethindrone and levonorgestrel. Both of the above groups of progestogens are devoid of the antimineralocorticoid activity of progesterone, which induces natriuresis and a compensatory activation of the renin-angiotensin-aldosteron system (RAAS) in the luteal phase of the menstrual cycle and during pregnancy. The introduction of drospirenone (DRSP), a novel 17α-spirolactone derivative, has provided a pharmacodynamic profile more closely related to endogenous progesterone than that of other synthetic progestogens in use today. DRSP displays progestational, antimineralocorticoid, and antiandrogenic activity and is devoid of any estrogenic, androgenic, glucocorticoid, and antiglucocorticoid activity.

The "progestogen tree" (Figure 1) identifies and categorizes steroid hormones derived from progesterone, the pure agonist and mother compound, which is represented by the trunk of the tree. The first antiandrogen, CPA, was synthesized in Berlin in the late 1950s, and was introduced into clinical use in the 1960s. Chlormadinone acetate, which can be used in oral contraceptives, and dienogest also have antiandrogenic action. Cyproterone acetate and dienogest are the most widely used antiandrogens in current clinical practice. This review discusses the role of antiandrogens such as CPA and dienogest in hormone replacement therapy (HRT) and provides a prospect of the newly developed DRSP.

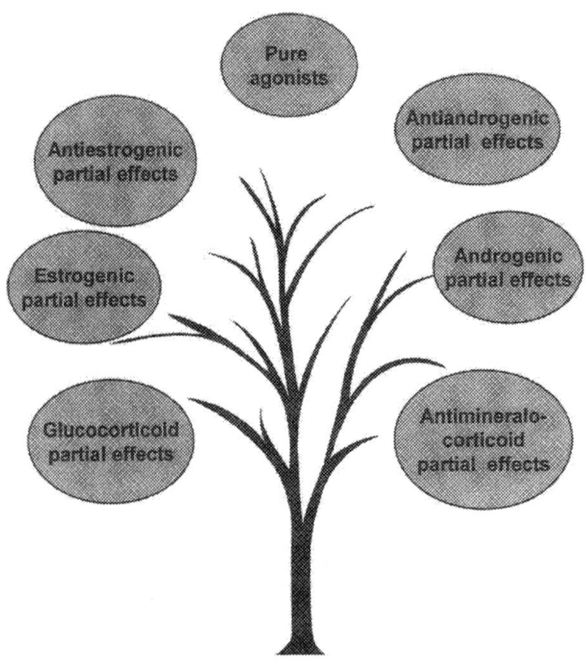

Figure 1. The "progestogen tree."

Hormonal Balance in the Perimenopause

The decrease in levels of estrogens and sex hormone binding globulin (SHBG) in the climacteric leads to an increase in the levels of free, biologically active androgens. The androgen-dominant hormonal status of the climacteric is associated with adverse metabolic effects. Decreases in levels of high density lipoprotein cholesterol (HDL-C) and increases in levels of low density lipoprotein cholesterol (LDL-C) and free fatty acids, for example, shift the lipid status of the climacteric towards atherogenicity. Other effects include loss of insulin receptors, which leads to incremental insulin resistance, hyperinsulinemia, and increased ovarian androgen production. An adequate clinical management of this biological transition is a first step into climacteric medicine and serves as an add-back in the prevention of frailty and disability of older age.

Antiandrogens: Cyproterone Acetate, Dienogest, Drospirenone

The most widely used antiandrogens in clinical practice are cyproterone acetate (CPA) and dienogest. CPA has 100% bioavailability, a short half-life (2-8 hours) and an elimination time of 60 hours. It is mostly albumin-bound, and is metabolized by 15β-hydroxylation, which distinguishes it from other hydroxyprogesterones (Table 1).

Dienogest is a 19-norprogestin with high bioavailability, and a short half-life (0.24 hours) and elimination time (6.3 hours). Serum levels after doses of 2-3 mg are approximately 50 ng/ml. It is 90% albumin-bound and, in contrast to other nortestosterones, is not bound by SHBG or corticosteroid binding globulin (CBG) (Table 1). Dienogest has a 17α-cyanomethyl group instead of the 17α-ethinyl group typical of the common 19-nortestosterone derivatives.

Cyproterone Acetate and HRT

COMBINING CPA WITH ESTRADIOL VALERATE

A sequential preparation is available consisting of 11 days of 2 mg estradiol valerate, followed by 10 days of 2 mg estradiol valerate with 1 mg CPA, followed by a 7-day drug-free interval.

THE BENEFICIAL EFFECTS OF ADDING CPA

CPA is a highly progestogenic compound that produces excellent endometrial transformation and good bleeding control (the latter is seen with CPA in a sequential preparation, but not in a continuous, combined formulation). It protects the endometrium, reduces menopausal symptoms, and may also protect the mammary glands because it is a progestogen-derived compound. CPA has no androgenic properties, and is therefore not associated with facial acne, glandular seborrhea, or androgenic alopecia. Above a certain dose, it has antiandrogenic effects on the skin and other androgen-sensitive epidermal structures.

Table 1. Hydroprogesterones and Nortestosterones

	Bioavailability %	Serum (ng/ml)	Half-life α/β (h)	Metabolism
Hydroxyprogesterones				
Chlormadinone acetate	100	4	2.4/89 albumin	Reduction 3-keto hydroxylation
Medroxyprogesterone acetate	100	12	2.2/33 albumin	Hydroxylation $C_{6\beta}$ and C_{12}
Cyproterone acetate	100	11	2-8/60 albumin	15β-hydroxylation
Megestrol acetate	100	7-24	—	Hydroxylation
Medrogesterone	100	10-15	4/36 albumin	Hydroxylation
Dydrogesterone	No central thermogenic or sedative effect		< 24 85% clearance	Restrosteric configuration ·no reduction 3-keto and ? [1] ·20-keto-hydroxylation
Nortestosterones				
Norethisterone	50-77	oral 5-10	2.5/8	Ring A reduction
Norethisterone acetate		Transdermal 0.5-1	36% SHBG 61% albumin	Aromatization (0.35%)
Levonorgestrel	100	3.5	1/24	Reduction
DL-norgestrel	D-N = inactive	Intrauterine 0.1-0.2; 50	48% SHBG 50% albumin	3-keto and ? [1]
Dienogest	High	50	0.24/6.3 90% albumin; no SHBG/CBG	Reduction 3-keto 17α cyanomethyl hydroxylation
Spirolactone	76 ± 13	3-5% free	1.6/27 albumin; no SHBG/CBG	Opening of the lactone ring to 4,5 dihydro-drosperinon e-3-sulfate

CPA does not counteract the estrogenic effects of estradiol valerate. This therapy is therefore highly estrogenic and has optimal effects on lipid metabolism and coronary heart disease risk, preserves bone and reduces osteoporotic fracture risk, maintains constant systolic and diastolic blood pressures (although there is a tendency for both to decrease), and supports female-type body fat distribution.

EVIDENCE OF DECREASED FRACTURE RISK

Komulainen and colleagues conducted a randomized study in nonosteoporotic postmenopausal women to compare the effects of this regimen on fracture risk with those of vitamin D3, calcium, and placebo [2]. After 4.3 years, the incidence of nonvertebral fracture was lower in women treated with this regimen compared with the other treatments.

EFFECTS ON BODY WEIGHT AND BODY FAT DISTRIBUTION

An increased body weight, particularly an increased central distribution of body fat, is recognized as an independent predictor of coronary heart disease in women [1,3-5]. The early postmenopausal period is associated with a progressive increase in body weight and body fat and a shift to a more central, android body fat distribution. Changes in body weight are an important concern for menopausal women. HRT has been thought to increase body weight; this concept greatly influences the acceptance of and compliance with HRT.

The effect of estradiol + CPA on body weight and body fat distribution (determined by dual energy X-ray) was compared with that of oral calcium (500 mg/day) in early postmenopausal women in a study by Gambacciani and colleagues in Italy [6]. This study showed that there was a significant increase in body weight in women who received oral calcium after 12 months (i.e. the controls, from 61.8 ± 2.1 kg to 63.3 ± 1.9 kg ($p = 0.05$)), but not in women who received estradiol + CPA (from 62.2 ± 1.6 kg to 62.7 ± 1.6 kg). Total body fat mass and fat mass in the trunk and arms were also significantly increased in the controls, but not in the women who received estradiol + CPA (Figure 2). The reverse was true for fat mass in the upper thighs.

The results indicate that estradiol with CPA can partially counteract the increase in body weight and body fat observed in postmenopausal women, and prevent the shift to a distribution of central, android body fat. The observed stabilization of body weight and body fat distribution can be seen as a further protective effect of HRT against coronary heart disease.

Dienogest and HRT

DIENOGEST: A HYBRID PROGESTOGEN

Dienogest has pharmacodynamic properties in common with 19-norprogestins (nortestosterones) and hydroxyprogesterones, so it is referred to as a hybrid progestogen (Table 2).

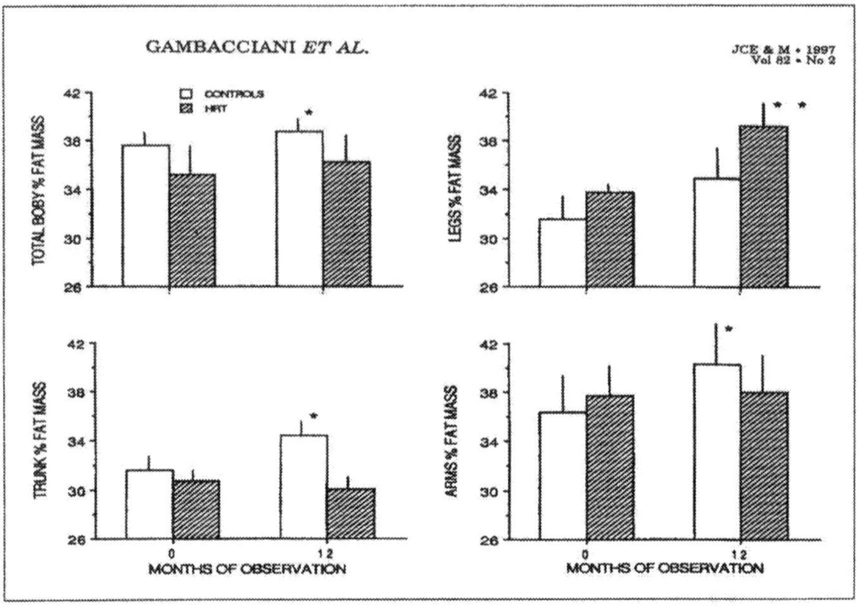

Figure 2. Body fat distribution with estradiol + CPA compared with controls.

Table 2. Dienogest: A "Hybrid" Progestogen

Similarities to 19-norprogestins	Similarities to progesterone derivatives	Specific properties of dienogest
·Short plasma half-life	·Weak antigonadatropic properties	·No interaction with specific transport proteins (SHBG, CBG)
·Good cycle control if used in OCs	·Antiandrogenic partial action	·Weak influence on drug metabolizing enzymes
·High transformatory effect on endometrium	·Antiproliferative effects (mamma in vitro)	·High concentration of unbound substance in serum
	·Dosages in milligram range	

Dienogest is similar to 19-norprogestins in that it has a short plasma half-life, and produces good cycle control and endometrial transformation. Similarities to hydroxyprogesterones include antigonadotropic, antiandrogenic, and antiproliferative effects. Specifically, dienogest does not interact with transport proteins, has only a weak influence on drug-metabolizing liver enzymes, and is present in high concentrations, unbound, in serum.

A fixed formulation containing 2 mg estradiol valerate and 2 mg dienogest is available for a 28-day continuous combined HRT regimen. One of the most important effects of HRT is the alleviation of menopausal symptoms, such as hot flushes. A randomized, controlled study showed that this regimen was as effective as continuous norethindrone acetate (1 mg) with 2 mg of estradiol at reducing the incidence of mild, moderate, and severe hot flushes after 1 month (Figure 3) [7].

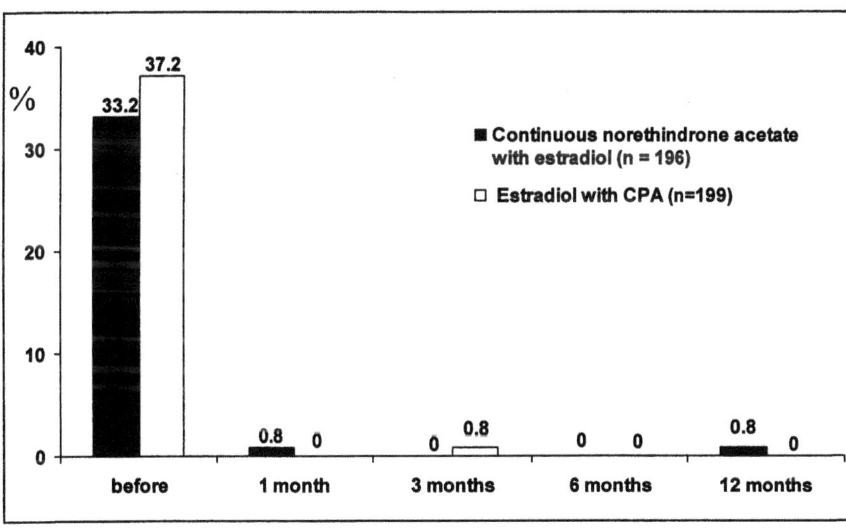

Figure 3. Efficacy of estradiol + CPA and continuous norethindrone + estradiol with respect to hot flushes.

These regimens are also comparable in terms of their effects on the endometrium. Analysis of endometrial biopsies after 12 cycles of treatment showed that the incidences of atrophic, proliferative, and secretory endometria were similar with both treatments (Figure 4) [8]. A total of 85-87% of women had atrophic endometria, there were few proliferative and secretory changes and there were no cases of hyperplastic regeneration. In addition, there were fewer days of bleeding during 12 cycles of treatment with dienogest compared with norethindrone regimen [7]. The incidence of adverse events also was similar [7]. The most common adverse events reported were breast problems, vaginal bleeding/dysmenorrhea and central nervous system/sensory events.

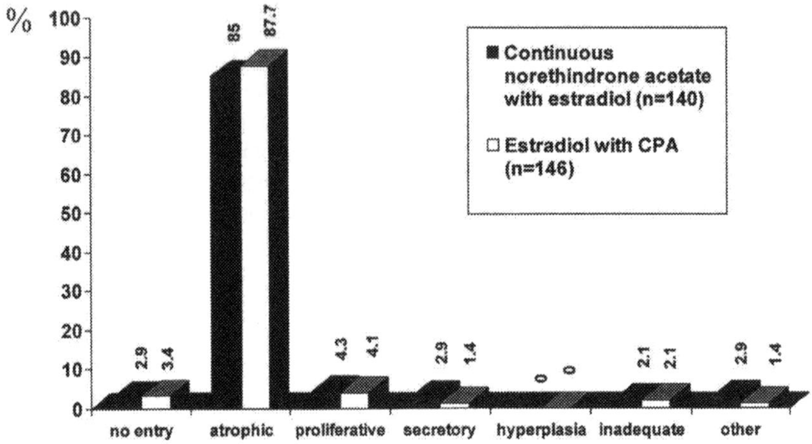

Figure 4. Results of endometrial biopsies after 12 cycles of treatment.

Dienogest and Vascular Function

Mück and colleagues from Tübingen conducted an interesting study in which they looked at factors beyond lipids as indicators of coronary heart disease risk, and investigated vascular function [9]. This open, randomized, parallel-group study compared the effects of dienogest + estradiol valerate on vascular function with 2 mg estradiol valerate alone during 3 months of treatment in postmenopausal women.

The end-point in the study was biochemical markers of vascular function in overnight urine collected at weeks 0, 5-7, and 11-12. The primary efficacy variables in the study (markers of vasorelaxation) were cyclic GMP (cGMP; a measure of endothelial nitric oxide production), 5-hydroxyindolacetic acid (5-HIAA; a measure of systemic serotonin levels), and the 6-ketoprostaglandin $F_{1\alpha}$/11-dihydroxythromboxane B_2 ratio ($PGF_{1\alpha}$/ $DHTXB_2$; a measure of regulation of the prostacyclin/thromboxane system). Secondary efficacy variables included relaxin and urodilatin (vasoactive peptides involved in regulation of kidney function and electrolytes).

Significant changes (all increases $p < 0.05$) compared with baseline were seen by the end of the study in urine levels of cGMP and 5-HIAA with both treatments, in PGF_{1}/$DHTXB_2$ with estradiol valerate and in urodilatin with dienogest + estradiol. Overall, the results of the study show that dienogest + estradiol valerate and estradiol valerate alone had similar effects on the vasoactive markers, which indicates that dienogest does not significantly alter the vasorelaxant effects of estradiol valerate.

DIENOGEST AND PSYCHIC AND SOMATIC STATUS

Saletu and colleagues studied the effects on sleep, psychophysiological and psychopathological parameters in a prospective, randomized, double-blind study in comparison to estradiol valerate and placebo [10,11]. Estradiol valerate alone improved subjective sleep quality; this effect was not counteracted by the addition of dienogest and ranged significantly beyond any placebo action [11]. This investigation has been extended to the assessment of periods of apnoe and hypopnoe (frequency per hour of sleep). Estradiol valerate in combination with dienogest will reduce the number of apnoe and hypopnoe episodes following two months of treatment in postmenopausal women. Thereby, known consequences of apnoe such as the psychic and psychosocial alterations of impaired sleep quality with resultant hemodynamic impact such as cardiac arrhythmia, hypertension, and multi-infarct dementia will be attenuated. The combination of estrogen and dienogest, therefore, appears to have an excellent effect on depressive attitudes according to psychiatric standard definitions.

THE MENTAL TONIC EFFECT

The analysis of electroencephalogram (EEG) parameters in women treated with dienogest + estradiol valerate or estradiol valerate alone showed that dienogest enhanced the vigilance, alertness, and awareness-promoting effects of estradiol in a dose-dependent manner. A positive effect on the early stages of information processing because of an improvement in vigilance was observed. Based on observed patterns, estradiol valerate may improve the stimulus evaluation time (i.e. classification speed) and dienogest may improve the cognitive information-processing capacity. This study indicates that dienogest potentiates the neurophysiological effects of estradiol, in contrast to the general perception of estrogen exerting a stimulatory and progesterone a rather sedative effect on the brain. Continuous combined HRT with dienogest therefore has an excellent mental tonic effect and may represent an option for HRT in postmenopausal women with mood complaints.

Drospirenone: Experience with Oral Contraception and the Prospects of Use as a Component for HRT

A multi-center open-label randomized study carried out in 25 European centers was to assess the contraceptive reliability, psychic control, and tolerance of a new monophasic oral contraceptive containing 30 μg ethinylestradiol and 3 mg drospirenone [12]. This comparative investigation utilized an equal dose of ethinylestradiol combined with 150 μg desogestrel. There were no pregnancies considered to have been the result of method failure. The subjective and objective tolerance was good in both groups. A statistically significant difference was found in body weight changes between the two groups. While there was an increase in mean body weight with ethinylestradiol/desogestrel from cycle 5 onward, the mean body weight per cycle in the ethinylestradiol/drospirenone group was more favorable, with a mean body weight remaining lower than baseline for the majority of the women.

The clinical profile of drospirenone as a contraceptive, besides reliability in phase-II and phase-III clinical trials, disclosed good bleeding control over up to 26 cycles; this includes a positive effect on withdrawal bleeding, reducing both the duration and the intensity of the bleed, when compared with normal menstruation. Spotting was only recorded in 6.7% of cycles, whilst breakthrough bleeding (heavy/normal bleeding) occurred in less than 0.5% of cycles. The effects on the endometrium were studied over 30 cycles in 40 young subjects; women were randomized to have an endometrial biopsy in either cycle 3 or 6, together with biopsies at baseline. When at baseline, most subjects showed secretory endometrium, while under treatment, the endometrium became moderately suppressed to atrophic. Thickness of the endometrium was reduced by about 50%. There was a potentially favorable increase in HDL-cholesterol, LDL-cholesterol remained close to baseline; estrogen-mediated increases in triglycerides were more marked with drospirenone, probably due to its lack of androgenic activity. All changes were within the reference ranges. The carbohydrate metabolism was investigated by oral glucose tolerance testing, and none of the changes induced were clinically significant. As far as hemostasis is concerned, there was a high rate of turnover of coagulation factors with drospirenone, but the very similar activation of coagulation and fibrinolysis indicated hemostatic equilibrium.

Of particular importance is the pharmacological profile that drospirenone shares with progesterone as being an antimineralocorticoid and thereby counteracting increases in aldosterone and other mineralocorticoids induced by estrogens. Since this property is, today, not displayed by any other synthetic progestogen, clinical studies were particularly designed to look at changes of body weight and blood pressure, both of which can be influenced by aldosterone levels. An increase in body weight during oral contraceptive use might, in part, be explained by fluid retention resulting from unopposed stimulation of the RAAS by estrogens including ethinylestradiol. The mean body weight fell with drospirenone by 0.78 kg, whereas it rose with desogestrel by 0.68 kg.

Blood pressure as monitored in almost 3,000 women altogether, did not change significantly. Overall, the results showed no unfavorable or negative trends in the value of mean systolic and diastolic blood pressure, which were slightly below baseline values. There were more individuals to display a decrease of systolic blood pressure of 10 mm Hg, when drospirenone is again compared to desogestrel in combination with ethinylestradiol [13].

Studies have also shown that drospirenone has beneficial effects on mild to moderate acne in young women, reflecting the antiandrogenic activity of its progestogenic components. Facial lesions (comedones, papules, pustules, and nodules) as well as sebum production were monitored to objectify the qualitative effects on acne and seborrhea.

There is indication of drospirenone as a combination progestogen with estradiol valerate to reproduce the favorable effects on blood pressure, body weight, and androgenic skin lesions in postmenopausal women (see contribution by R. Lobo, this conference).

Summary of Clinical Experience with Antiandrogenic Progestogens

A considerable amount of data have so far been collected on the clinical use of antiandrogenic progestogens, such as cyproterone acetate and dienogest, in HRT [1,6,14]. These data can be summarized as follows.

Antiandrogenic progestogens have beneficial effects on skin disorders related to hormonal deficiency and imbalance, for example, they are associated with less seborrhea, acne, hirsutism, and androgenic loss of hair, and increased skin collagen content. These compounds do not counteract estrogenic effects on lipid metabolism, and therefore they are associated with increased levels of HDL-C, SHBG and triglycerides [14].

Antiandrogenic progestogens are associated with reduced postmenopausal nonvertebral fracture incidence, and systolic and diastolic blood pressures are either stabilized, or slightly decreased. There is evidence for the estrogenic type of body fat distribution with these compounds, and no significant weight increase or the potential of significant individual weight loss, which is important for compliance with therapy. The extent of bleeding control is dependent on the type and mode of application.

Continuous combined HRT with antiandrogenic progestogens appears to have an excellent mental tonic effect and may represent an elective HRT in postmenopausal women with mood defects as well as blood pressure and body weight problems.

Conclusion

With its highly specific characteristics, HRT with antiandrogenic progestogens preserves metabolic estrogenicity and improves vigilance, mood disorders, blood pressure, and body weight. These treatments therefore widen individual therapeutic options for HRT in peri- and postmenopausal women.

References

1. Lapidus L, Bengtsson C, Larsson B, et al. Distribution of adipose tissue and risk of cardiovascular disease and death: A 12 years follow up of participants in the population study of women in Gothenburg, Sweden. Br Med J 1984;289:1257-61.
2. Komulainen MH, Kroger H, Tuppurainen MT, et al. HRT and vitamin D in prevention of non-vertebral fractures in postmenopausal women; a 5 year randomized trial. Maturitas 1998;31:45-54.
3. Evans DJ, Hoffman RG, Kalkhoff RK, Kissebah AH. Relationship of body fat topography to insulin sensitivity and metabolic profiles in postmenopausal women. Metabolism 1983; 33:68-75.
4. Evans DJ, Hoffman RG, Kalkhoff RK, Kissebah AH. Relationship of androgenic activity to body topography, fat cell morphology and metabolic aberrations in premenopausal women. J Clin Endocrinol Metab 1983;57:304-10.
5. Haarbo J, Hassager C, Schlemmer A, et al. The influence of smoking, body fat distribution, and alcohol consumption on serum lipids, lipoproteins, and apolipoproteins in early postmenopausal women. Atherosclerosis 1990;84:239-44.

6. Gambacciani M, Ciaponi M, Cappagli B, et al. Body weight, body fat distribution, and hormonal replacement therapy in early postmenopausal women. J Clin Endocrinol Metab 1997;82:414-17.
7. Gräser T, Koytchev R, Müller A, et al. Comparison of the efficacy and endometrial safety of two estradiol valerate/dienogest combinations and Kliogest® for continuous combined hormone replacement therapy in postmenopausal women. Climacteric 2000;3:109-18.
8. Gräser T, Koytchev R, Römer T, et al. Dienogest as a progestin for hormone replacement therapy. Drugs of Today 1999;35(Suppl.C):115-26.
9. Mück AO, Seeger H, Lüdtke R, et al. Changes in biochemical, vasoactive markers during postmenopausal hormone replacement therapy: Estradiol versus estradiol/dienogest. Submitted to Maturitas.
10. Pietzcker A, Gebhardt R, Strauss A, Stoeckel M, Langer C, Freudenthal K. The syndrome scales in the AMDP system. In: Bobon D, et al, editors. The AMDP system in pharmacopsychiatry. Basel: Karger, 1983.
11. Saletu B, Anderer P, Gruber D, et al. Effect of estrogen on vigilance and cognition. Eur Arch Psychiatry Clin Neurosci 2000;250(Suppl.1):46 (abstract).
12. Foidart J-M, Wuttke W, Bouw M, Gerlinger C, Heithecker R. A comparative investigation of contraceptive reliability, cycle control and tolerance of two monophasic oral contraceptives containing either drospirenone or desogestrel. Eur J Contraception Reprod Health Care 2000;5:124-34.
13. Fuhrmann U, Krattenmacher R, Slater EP, Fritzemeier K-H. The novel progestin drospirenone and its natural counterpart progesterone: Biochemical profile and antiandrogenic potential. Contraception 1996;54:243-51.
14. Husmann F. Klinische Erfahrungen mit Climen® bei peri- und postmenopausalen Frauen. Zentralbl Gynakol 1997;119:123-27.

Sex Steroid-Sensitive Reproductive Tissues in Women During Reproduction and Menopause

Frederick Naftolin, Paulo Rinaudo, Fadi Abushahin, and Eddie Sze

Introduction

Reproduction is the forge of Darwinian evolution, and, reproductive fitness (positive adaptation for reproductive success) is directly and deeply ingrained in our genomic fabric. During the evolution of species from aquatic to terrestrial existence there was an internalization of the reproductive processes. This entailed the development of the contemporary urogenital tract through which retention of access from the exterior to the workings of the internalized reproductive processes occurs. The ancient excretory ducts were a natural venue for this since they were developed to provide an interface between the interior milieu and outside conditions [1]. Thus, even though sperm and eggs develop and fertilize inside the body there remains a pathway to and from the exterior in both male and female genital tracts. This pathway is used in males to emit sperm deeply in the vagina and in females to allow the timely ingress of sperm and egress of the fetus and placenta. Since there is an enormous difference between the size of the gametes and each fully developed fetus there must be mechanisms to allow the involved tissues to accommodate the changes in size without sustaining damage. This is part of the development of steroid-sensitive mechanisms such as the management of the interface between the interior of the genitourinary tract and the exterior that have evolved to foster reproduction. These include specialization of the epithelium, stroma, and immune system to maintain the integrity of the genital tract and its adaptation to injury, the response to the urogenital flora and the immune-privileged status of the genetically heterogeneous fetus, etc. Sex steroids that act primarily through nuclear receptors regulate most of these adaptations. In this brief review we describe some of the mechanisms and clinical effects with which evolution has supported internalized extra-corporeal reproduction, and, the results of maintaining these reproductively adaptive responses after menopause, during the postreproductive period. Because of the context of this review, we will concentrate on the role of sex steroids in maintaining healthy and functional tissues in mammals [2]. Space limitations also limit the consideration of the important roles of protein and peptide regulators such as relaxin, angiotensin, and numerous cytokines and growth factors [3].

Old Wine in New Bottles

The evolutionary basis of the genital tract in terrestrial species is that the union of gametes has become an internal phenomenon, but retains many characteristics of extra-corporeal reproduction. In fact our gametes float in peritoneal and seminal fluids, and the embryo drifts in sea-like tubal fluid into the uterus where it will implant in the endometrium. In humans the endometrial lining is thick and thus adapted to accept human placenta, which is the most invasive placenta in nature. Throughout the genital tract intercellular tight junctions have evolved to keep the "exterior-like milieu" from mixing with the internal milieu. Like so many things in nature and evolution, this reuse of ancient excretory tracts results from the Darwinian appropriation of ancient mechanisms that were evolved for other purposes: in this case, living in harmony with an aquatic-like environment and its contents. A cartoon of that relationship and some of the regulatory mechanisms is found in Figure 1.

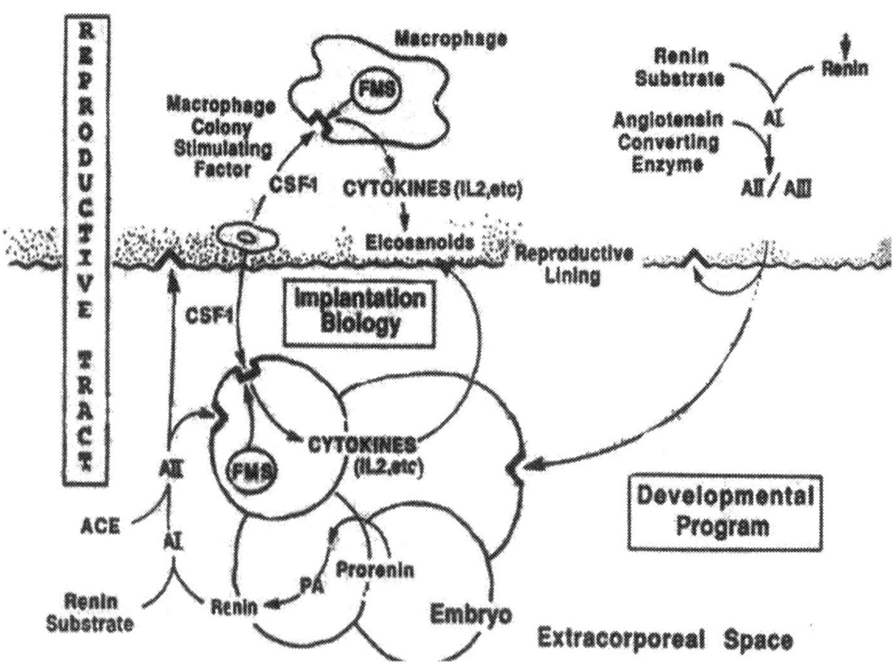

Figure 1. The interface between seawater-like luminal fluid of the genital tract and the blood is regulated by the renin-angiotensin system and leukocytes, especially macrophages. Modified from Lavy, et al.

The action of sex steroids generally requires nuclear receptors, although this is complicated by the cofactors necessary for steroid regulation of gene expression. As well, there are non receptor-mediated actions of steroids. Indirect steroid actions also play important roles via cytokines, growth factors, etc. Changing levels of sex steroids result in changes in the epithelium and stroma of the genital tract, as well as the skin, etc. [2]. These include changes in epithelial cell type and the thickness, hydration, strength, elasticity, glycoseaminoglycans (GAGs), collagen, and cellular composition in these tissues [3]. An example of different sex hormones-sensitive tissues in the genital tract and their functions can be seen in Figure 2.

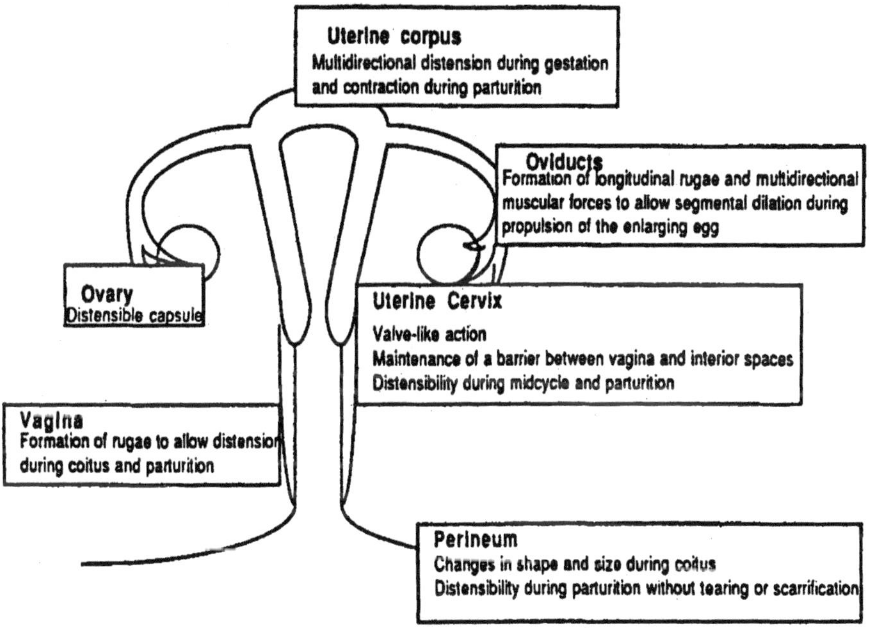

Figure 2. Examples of estrogen-sensitive genital tissues. Modified from Naftolin, et al.

In genital tract tissues estrogen and progesterone act primarily via the estrogen receptors (ER) and progesterone receptors (PR) that regulate gene transcription. Both receptors are regulated by progesterone via progesterone receptors (PR). This is the classical formulation of the interaction between estrogen and progesterone that is well known and described in Figure 3

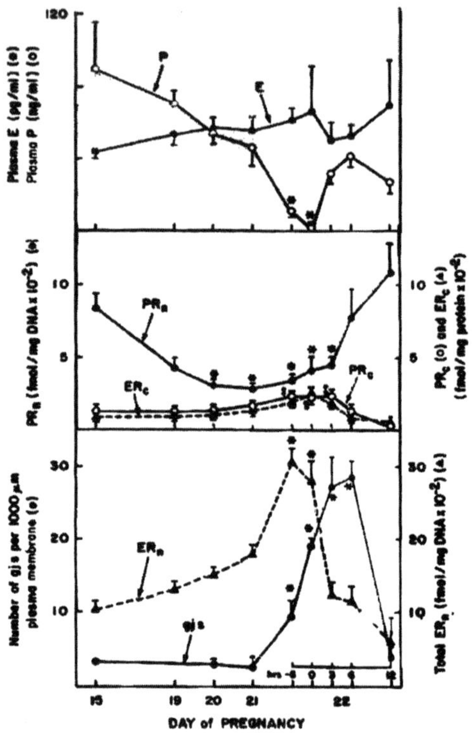

Figure 3. Rat pregnancy is sustained by progesterone and estradiol from the corpus luteum and labor follows the fall in progesterone. Modified from Saito, et al.

In addition, it has become clear that both estradiol and progesterone can cause differentiation that leads to apoptosis [4,5].

The immune system affects the phenotype and function of sex steroid-sensitive tissues. Sex steroids regulate immune function, including cytokines and growth factors that regulate immune cells and fibroblast function [6)] Sex steroids also regulate other enzymes that control collagen synthesis and breakdown (Figure 4; ref. 7) as well as differential glycosaminoglycan (GAG) production (Figures 5,6; ref. 8). Sex steroids regulate the development of gap junctions in the genital tract [9,10]. Actual or functional withdrawal of progesterone at the end of pregnancy plays an important role in the initiation of labor in rats [9] and in primates [11], respectively. As Liggins has indicated, the changes seen in the genital tract, particularly the cervix at the time of parturition are largely, if not wholly, those that are represented in an inflammatory reaction [12]. In fact, macrophages are among the main players in such reactions. They are increasingly known to play a role in non-immune regulation, in addition to their traditional roles in immune regulation. The contemporary portrait of the macrophage stresses its induction of cytokines and growth factors, its ability to produce estrogen via the enzyme aromatase and the presence of estrogen receptors. This completes the picture of macrophage autocrine regulation and supplements the effects of hormones that may come from other sites such as the ovary or placenta or administration of hormones [6].

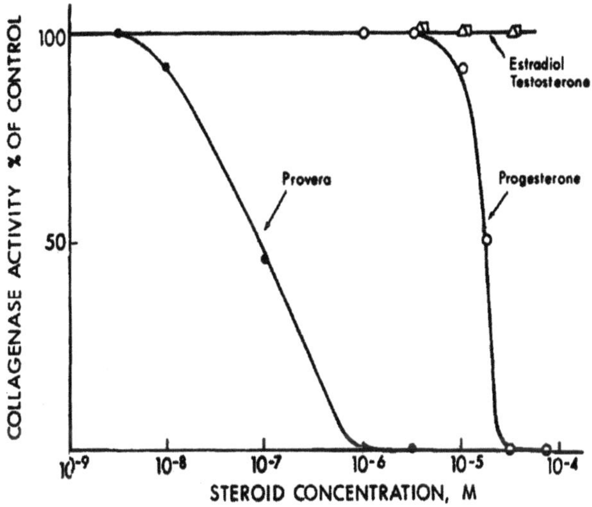

Figure 4. Effects of steroid hormones on collagenase produced by rat uterine explant cultures. Modified from Jeffreys.

Estradiol and Progesterone Regulation of the Genital Tract During Pregnancy and Parturition

It is instructive to follow the effects of estrogen and progesterone during pregnancy [9] when sex steroid-induced changes foster the growth of a hypertrophic/ hyperplastic, elastic uterine fundus capped by a small (inelastic) uterine cervix. Although both estrogen and progesterone are elevated during this period, progesterone dominates and the result is to make the smooth muscle-containing uterine fundus grow and stretch and to accept the developing fetus and placenta while the collagenous non-muscular cervix is small and unyielding keeping the fetus inside. The approach of parturition requires role reversal, with the fundus contracting and lessening its bulk while the cervix becomes boggy and bulky and elastic. Tissue bulk is needed for the massive extensibility needed to accommodate the exiting fetus and placenta. The bogginess reflects the increase in water and breakdown in collagen and other connective tissue components within the cervix [13]. The vagina and vulva also become greatly elastic while pelvic muscles and fascia provide both the accommodating elasticity and directional stiffness necessary to guide the descending fetus. These tissues have undergone hydration and increased extensibility due to collagen fibril breakdown and the increase of hydrophilic glycosaminoglycans. Biopsies show that they have a higher percentage of hydroxyproline to total protein and lower percentage of soluble hydroxyproline to total hydroxyproline than do non-pregnant women [14]. This is further evidence that tissues have become hydrated and that their total cross-linked collagen per gram of tissue has decreased even though the total amount of collagen in the cervix is increased (Figure 5).

Perhaps most important in the extensibility of the connective tissues is the decrease in collagen cross-linking that allows for sliding of collagen fibers over one another [7,15]. Jeffrey [7]has shown that estradiol and testosterone induce high levels of collagenase, while progesterone and medroxy progesterone (Provera®) diminish the levels of collagenase (Figure 4).

During rat pregnancy progestin dominance is reversed at term (Figure 3). The result is increased ER expression, which is accompanied by extrusion of hyaluronic acid and other hydrophilic GAG's, collagen breakdown and clearance, cervical elasticity and the formation of myometrial gap junctions (Figures 5,6; ref. 9).

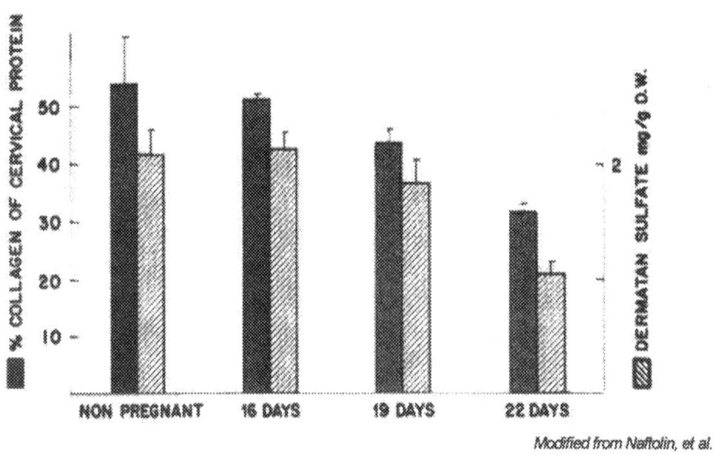

Figure 5. As pregnancy proceeds the rat cervix loses both collagen and predominance of less hydrophyllic GAG's.

In addition to the shift from a progesterone-dominated to an estrogen-dominated state, strategic increases in hormones like relaxin also support these changes [16]. Failure to develop elastic reproductive tract tissues that have a bland response to injury could result in tearing and other disruption, hemorrhage, scarring or other impediments to successful reproduction. Those who lacked these responses to sex steroids were bred out during evolution and an estrogen-dependent bland (inflammation without scarring) reaction to injury in the genital tract and other sex steroid-responsive tissues evolved as the dominant adaptation to mammalian reproduction Table 1.

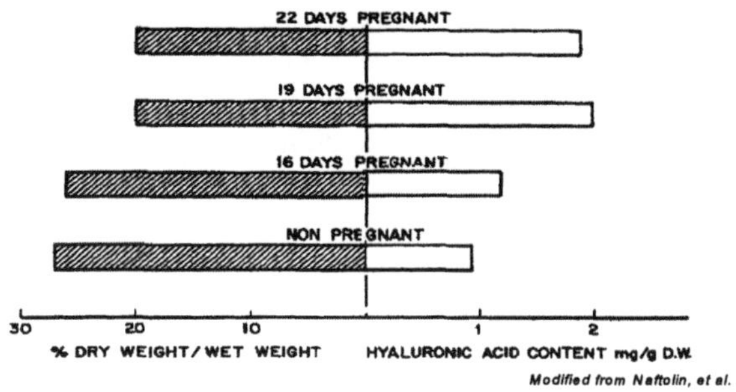

Figure 6. Rat cervix wet/dry weight (%) and hyaluroninc acid during pregnancy.

The most extreme example of this tissue specialization is the so-called "sex skin", which is well known to observers of primates in zoos. The hydration and swelling is caused by the preovulatory peak of estrogen at midcycle and can be quite spectacular, adding the evolutionary advantage of recognition of females in "heat" (Figure 7) at a distance.

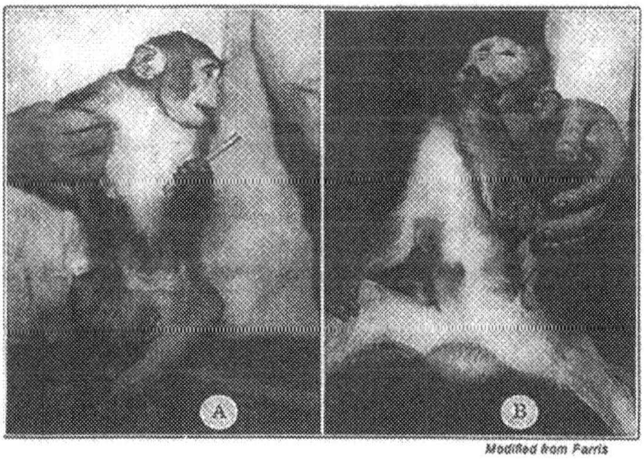

Figure 7. A. A year-and-a-half-old monkey at the time of first menstruation. Note the two small swelling in pubic region, the first indication of sex skin development. B. The same monkey two cycles later.

Sex skin is not limited to the genitalia. It occurs to a greater or lesser degree in other areas of the body in primates and other orders. Figure 8 shows sex skin swelling on the extremities and back of a female monkey. This appearance is due to hydration of these tissues that is in part due to expression of hydrophilic GAGs under the influence of estrogen in a manner similar to the changes in the uterine cervix at term. In an extension of the above evolutionarily adaptive characteristics in women the mucus membranes and skin reflect the levels of estrogen during the climacteric.

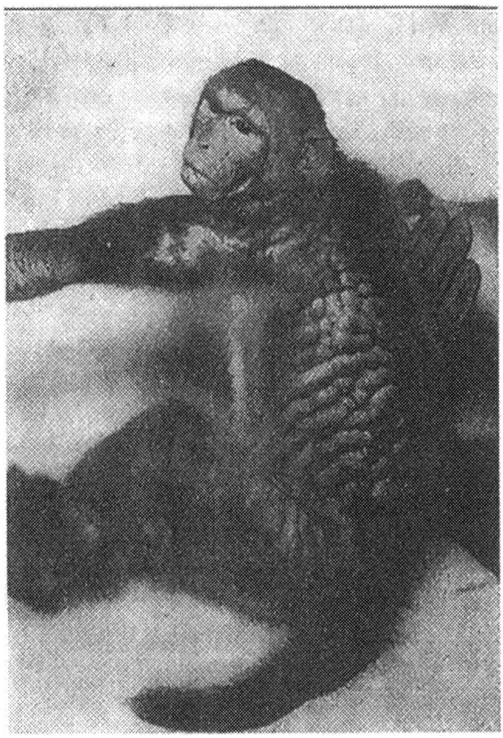

Modified from Farris

Figure 8. Sex skin extends to the back and less to the limbs. In monkeys it becomes more dramatic with age.

Table 1. The role of estrogen-sensitive tissues in the reproductive tract.

Estrogen-sensitive stroma-epithelial combinations are present throughout the body. In the case of the reproductive tract they form the major structures and also allow accommodation to extremes of shape, size, and resistance which are required to suit the demands of reproductive function. These characteristics, which come about as a result of the sensitivity of the stroma and epithelium to sex steroid action, include changes in cell number and size as well as in the composition of the extracellular matrix (collagen, glycosaminoglycans, and water).

Characteristics of estrogen-sensitive tissue	
1.	Elasticity
	Strength
	Reconstruction
	Extensibility
2.	Bland healing response
	Minimal scarring
	No keloid formation
3.	Water imhibition-swelling
4.	Hypertrophy/hyperplasia-structural mass
5.	Specialized cell-cell interactions

Modified from Naftolin, et al.

Estrogen Withdrawal and Estrogen Deficiency

The common urogenital complaints in estrogen-deficient women (medical treatment, menopause, surgical or therapeutic ovariectomy) can be mainly explained as effects on these tissues that prove the role of estrogen (Table 2).

It is interesting that a number of these symptoms and signs are also seen in hypoestrogenic pre-pubertal girls who have irritated or put a foreign body into the vagina/vulva. In addition, pre-pubertal girls also fail to have a bland response to injury. Administration of estrogen in pre-pubertal and postmenopausal females reverses these problems.

Table 2. Common genitourinary complaints in estrogen-deficient women.

Common genitourinary complaints in estrogen-deficient women
• Vaginal dryness and irritation
• Infection and scratching leading to scarring
• Vulvovaginal pruritis
• Vaginitis
• Malodorous discharge
• Dyspareunia
• Postcoital bleeding
• Dysuria
• Urinary frequency and urgency
• Frequent urinary tract infections
• Urinary stress incontinence

Modified from Bachmann

In aging women the loss of estrogen results in diminished skin thickness/turgor, as shown in Figure 9. For the same reason decreased skin thickness correlates positively with decreased bone density and both deficits are reversed by hormone replacement.

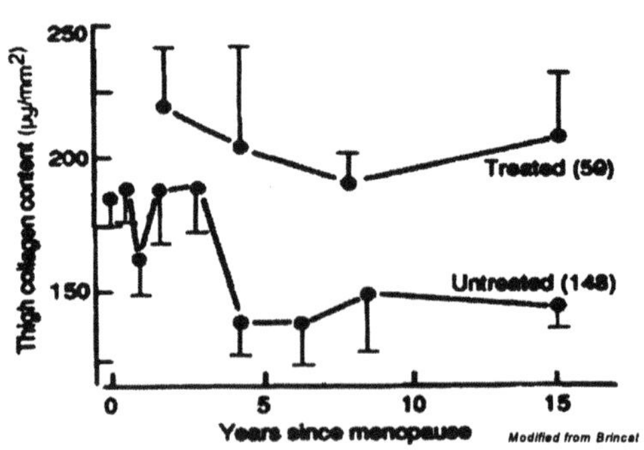

Figure 9. In aging women the skin thickness is correlated with bone density.

As shown in numerous publications, hormone replacement therapy causes an increase in bone mass and in skin thickness while adrenocorticosteroids do the opposite [17].

It is interesting that while estrogen increases the enzymes that degrade collagen and increases muccopolysaccharides, adrenocorticosteroids stabilize zymogens to diminish these functions [7]. The changes in thickness represent maintenance of both the hydration of the tissues and the total amount of collagen in the skin (Figure 10).

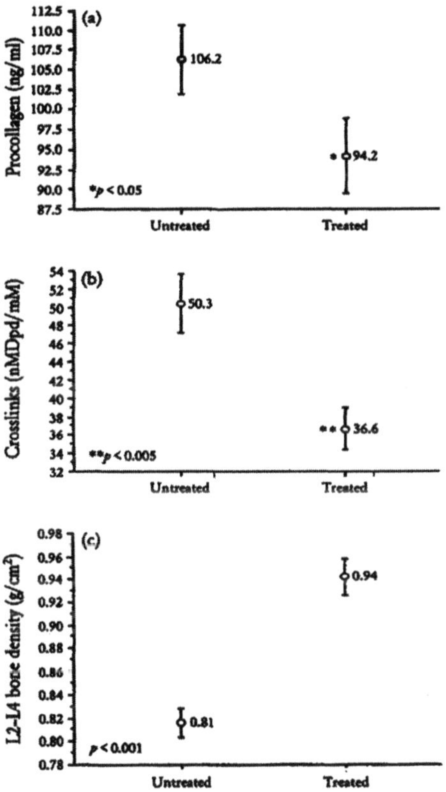

Modified from Brincat

Figure 10. Plot of collagen content at the thigh region versus years since menopause in untreated and estrogen-treated postmenopausal women.

On further examination, increased collagen turnover as indicated by decreased procollagen and cross-linking in skin collagen has been shown and correlated with replacement of bone mineral mass by hormone replacement therapy (Figure 11).

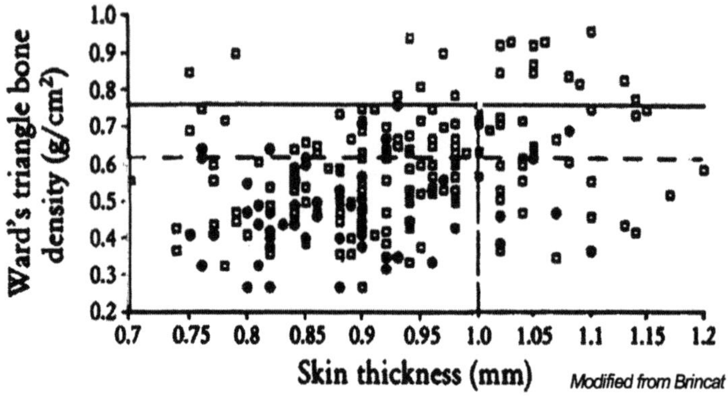

Figure 11. HRT Decreases procollagen and crosslinks in collagen in skin while building bone.

Further Context for the Evolutionary Viewpoint in Understanding Sex Steroid Regulation of Tissues in Women

Menopause is the post reproductive period, when there are no more follicles to produce estrogen in the ovaries and the levels of estrogen are markedly reduced. Because it is post reproductive, there is no Darwinian adaptive response specific to the menopause [18]. Therefore, the woman will respond to the fall in sex steroids in a way that is largely similar to her response to the fall of sex hormone after delivery, in the puerperium. But, the adaptive responses to the fall of estrogen and progesterone during the puerperium which are directed to the success of reproduction will be maladaptive during the climacteric and contribute to the untoward effects of the menopause.

A multi-system comparison between the responses to falling sex steroids in the puerperium and at menopause is shown in (Table 3).

Conclusions

While a number of targeted studies have aimed at categorizing the components and changes in sex steroid-sensitive tissues such as the genital tract, a global approach to this issue is needed. From the available information it is clear that the evolutionary mechanisms that provided for increased safety and efficiency of reproduction in mammals, particularly primates, continue to function during the post-reproductive years. This results in many of the adverse outcomes associated with the climacteric. In the past century the life span in industrialized countries doubled. We now have a large and growing population of post-reproductive women. It is necessary to understand the basis of the physical and mental changes that they will undergo during the climacteric. Only then will our preventative and therapeutic interventions be rational and correct.

Table 3. Adaptive and Maladaptive Responses to Falling Sex Steroids

Adaptive during reproductive era	Affected cells/system	Maladaptive during postreproductive era
Organ dependent changes in immune response	Immunocytes	Failure of immune privilege may ↓ breast cancer and ↑ CNS dystrophy
Fat up in blood to make milk	Lipoprotein lipase ↑	Atherosclerosis
Maintenance of blood flow to critical organs	Arterial tone increased	Atherosclerosis
Sex skin loses elasticity Thinner mucosa	Sex skin function fails	Scarring and genital atrophy
Increased vigilance	Sleep pattern disintegrates	Insomnia Poor performance
Radiation of body heat to the suckling infant	Vasomotor control set point changes, oxytocin changes	Hot flushes
Mobilization of calcium for milk	Cell cycle favors bone loss	Osteoporosis/fracture
Concentration defects Cognitive defects Decreased immune-brain barrier	Central nervous system	Memory defects Dystrophies

References

1. Naftolin F, Lavy G, Palumbo A, DeCherney AH. Poissons, grenouilles, femmes et hommes: The appropriation and retention of archetypical systems for reproduction. Gynecol Endocrinol 1988;2:265-73.
2. Brincat M.P, Galea R. The skin and hormone replacement therapy. In: Brincat M, editor. Hormone replacement therapy and the skin. The Parthenon Publishing Group, 2001:1-17.
3. Lavy G, Whitten PL, Naftolin F. Introduction to vertebrate reproductive endocrinology. In: Pang PKT, Schreibman MP, editors. Vertebrate endocrinology: Fundamentals and biomedical implications. New York: Academic Press, 1991:1-22.
4. Nilsen J, Mor G, Naftolin F. Estrogen-regulated developmental neuronal apoptosis is determined by estrogen receptor subtype and the Fas/Fas ligand system. J Neurobiol

2000;43:64-78.
5. Song J, et al. Fas mediated endometrial remodeling. J Mol Human Reprod 2002; in press.
6. Mor G, Naftolin F. Oestrogen, menopause and the immune system. J British Menopause Society 1998;S1:4-8.
7. Jeffrey J, Koob T. Endocrine control of collagen degradation in the uterus. In: Naftolin F, Stubblefield P, editors. Dilatation of the uterine cervix. New York:Raven Press, 1980:135-45.
8. Cabrol D, Huszar G, Romero R, Naftolin F. Gestational changes in the rat uterine cervix: protein, collagen and glycosaminoglycan content. In: Ellwood D, Anderson A. The cervix in pregnancy and labour. Edinburgh, Scotland: Churchill Livingstone, 1981:34-56.
9. Saito Y, Sakamoto H, MacLusky NJ, Naftolin F. Gap junctions and myometrial steroid hormone receptors in pregnant and postpartum rats: A possible cellular basis for the progesterone withdrawal hypothesis. Am J Obstet Gynecol 1985 Mar 15;151(6):805-12.
10. Garfield RE, et al. Control of myometrial contractility: role and regulation of gap functions. Oxf Rev Reprod Biol 1998;10:436-90.
11. Haluska GJ, et al. Progesterone receptor localization and isoforms in myometrium, decidua and fetal membranes from rhesus macaques: Evidence for functional progesterone withdrawal at parturition. J Society for Gynecologic Investigation 2002, in press.
12. Liggens GC. Cervical ripening as an inflammatory reaction. In: Ellwood D, Anderson A, editors. The cervix in pregnancy and labour. Churchill Livingstone, 1981:1-9.
13. Huszar G, Cabrol D, Naftolin F. The relationship between myometrial and cervical functions in pregnancy and labor. In: Huszar G, editor. The physiology and biochemistry of the uterus in pregnancy and labor. Boca Raton: CRC Press, 1986:287-306.
14. Kleissl HP, VanderRest M, Naftolin F, Glorieux FH, DeLeon A. Collagen changes in the human uterine cervix at parturition. Am J Obstet Gynecol 1978;130(7):748-53.
15. Poole A. Proteinases of connective tissues. In: Naftolin F, Stubblefield P, editors. Dilatation of the uterine cervix. New York:Raven Press, 1980:113-31.
16. Ivell R. This hormone has been relaxin' too long! Science 2002 Jan 25;295(5555):637-38.
17. Muscat Baron Y. Corticosteroids, skin and hormone replacement therapy. In: Brincat M, editor. Hormone replacement therapy and the skin. The Parthenon Publishing Group, 2001:111-20.
18. Naftolin F, et al. An evolutionary perspective on the climacteric and menopause. J North American Menopause Society 1994;1(4):223-25.

DOES MENOPAUSE INCREASE THE INCIDENCE OF CORONARY HEART DISEASE?

Yvonne T. van der Schouw

Introduction

In Westernized societies, most women die from coronary heart disease. Importantly, premenopausal women are at lower risk relative to men of comparable age and postmenopausal women [1,2]. Protection by endogenous oestrogens is a likely explanation, yet the question whether menopause increases the incidence of coronary hear disease has still not been answered satisfactorily yet.

A now famous paper was written by Tracey as early as 1966 in the *Journal of Chronic Diseases*, entitled "Sex differences in coronary artery disease: Two opposing views" [3]. He raised the point that, according to the type of analysis of vital statistics data, a sudden increase in coronary disease susceptibility of women takes place after menopause or not. In 1998, this discussion was revived again [4]. Turnstall-Pedoe argued that increases in risk after menopause are an artifact of the way vital statistics data are presented, such as by displaying crude disease rates compared to age-specific rates or by plotting the data in semi-logarithmic graphs. When the same data are presented, for example as ratios of male-to-female mortality rates, there is no rebound acceleration in risk in women at or after the age of 50.

Later in 1998 this viewpoint was refuted again by some researchers with the argument that Tunstall-Pedoe held a wrong assumption of increased acceleration of coronary heart disease risk. Increased acceleration of risk implies a continuous increase of the relative risk. However, this is seldom the case, not even for hypertension and smoking. The effect of age at menopause on cardiovascular mortality had been estimated as an 2% increased risk per year [5]. If one superimposes this risk on a curve showing death rates presuming women spend their entire life in a premenopausal state, there is hardly any infliction visible, although it certainly is there, because it was modeled so. At least these data show that vital statistics are not the source providing the easy answers.

Early Studies

The earliest studies that looked at effects of early menopause originate from the fifties and sixties. Several authors looked at autopsy material, such as coronary arteries or checked autopsy records of oophorectomized women. Several of them found oophorectomized women to have more severe atherosclerosis than women with their ovaries still intact [6-8]. A figure from the study by Rivin et al. is representative for the main findings of all three papers:

(1) At all ages, males have the highest incidence of severe atherosclerosis;
(2) Oophorectomized women are next, particularly at older ages;
(3) Women with their ovaries intact are at low risk of atherosclerosis; and
(4) Female breast cancer patients, whom were considered to be in a hyper-estrogenic state by the authors, did indeed have the lowest prevalence of atherosclerosis.

In the same period, several follow-up studies and case-control studies on coronary heart disease in oophorectimized women were published [9-14]. Several authors went back to the archives to trace women who underwent bilateral oophorectomy in the past, and tried to find out what had happened to these women. They compared their findings with data from women with unilateral oophorectomy, or from a more general population. At that time it was still very uncommon to prescribe HRT in those women. All studies presented a higher incidence of coronary heart disease in the oophorectimized women.

Although many studies were positive, at least 6 studies are published that did not find associations between oophorectomy and heart disease risk [15-20]; therefore, these early studies are not entirely conclusive. It has to be kept in mind that none of those early studies performed any adjustments for potential confounders. Also the numbers in the studies were often limited, so the power to detect small associations is rather modest.

Prospective Studies

Two reports have been published from the Framingham Heart Study. The first compared 20-year risks of cardiovascular diseases, coronary heart diseases, and other vascular diseases between pre-and postmenopausal women in 4 age groups [21]. In all, postmenopausal women had a higher incidence of all types of heart disease than premenopausal women. The differences were not statistically significant due to the relatively small number of cases in the various categories. Two years later a re-analysis of the data was performed after almost all women had become menopausal [2]. In this analysis postmenopausal was defined as not having menstruated for at least 12 months. Again it was found that postmenopausal women had an increased risk of heart disease, which was now somewhat more pronounced because perimenopausal women were not included in the postmenopausal group and because of the longer follow-up. To my knowledge, this was the first study that adjusted for age and smoking behavior.

The Nurses' Health Study also yielded several reports on menopause and heart disease. The earliest is from 1981 and presents data of a case-control analysis within the baseline data of the Nurses' Health Study cohort, comprising 279 cases and 5,580 age-matched controls [22]. The authors found a clear increasing risk of myocardial infarction (MI) with decreasing age at bilateral oophorectomy. Natural menopause before the age of 35 was also associated with increased MI risk, but natural menopause at later ages was not. However, the numbers of women in the subgroups of age at menopause were quite small.

The first follow-up data from this cohort were based on 6 years of follow-up [1]. After controlling for age and cigarette smoking, women who had had a natural menopause and who had never taken replacement estrogen had no appreciable increase in the risk of coronary heart disease, as compared with premenopausal women. (adjusted rate ratio, 1.2; 95% confidence limits, 0.8 and 1.8). Women who had undergone bilateral oophorectomy and who had never taken estrogens after menopause had an increased risk, with a rate ratio of 2.2, which was statistically significant. The use of estrogens in the postmenopausal period appeared to eliminate this increased risk among these women as compared with premenopausal women (rate ratio, 0.9).

In Utrecht we had data of the Diagnostich Onderzoek Mammacarcinoom (DOM) cohort available, a cohort of 15,000 women aged 50 to 65 at enrollment in an experimental breast cancer screening program in the late 1970s. We hypothesized that if menopause was a risk factor for heart disease, than the later women become menopausal, the longer they profit from their endogenous estrogens, and the lower their cardiovascular risk. For the DOM-cohort, no incidence data are available, but vital status and causes of death were collected until 1995. When adjusted for age, we found that overall each year that the menopause is delayed decreases the annual risk of cardiovascular death by 2%. This effect was somewhat more pronounced for women with bilateral oophorectomy. The effect decreased with increasing chronological age; in 80-year-olds we could not find an effect of early menopause any longer. Adjustment for other risk factors, such as smoking did not alter the results [5]. Although the interaction was not statistically significant, the effect of early menopause seemed confined to nonsmokers.

One year later data from a large Norwegian breast cancer screening cohort were published. Through a unique official personal registration number, it was possible to link the cohort data with the vital status and cause of death information at the Norwegian Central Bureau of Statistics. Basically, this group found results similar to the our own data: coronary heart disease mortality risk decreased with increasing age at menopause. Especially in women aged 70 and younger an almost 60% reduced risk was found for women with a late menopause compared to the earliest menopausal women [23].

Glinda Cooper and co-workers had the opportunity to work with data from a cohort with very detailed information on menstrual cycles that was set up in 1934 by Alan Treloar, which was followed for over 50 years. Although there were only 45 cases in this cohort, the age-adjusted rate ratios show a clear age-adjusted association between age at menopause and risk of coronary heart disease. This was found for natural menopause as well as menopause because of bilateral oophorectomy [24].

Data from the Nurses' Health Study have also been analyzed for the women who were naturally postmenopausal at baseline who never used HRT and were at baseline free from cardiovascular disease. The relative risk for a one-year decrease in age at natural menopause was 1.03, quite comparable to the previous Dutch findings. In contrast, however, was the finding that the results seemed only present in the smoking women. The authors suggest that residual confounding by smoking might be the cause of these results [25].

In 1989 it had already been reported that in Californian Seventh-Day Adventists early menopause seemed to be associated with coronary heart disease mortality [26]. In 1999 a re-analysis of these data was published, with substantially more cases and longer follow-up. The observed association between age at natural menopause and coronary heart disease mortality was stronger in the youngest women, as was found twice before. Surprisingly, the authors found the risk of coronary heart disease mortality to decrease with increasing age at menopause, but to increase again in the highest age at menopause group. It is not quite clear how to interpret this unexpected finding [27].

A recent Italian case-control study did not find any meaningful association between age at natural menopause. In their analyses, HRT-users were included and HRT-use was adjusted for. For current oral contraceptive or HRT users, however, it is difficult to determine the true age at natural menopause, which might have diluted the results [28]. In their discussion, the authors conclude that the overall literature is compatible with a modest effect of early menopause on coronary heart disease risk, despite their own null findings.

Atheroslcerosis

The hypothesis that loss of ovarian function and subsequent deficiency of estrogen may promote cardiovascular disease would gain strength if an association would also be found with atherosclerosis. Presence of aortic calcification on X-rays of the lumbar spine have been compared between pre- and postmenopausal women. For naturally postmenopausal as well as oophorectomized women, a clear age-adjusted increase of calcifications with increasing time since menopause was found [29].

Recently, a study was published that looked at carotid intima media thickness, which is a currently very well-accepted measure of generalized atherosclerosis. In the Norwegian Tromsø study with a cross-sectional design, dose-response relationships were found for age at menopause with caritid intima media thickness, but also with prevalence of carotid atherosclerosis [30].

Conclusion

In conclusion, the findings are in general compatible with a modest effect of early menopause on coronary heart disease. That this modest effect is yet relevant, can be concluded from the fact that menopausal status has been included in the coronary risk functions for women, derived from the Framingham Heart Study. Last year, the risk functions were updated with more persons, including participants of the Framingham Offspring Cohort, and with longer follow-up [31]. Who would dare to deny the importance of menopause for coronary heart disease risk now that the well-respected Framingham risk functions have included it?

References

1. Colditz GA, Willett WC, Stampfer MJ, Rosner B, Speizer FE, Hennekens CH. Menopause and the risk of coronary heart disease in women. N Engl J Med 1987;316:1105-10.

2. Gordon T, Kannel WB, Hjortland MC, McNamara PM. Menopause and coronary heart disease: The Framingham study. Ann Intern Med 1978;89:157-61.
3. Tracey RE. Sex differences in coronary artery disease: Two opposing views. J Chron Dis 1966;19:1245-51.
4. Tunstall-Pedoe H. Myth and paradox of coronary risk and the menopause. Lancet 1998; 351:1425-27.
5. Schouw van der YT, Graaf van der Y, Steyerberg EW, Eijkemans MJC, Banga JD. Age at menopause as a risk factor for cardiovascular mortality. Lancet 1996;347:714-18.
6. Wuest JH, Dry TJ, Edwards JE. The degree of coronary atherosclerosis in bilaterally oophorectomized women. Circulation 1953;8:801-8.
7. Rivin AU, Dimitroff SP. The incidence and severity of coronary atherosclerosis in estrogen-treated males, and in females with a hypoestrogenic or a hyperestrogenic state. Circulation 1954;9:533-39.
8. Parrish HM, Carr CA, Hall DG, King TM. Time interval from castration in premenopausal women to development of excessive coronary atherosclerosis. Am J Obstet Gynecol 1967; 99:155-62.
9. Oliver MF, Boyd GS. Effect of bilateral ovariectomy on coronary artery disease and serum lipid levels. Lancet 1959;ii:690-94.
10. Robinson RW, Higano N, Cohen WD. Increased incidence of coronary heart disease in women castrated prior to the menopause. Arch Intern Med 1959;104:908-13.
11. Ask-Upmark E. Life and death without ovaries. Acta Med Scand 1962;172:129-35.
12. Johansson BW, Kaij L, Kullander S, Lenner H-C, Svanberg L, Astedt B. On some late effects of bilateral oophorectomy in the age range 15-30 years. Acta Obstet Gynecol Scand 1975;54:449-61.
13. Winkelstein W, Stichever MA, Lilienfield AM. Occurrence of pregnancy, abortion and artificial menopause among women with coronary artery disease. J Chron Dis 1958;7:273-86.
14. Oliver MF. Ischaemic heart disease in young women. Br Med J 1974;4:253-59.
15. Glendy RE, Levine SA, White PD. Coronary disease in youth: Comparison of 100 patients under 40 with 300 persons past 80. J Am Med Assoc 1937;109:1775-78.
16. Randall CL, Paloucek FP, Graham JB, Graham S. Causes of death in cases of preclimacteric menorrhagia. Am J Obstet Gynecol 1964;88:880-97.
17. Furman RH. Are gonadal hormones (estrogens and androgens) of significance in the development of ischemic heart disease? Ann N Y Acad Sci 1968;149:822-33.
18. Heller RF, Jacobs HS. Coronary heart disease in relation to age, sex, and the menopause. Br Med J 1978;1:472-74.
19. Alderson MR, Jackson SM. Long term follow-up of patients with menorrhagia treated by irradiation. Br J Radiol 1971;44:295-98.
20. Manchester JH, Herman MV, Gorlin R. Premenopausal castration and documented coronary atherosclerosis. Am J Cardiol 1971;28:33-37.
21. Kannel WB, Hjortland MC, McNamara PM, Gordon T. Menopause and the risk of cardiovascular disease: The Framingham study. Ann Intern Med 1976;85:447-52.
22. Rosenberg L, Hennekens CH, Rosner B, Belanger C, Rothman KJ, Speizer FE. Early menopause and the risk of myocardial infarction. Am J Obstet Gynecol 1981;139:47-51.
23. Jacobsen BK, Nilssen S, Heuch I, Kvale G . Does age at natural menopause affect mortality from ischemic heart disease? J Clin Epidemiol 1997;50:475-79.
24. Cooper GS, Ephross SA, Weinberg CR, Baird DD, Whelan EA, Sandler DP. Menstrual

and reproductive risk factors for ischemic heart disease. Epidemiology 1999;10:255-59.
25. Hu FB, Grodstein F, Hennekens CH, et al. Age at natural menopause and risk of cardiovascular disease. Arch Intern Med 1999;159:1061-66.
26. Snowdon DA, Kane RL, Beeson WL, et al. Is early menopause a biological marker of health and aging? Am J Public Health 1989;79:709-14.
27. Jacobsen BK, Knutsen SF, Fraser GE. Age at natural menopause and total mortality and mortality from ischemic heart disease: The Adventist Health Study. J Clin Epidemiol 1999;52:303-7.
28. Fioretti F, Tavani A, Gallus S, Franceschi S, La Vecchia C. Menopause and risk of non-fatal acute myocardial infarction: An Italian case-control study and a review of the literature. Hum Reprod 2000;15:599-603.
29. Witteman JCM, Grobbee DE, Kok FJ, Hofman A, Valkenburg HA. Increased risk of atherosclerosis in women after the menopause. Br Med J 1989;298:642-44.
30. Joakimsen O, Bonaa KH, Stensland-Bugge E, Jacobsen BK. Population-based study of age at menopause and ultrasound assessed carotid atherosclerosis: The Tromso Study. J Clin Epidemiol 2000;53:525-30.
31. d'Agostino RB, Russell MW, Huse DM, et al. Primary and subsequent coronary risk appraisal: New results from the Framingham study. Am Heart J 2000; 39:272-81.

REDUCING CARDIOVASCULAR RISK IN POSTMENOPAUSAL WOMEN: ESTROGEN OR STATINS?

Richard O. Cannon, III

Introduction

Before menopause, low-density lipoprotein (LDL) cholesterol levels in blood are lower and high-density lipoprotein (HDL) cholesterol levels are higher compared with those in men of the same age. After menopause, LDL cholesterol levels rise and may exceed those of age-matched men, with a shift to smaller, more dense (and potentially more atherogenic) particle sizes, and HDL cholesterol levels decline [1-2]. Prospective population-based observational studies including women have reported a positive association between total cholesterol levels and coronary heart disease risk, and an inverse association between HDL cholesterol levels and risk. In the Framingham cohort, women whose ratio of total to HDL cholesterol was between 5.5 and 7.4 had twice the risk of coronary heart disease compared with women whose ratio of these cholesterol values was less than 3.5: women whose ratio was between 7.5 and 9.4 had 4 times the risk, and women whose ratio was greater than 9.5 had 5 times the risk of coronary heart disease events [3]. The combination of high LDL with low HDL cholesterol levels (resulting in high ratios of total to HDL cholesterol) is commonly found in the "metabolic syndrome" associated with central obesity, hypertension and adult-onset diabetes. High levels of triglycerides (also a feature of the metabolic syndrome) also appear to be a marker of cardiovascular risk in women, and to a greater degree than in men [4-6].

Cardiovascular Effects of Statin Therapy in Women

Angiographic studies of effects of various lipid-lowering therapies conducted in the 1980s had suggested treatment-related reduction in cardiovascular risk, despite rather small effects on coronary atherosclerosis progression. The most potent of these therapies is an HMG-CoA reductase inhibitor (commonly referred to as "statin") that blocks the enzyme catalyzing the rate-limiting step in cholesterol synthesis. Depending on the preparation and dose of statin used, reduction in LDL cholesterol levels by over 50% may be achieved. Reduction in apolipoprotein B levels indicates that statin therapy actually reduces the number of LDL particles in blood. Statins also increase levels of HDL cholesterol and reduce levels of triglycerides to varying degrees, but have no effect on levels of another atherogenic lipoprotein, lipoprotein(a).

Several randomized, placebo-controlled clinical trials have shown reduction in cardiovascular events associated with statin therapy in women with atherosclerosis. In the Scandinavian Simvastatin Survival Study, 4,444 patients with coronary artery disease who had LDL cholesterol levels averaging 188 mg/dL were randomized to simvastatin versus placebo, in addition to diet and conventional anti-anginal therapy [7]. After a median of 5.4 years of treatment, the simvastatin group had a 35% reduction in LDL and 8% increase in HDL cholesterol compared with pretreatment levels, and a 30% reduction in total mortality, due primarily to fewer fatal cardiac events (myocardial infarction and sudden death) compared with the placebo group. Of the 827 women in the study, those randomized to simvastatin had a 35% lower risk of major coronary events (coronary death, myocardial infarction, resuscitation from cardiac arrest) compared with placebo-treated women, although total mortality was not reduced with simvastatin therapy in this relatively small subgroup. The Cholesterol and Recurrent Events (CARE) trial of post-infarct patients (average LDL cholesterol 139 mg/dL), which included 576 women, reported a 50% reduction in coronary heart disease events in women randomized to pravastatin compared with placebo-treated women [8]. In the Long Term Intervention with Pravastatin In Ischemic Disease (LIPID) trial of patients with atherosclerotic cardiovascular disease (average LDL cholesterol 150 mg/dL), which included 1,518 women, those women randomized to pravastatin had an 11% lower risk of cardiovascular events compared with placebo-treated women [9].

The Air Force/Texas Coronary Atherosclerosis Prevention Study (AFCAPS/TexCAPS) enrolled apparently healthy subjects (including 997 women) with ratios of total to HDL cholesterol ≥ 5 [10]. Women randomized to lovastatin had a 46% reduction in cardiovascular events compared with placebo-treated women in this primary prevention trial. However, the absolute risk was low in the women participants, such that 80 women required statin treatment for 5 years in order to prevent one event.

Statin lipid-lowering therapy may also reduce the risk of stroke. In a meta-analysis of 16 clinical trials that included almost 39,000 patients in which almost 900 strokes were recorded, statin therapy was associated with reduced risk of ischemic (but not hemorrhagic) stroke in those patients with coronary artery disease [11]. Few patients in these trials had a history of stroke, therefore statin effects on recurrent stroke risk is unknown. The statin effect on stroke does not appear to be limited by age, but whether this class of drugs actually reduces stroke mortality is unclear [12]. In this analysis of trials using pravastatin (CARE and LIPID), the reduction in stroke risk was not significant for women, although the relatively small number of women in these trials resulted in large confidence limits. Further clinical trials with inclusion of significant numbers of women are clearly needed to better define the effect of statin therapy on stroke risk.

Mechanisms of Statin Effects on Cardiovascular Risk Reduction

Angiographic studies have shown that statin therapy causes only minimal reduction in plaque size and number of new plaques during of the time course of the study compared with placebo-treated patients. The Canadian Coronary Atherosclerosis Intervention Trial reported the results of lovastatin 40 to 80 mg daily versus placebo for 2 years on the angiographic progression of disease separately for women and for men [13]. The 25 women in the lovastatin group had significantly less progression (worsening of the minimum diameter of 1 or more stenoses ≥ 0.4 mm) compared with the 29 women in the placebo group: 7 of 25 versus 17 of 29). Further, new lesions developed in 1 lovastatin-treated woman, versus 13 in the placebo group.

Patients with atherosclerosis or its risk factors commonly have evidence of endothelial dysfunction of the coronary circulation, as evidenced by constrictor responses of coronary artery segments to acetylcholine [14]. These responses are compatible with deficient nitric oxide synthesis or release by the endothelium of those segments. In recent years, several groups have reported that patients with coronary endothelial dysfunction are at increased risk for cardiac events including myocardial infarction, unstable angina pectoris, need for revascularization, and cardiac-related death [15,16]. Statins have been shown to improve coronary artery endothelium-dependent responsiveness to acetylcholine, consistent with improved nitric oxide release, in randomized, placebo-controlled clinical trials that included women with coronary artery disease [17,18]. Statins reduce cholesterol content of LDL particles, possibly rendering this lipoprotein less susceptible to oxidation that would otherwise result in macrophage uptake and foam cell formation [19]. Additional benefits of statin therapy may be independent of lipid-lowering effects of this drug. Thus, cell culture experiments suggest that statins may stabilize eNOS mRNA by blocking the synthesis of isoprenoid intermediates from mevalonate (farnesyl phosphate and geranylgeranyl phosphate), which in turn prevents their attachment to intracellular signaling molecules [20]. An additional lipid-independent benefit of statins to atherosclerotic arteries may be reduction in vascular inflammation, as evidenced by inhibition of expression of cell adhesion molecules on monocytes with reduced binding to endothelial cells in culture [21], and by reduction in levels of C-reactive protein in clinical trials of statin therapy [22,23].

Lipoprotein and Cardiovascular Effects of Hormone Replacement Therapy

Oral administration of estrogen preparations to postmenopausal women reduces LDL cholesterol levels by 10-15% [24,25], probably as a result of increased expression of LDL receptors on hepatocytes [26], and similarly reduces levels of the structurally related lipoprotein(a) [27]. HDL levels are increased by approximately 15%, due to increased synthesis of apolipoprotein A-I and decreased hepatic lipase activity. The combination of estrogens and statin therapies for hypercholesterolemic postmenopausal women seems particularly appealing, with greater reduction in LDL and lipoprotein(a) and greater increase in HDL than achieved with statin therapy alone [28]. Estrogen therapy also protects LDL from oxidation [29], enhances fibrinolysis [30], and improves coronary endothelium-dependent responses to acetylcholine consistent with enhanced nitric oxide synthesis and release [31]. In a primate model of atherosclerosis, estrogen administration to ovariectomized animals reduced the extent of atherosclerosis in the coronary arteries [32].

However, despite these beneficial effects of estrogen in experimental settings and prospective observational studies reporting reduced risk of cardiovascular events in postmenopausal women on hormone replacement therapy compared with estrogen nonusers [33], randomized, double-blind, placebo-controlled clinical trials of hormone therapy in postmenopausal women with coronary artery disease have not shown cardiovascular benefit. Thus, after 4.1 years of follow-up in the Heart and Estrogen/progestin Replacement Study (HERS) with 2,763 women, those randomized to active treatment (conjugated equine estrogens 0.625 mg and medroxyprogesterone acetate 2.5 mg daily) had similar rates of cardiovascular events as placebo-treated women (approximately one-half of study participants received lipid-lowering therapy) [34]. In the Estrogen Replacement and Atherosclerosis (ERA) trial of 309 women with coronary artery disease, those women randomized to conjugated equine estrogens 0.625 mg daily, either alone or combined with medroxyprogesterone acetate 2.5 mg daily, showed no evidence of altered progression of atherosclerosis by coronary angiography compared with placebo-treated women [35]. In this clinical trial, about one-third of study participants were treated with lipid-lowering therapy.

An observation in HERS that has prompted considerable discussion was the 50% higher incidence of nonfatal myocardial infarction and cardiovascular death during the first year following randomization in hormone-treated women, with fewer events during years 3 and 4 compared with placebo-treated women. Concern regarding hormone therapy-induced events soon after initiation of therapy is supported by a report of 2,489 postmenopausal women in the Nurses' Health Study cohort who had evidence of coronary artery disease, in which a 25% increased risk of myocardial infarction or coronary heart disease death was observed within the first year after initiation of hormone therapy compared with nonusers of hormones [36]. In a recent report, investigators of the Coumadin Aspirin Reinfarction Study (CARS) examined the study database, which included 1,857 postmenopausal women, and found the 111 women who began hormone therapy after their myocardial infarction had a higher incidence of cardiovascular events, especially unstable angina, compared with women not on hormone therapy during the year following their infarction [37].

The early risk of cardiovascular events after initiation of hormone therapy noted in HERS and in the observational studies of women with coronary artery disease has also been noted in apparently healthy postmenopausal women. The Women's Health Initiative, sponsored by the National Institutes of Health, includes 27,00 women randomized to hormone therapy appropriate to their uterine status, or placebo. Last year, investigators of this clinical trial issued a press release reporting an increased incidence of cardiovascular risk (including venous and arterial events) among those women randomized to hormone therapy within the first two years of randomization [38].

The early cardiovascular event risk associated with initiation of hormone therapy has generated concerns regarding possible prothrombotic effects of estrogen. Estrogen administration increases levels of factor VII and X in serum, decreases levels of anti-thrombin III, and increases indices of coagulation activation [39-41]. In the venous circulation, observational studies and the HERS randomized clinical trial indicate a 3-fold increased risk of thromboembolic events associated with hormone therapy use [42-44]. In arteries, estrogen may provoke thrombus formation leading to myocardial infarction or stroke by coagulation activation on the surface of atherosclerotic plaques with exposed connective tissue or enhanced tissue factor release by activated macrophages. Estrogen may also aggravate arterial inflammation, now recognized to be an integral component of the progression and clinical expression of atherosclerosis, as evidenced by increases in levels of C-reactive protein [45]. Although likely a first pass effect of orally administered estrogen on the hepatic synthesis of this protein, elevated levels of C-reactive protein could have deleterious effects on vascular inflammation by inducing the synthesis of cytokines, inflammatory cell adhesion molecules, and tissue factor in macrophages and within the endothelium [46-48]. Tissue factor activates the extrinsic coagulation cascade, providing a link between inflammation and thrombosis. Further, C-reactive protein may contribute to atherosclerosis progression by facilitating uptake of lipoproteins by macrophages, thus accelerating foam cell formation [49]. Hormone therapy also increases levels in serum of matrix metalloproteinase-9, the increased synthesis of which within the vessel wall could digest and weaken fibrous caps of vulnerable plaques, thus provoking thrombosis [50].

As opposed to oral estrogens, transdermal administration of estrogen has minimal effects on coagulation activation [40,41] and has been reported to lower levels of C-reactive protein in postmenopausal women [51,52]. However, potentially atherogenic lipoproteins are unaltered by this route of administration [24], and thus transdermal estrogen may not provide an advantage over oral estrogen for reducing cardiovascular risk.

Recommendation of American Heart Association Advisory Panel

Because of concerns raised in HERS and in observational studies of postmenopausal women with coronary artery disease, the American Heart Association Advisory Panel recommends against initiating hormone therapy in women with known atherosclerotic cardiovascular disease [53]. If such a woman is already taking hormone therapy, continuation of hormone use should not be for the purpose of secondary prevention, and should be interrupted if the woman is hospitalized for an acute cardiovascular event (as well as anticipated prolonged immobilization). With regards to primary prevention, recommendations cannot be made until clinical trial data become available. Thus, decisions to use hormone therapy should be predicated at the present time on accepted indications, such as menopausal symptoms and osteoporosis prevention. Instead, women (and men) should be encouraged to make lifestyle choices including diet, exercise, and smoking cessation that may reduce their risk of cardiovascular disease. Greater use of lipid-lowering therapy, especially statins, in accordance the recently released update of the National Cholesterol Education Program is also likely to reduce death and disability from myocardial infarction and stroke.

References

1. Stevenson JC, Crook D, Godsland IF. Influence of age and menopause on serum lipids and

lipoproteins in healthy women. Atherosclerosis 1993;98:83-90.
2. Campos H, McNarara SR, Wilson PWF, Ordovas JM, Schaefer EJ. Differences in low density lipoprotein subfractions and apolipoproteins in premenopausal and postmenopausal women. J Clin Endocrinol Metab 1988;67:30-35.
3. Kannel WB, Wilson PW. Efficacy of lipid profiles in prediction of coronary disease. Am Heart J 1992;124:768-74.
4. Sprecher DL, Pearce GL, Cosgrove DL, et al. Relation of serum triglyceride levels to survival after coronary bypass grafting. Am J Cardiol 2000;86:285.
5. Assmann G, Cullen P, Schulte H. The Munster Heart Study (PROCAM). Results of follow-up at 8 years. Eur Heart J 1998;19(suppl):A2.
6. Hokanson JE, Austin MA. Plasma triglyceride level is a risk factor for cardiovascular disease independent of high-density lipoprotein cholesterol level: A meta-analysis of population-based prospective studies. J Cardiovasc Risk 1996;3:213.
7. Scandinavian Simvastatin Survival Study Group. Randomized trial of cholesterol lowering in 4444 patients with coronary heart disease: The Scandinavian Simvastatin Survival Study (4S). Lancet 1994;344:1383-89.
8. Sacks FM, Pfeffer MA, Moye LA, et al. The effect of pravastatin on coronary events after myocardial infarction in patients with average cholesterol levels. N Engl J Med 1996;335: 1001-9.
9. LIPID Study Group. Prevention of cardiovascular events and death with pravastatin in patients with coronary heart disease and a broad range of cholesterol levels. N Engl J Med 1998:339:1349-57.
10. Downs JR, Clearfield M, Weis S, et al. Primary prevention of acute coronary events with lovastatin in men and women with average cholesterol levels: Results of AFCAPS/TexCAPS. JAMA 1998: 279:1615-22.
11. Di Mascio R, Marchioli R, Tognoni G. Cholesterol reduction and stroke occurrence: An overview of randomized clinical trials. Cerebrovascular Dis 2000;10:85-92.
12. Byington RP, Davis BR, Plehn J, et al Reduction of stroke events with pravastatin: The Prospective Pravastatin Pooling (PPP) Project. Circulation 2001;103:387-92.
13. Waters D, Higginson L, Gladstone P, et al. Effects of monotherapy with an HMG-CoA reductase inhibitor on the progression of coronary atherosclerosis as assessed by serial quantitative angiography. The Canadian Coronary Atherosclerosis Intervention Trial. Circulation 1994;89:959-68.
14. Quyyumi AA, Dakak N, Andrews NP, et al. Nitric oxide in the coronary circulation. Impact of risk factors for coronary atherosclerosis. J Clin Invest 1995;95:1747-55.
15. Al Suwaidi J, Hamasaki S, Higano ST, Nishimura RA, Holmes DR Jr, Lerman A. Long-term follow-up of patients with mild coronary artery disease and endothelial dysfunction. Circulation 2000;100:948-54.
16. Schachinger V, Britten MB, Zeiher AM. Prognostic impact of coronary vasodilator dysfunction on adverse long-term outcome of coronary artery disease. Circulation 2000; 101:1899-1906.
17. Treasure CB, Klein JL, Weintraub WS, et al. Beneficial effects of cholesterol-lowering therapy on the coronary endothelium in patients with coronary artery disease. N Engl J Med 1995;332:481-87.
18. Anderson TJ, Meredith IT, Yeung AC, Frei B, Selwyn AP, Ganz P. The effect of cholesterol-lowering and antioxidant therapy on endothelium-dependent coronary vasomotion. N Engl J Med 1995;332:488-93.

19. Giroux LM, Davignon J, Naruszewicz M. Simvastatin inhibits the oxidation of low-density lipoproteins by activated human monocyte-derived macrophages. Biochim Biophys Acta 1993;1165:335-38.
20. Laufs U, Liao JK. Post-transcriptional regulation of endothelial nitric oxide synthase mRNA stability by Rho GTPase. J Biol Chem 1998;273:24266-71.
21. Weber C, Erl W, Weber K. HMG-CoA reductase inhibitors decrease CD 11b expression and CD11b-dependent adhesion of monocytes to endothelium and reduce increased adhesiveness of monocytes isolated from patients with hyperlipidemia. J Am Coll Cardiol 1997;30:1212-17.
22. Ridker PM, Rifai N, Pfeffer MA, Sacks F, Braunwald E, for the Cholesterol and Recurrent Events (CARE) Investigators. Long-term effects of pravastatin on plasma concentration of C-reactive protein. Circulation 1999;100:230-35.
23. Ridker PM, Rifai N, Lowenthal SP. Rapid reduction in C-reactive protein with cerivaststin among 785 patients with primary hypercholesterolemia. Circulation 2001;103:1191-93.
24. Walsh BW, Schiff I, Rosner B, Greenberg L, Ravnikar V, Sacks FM. Effects of estrogen replacement on the concentrations and metabolism of plasma lipoproteins. N Engl J Med 1991;325:1196-1204.
25. The Writing Group for the PEPI Trial. Effects of estrogen or estrogen/progestin regimens on heart disease risk factors in postmenopausal women: The Postmenopausal Estrogen/Progestin Interventions (PEPI) Trial. JAMA 1995;273:199-208.
26. Windler E Kovanen PT, Chao YS, Brown MS, Havel RJ, Goldstein JL. The estradiol-stimulated lipoprotein receptor of rat liver. J Biol Chem 1980;225:10464-71.
27. Sacks FM, McPherson R, Walsh BW. Effect of postmenopausal estrogen replacement on Lp(a) lipoprotein concentrations. Arch Intern Med 1994;154:1106-10.
28. Koh KK, Cardillo C, Bui MN, et al. Vascular effects of estrogen and lipid-lowering therapies in hypercholesterolemic postmenopausal women. Circulation 1999;99:354-60.
29. Sack MN, Rader DJ, Cannon RO III. Oestrogen and inhibition of oxidation of low-density lipoproteins in postmenopausal women. Lancet 1994;343:269-70.
30. Koh KK, Mincemoyer R, Bui MN, et al. Effects of hormone replacement therapy on fibrinolysis in postmenopausal women. N Engl J Med 1997;336:683-90.
31. Gilligan DM, Quyyumi AA, Cannon RO. Effects of physiological levels of estrogen on coronary vasomotor function in postmenopausal women. Circulation 1994;89:2545-51.
32. Adams MR, Kaplan JR, Manuck SB, et al. Inhibition of coronary artery atherosclerosis by 17-beta estradiol in ovariectomized monkeys. Lack of an effect of added progesterone. Arteriosclerosis 1990;10:1051-57.
33. Stampfer MJ, Colditz GA, Willett WC, et al. Postmenopausal estrogen therapy and cardiovascular disease: 10-year follow-up from the Nurses' Health Study. N Engl J Med 1991;325:756-62.
34. Hulley S, Grady D, Bush T, et al. Randomized trial of estrogen plus progestin for secondary prevention of coronary artery disease in postmenopausal women. JAMA 1998; 280:605-13.
35. Herrington DM, Reboussin DM, Brosnihan KB, et al. Effects of estrogen replacement on the progression of coronary artery atherosclerosis. N Engl J Med 2000;343:522-29.
36. Grodstein F, Manson JE, Stampfer MJ. Postmenopausal hormone use and secondary prevention of coronary events in the Nurses' Health Study. A prospective, observational study. Ann Intern Med 2001;135:1-8.
37. Alexander KP, Newby IK, Hellkamp AS, et al. Initiation of hormone replacement therapy

after acute myocardial infarction is associated with more cardiac events during follow-up. J Am Coll Cardiol 2001:38:1-7.
38. Statement from Claude Lenfant, MD, NHLBI Director on preliminary trends in the Women's Health Initiative. NHLBI Communications Office, April 3, 2000.
39. Caine YG, Bauer KA, Barzegar S, et al. Coagulation activation following estrogen administration to postmenopausal women. Thromb Haemost 1992;68:392-95.
40. Kroon U-B, Silfverstolpe G, Tengborn L. The effects of transdermal and oral conjugated estrogens on Haemostasis variables. Thromb Haemost 1994;71:420-23.
41. Scarabin PY, Alhenc-Gelas M, Plu-Bureau G, Taisne P, Agher R, Aiach M. Effects of oral and transdermal estrogen/progesterone regimens on blood coagulation and fibrinolysis in postmenopausal women. A randomized controlled trial. Arterioscler Thromb Vasc Biol 1997;17:3071-78.
42. Daly E, Vessey MP, Hawkins MM, Carson JL, Gough P, Marsh S. Risk of venous thromboembolism in users of hormone replacement therapy. Lancet 1996;348:977-80.
43. Jick H, Derby LE, Myers MW, Vasilakis C, Newton KM. Risk of hospital admission for idiopathic venous thromboembolism among users of postmenopausal oestrogens. Lancet 1996;348:981-83.
44. Grodstein F, Stampfer MJ, Goldhaber SZ, et al. Prospective study of exogenous hormones and risk of pulmonary embolism in women. Lancet 1996;348:983-87.
45. Cushman M, Legault C, Barrett-Connor E, et al. Effect of postmenopausal hormones on inflammation-sensitive proteins. The postmenopausal Estrogen/progestin Interventions (PEPI) Study. Circulation 1999;100:717-22.
46. Gabay C, Kushner I. Acute-phase reactants and other systemic responses to inflammation. N Engl J Med 1999;340:448-54.
47. Cermak J, Key NS, Bach RR, Balla J, Jacob HS, Vercellotti GM.. C-reactive protein induces human peripheral blood monocytes to synthesize tissue factor. Blood 1993;82:513-20.
48. Pasceri V, Willerson JT, Yeh ETH. Direct proinflammatory effect of C-reactive protein on human endothelial cells. Circulation 2000;102:2165-68.
49. Zwaka P, Hombach V, Torzewski J. C-reactive protein-mediated low density lipoprotein uptake by macrophages. Implications for atherosclerosis. Circulation 2001;103:1194-97.
50. Zanger D, Yang BK, Ardans J, et al. Divergent effects of hormone therapy on serum markers of inflammation in postmenopausal women with coronary artery disease on appropriate medical management. J Am Coll Cardiol 2000;36:1797-1802.
51. Satter N, Small M, Lumsden M-A. Hormone replacement and sensitive C-reactive protein concentrations in women with type-2 diabetes. Lancet 1999;354:487-88.
52. Modena MG, Fontanesi L, le Noci A, et al. Effects of hormone replacement therapy on C-reactive protein in healthy postmenopausal women: Comparison between oral and transdermal administration. (Abstract) J Am Coll Cardiol 2001;37:254A.
53. Mosca L, Collins P, Herrington DM, et al. Hormone replacement therapy and cardiovascular disease. A statement for healthcare professionals from the American Heart Association. Circulation 2001;104:499-503.

Effects of Estrogen Replacement in Women with Coronary Disease

David M. Herrington and Karen Potvin Klein

Introduction

Postmenopausal hormone replacement therapy (HRT) has been recommended for the secondary prevention of coronary heart disease (CHD) in women due to observational and experimental studies showing favorable effects on cardiovascular parameters [1-5]. But in 1998, the Heart and Estrogen/progestin Replacement Study (HERS) found no overall effect of 4.1 years of estrogen plus progestin on the risk of nonfatal myocardial infarction (MI) and CHD death in a randomized clinical trial of 2,763 women with established coronary disease [6]. Further, there was evidence of an increased risk in Year 1 of HERS that was offset by a trend toward risk reduction in Years 2-5, producing an overall null effect. More recently, the Estrogen Replacement and Atherosclerosis (ERA) trial, a double-blind, randomized, three-arm angiographic trial of 309 women with heart disease, found no effect of estrogen alone or estrogen plus progestin on progression of coronary artery atherosclerosis [7]. Currently, much effort is being devoted to understanding why estrogen seems ineffective for secondary prevention of CHD. This article will briefly review the results from the HERS and ERA trials as well as other clinical studies of estrogen and CHD.

Summary of the HERS Results

HERS was the first multi-center randomized clinical trial (N = 2,763) evaluating the effects of HRT in women known to have CHD. After a mean of 4.1 years of treatment (0.625 mg/d oral conjugated equine estrogen [CEE] plus 2.5 mg/d medroxyprogesterone acetate [MPA]), the overall rate of CHD events (nonfatal MI and CHD death) was unchanged compared to placebo [6]. Surprisingly, a statistically significant increase in CHD events was found in Year 1 in the treatment group compared to the placebo group, a trend that gradually decreased over time. Thus, not only did HRT provide no CHD benefit in HERS, the evidence suggested that HRT could even increase CHD risk in some users early after initiating therapy.

EVIDENCE OF EARLY RISK

In the light of the HERS results, some researchers have re-examined HRT use and CHD risk in previously reported cohorts. Evidence from the Nurses' Health Study [8,9], Coronary Drug Project [10], and the Puget Sound Group Health Cooperative [11] all supports the pattern seen in HERS of early increased cardiovascular risk associated with HRT use. Furthermore, preliminary data from the ongoing Women's Health Initiative also show a similar trend (available online at http://www.nhlbi.gov/whi/hrt-en-htm) (Figure 1).

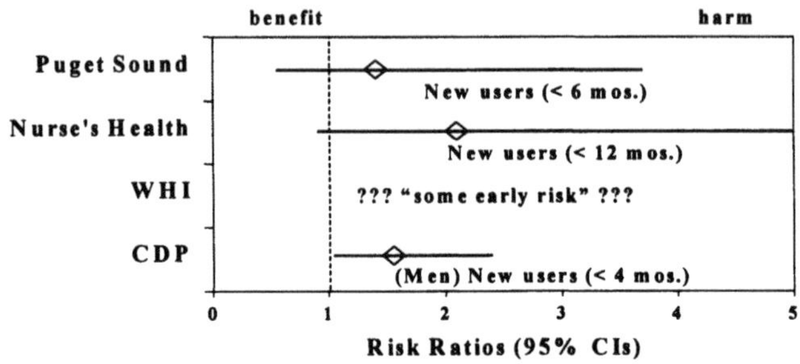

Figure 1. Risks for cardiovascular events among new users of hormone therapy. CDP = Coronary Drug Project; CIs = confidence intervals; WHI = Women's Health Initiative.

POTENTIAL MECHANISMS

Several hypotheses have been proposed to explain how HRT could confer an early increased risk of cardiovascular events. Areas under scrutiny include: HRT's effects on the thrombosis/coagulation pathways, how polymorphisms in thrombosis-related genes may affect risk for estrogen-associated thrombosis, whether estrogen has a proinflammatory effect, the influence of concomitant medications (especially HMG-CoA reductase inhibitors, or statins), and the role of estrogen-associated hypertriglyceridemia. Each area will be briefly discussed below.

Prothrombotic effects. Earlier reports have documented a two- to fourfold increase in risk for venous thromboembolism in HRT users compared with nonusers [2,12,13], and this trend was also seen in HERS (relative risk 2.7, 95% confidence intervals 1.4-5.0) [14]. The greatest risk was again in the first year of treatment, and paralleled the results for arterial thrombotic (CHD) events previously described. The ways in which estrogen may potentiate a thrombotic event are not yet clear.

Genetic polymorphisms. There is convincing evidence that Factor V Leiden [15-17] and the prothrombin 20210G→A mutations [18-20] increase the risk of arterial or venous thrombotic events in the presence of endogenous or exogenous estrogen. Recent data from the Puget Sound Group Health Cooperative found a significant interaction among HRT use, the prothrombin 20210G→A mutation, and risk for nonfatal myocardial infarction [21]. Furthermore, preliminary data from a subset of the HERS cohort indicate that among HRT users with the Factor V Leiden mutation, the adjusted odds ratio for a venous thromboembolic event was 12.74 ($p = 0.0015$) versus women on placebo without the mutation (Herrington DM, unpublished data).

Estrogen as a proinflammatory agent. Elevated levels of C-reactive protein (CRP), an inflammatory marker, have been associated with increased risk for CHD events [22]. Furthermore, several studies have found a relationship between estrogen use and increases in CRP[23,24]. Interestingly, one small study found that estrogen treatment increased levels both of CRP and of interleukin-6 [25].

Concomitant medications. Additional data from HERS suggest that concurrent use of statins may also affect the pattern of early CHD risk with HRT. After 1 year of treatment, the relative hazard among nonstatin users at baseline was markedly higher than for statin users at baseline (relative hazard 1.75 versus 1.34), although no significant statin/HRT interaction was found ($p = 0.57$) [26].

Estrogen-induced hypertriglyceridemia. In a recent meta-analysis (N = 10,864), women with hypertriglyceridemia were found to be at significantly greater risk for cardiovascular events than women with normal triglycerides (multivariate summary R = 2.24; 95% confidence intervals 1.05-1.28) [27]. Estrogen has been linked to smaller, more atherogenic LDL particles [28,29], but it is possible that in some subjects atherogenicity is independent of LDL size [30].

Results of Other Clinical Trials of HRT

Additional information generated by clinical trials after HERS has now become available for consideration. A summary of each trial now reported in full is presented in Table 1.

SECONDARY PREVENTION TRIALS

The ERA Trial. The Estrogen Replacement and Atherosclerosis (ERA) study was a three-arm, randomized, placebo-controlled, double-blind, angiographic endpoint trial of 309 postmenopausal women with angiographically confirmed CHD. After a mean follow-up of 3.2 years, there was no significant difference in atherosclerosis extent among the treatment arms (CEE alone versus placebo or CEE plus MPA versus placebo) in the angiographically determined progression of coronary atherosclerosis [7]. Treatment also had no effect on several secondary angiographic endpoints, although favorable effects on lipids were observed. Thus, the lack of effect of either treatment regimen suggests that the addition of MPA to CEE, the regimen used in HERS, may not explain the trial's overall null effect.

The PHASE Trial. The recently completed Papworth HRT Atherosclerosis Study Enquiry (PHASE) was another randomized, angiographic endpoint study of HRT and coronary artery disease (N = 255). Subjects received either transdermal 17β-estradiol 2 mg/day (plus 4 mg/day of cyclic norethindrone acetate in women with an intact uterus) or placebo for 3 years. Event rates (for unstable angina, MI, or death) were higher in the HRT group versus the control group, especially the first two years; however, this was not statistically significant [31]. This preliminary report suggests that route of administration is also not involved in HRT's lack of effect on atherosclerosis progression.

The WEST Trial. A recently completed clinical trial called The Women's Estrogen for Stroke Trial (WEST) (N = 652) evaluated the effect of 1 mg/day 17β-estradiol in women with a documented stroke or transient ischemic attack on the combined outcome of stroke or death. After an average of 2.7 years of follow-up, preliminary results indicate no effect of treatment on the primary outcomes (combined outcome: 27.6% in estradiol group versus 27.7% in the placebo group; $p = 0.80$) [32]. This too is consistent with the HERS and ERA results on CHD and coronary atherosclerosis progression, respectively.

PRIMARY PREVENTION TRIALS

The PHOREA Trial. In another recently reported clinical trial of HRT, the Postmenopausal Hormone Replacement against Atherosclerosis (PHOREA) study, two HRT regimens containing low and standard doses of progestin did not slow progression of carotid atherosclerosis (measured as intima-media thickness) in women without evidence of coronary heart disease [33]. The preparations used were 1 mg/d 17β-estradiol and 0.025 mg gestodene added for 10 days/month or continuously in every third 4-week cycle. This short-term, primary prevention study was different in emphasis from HERS and ERA; nonetheless, the results parallel those of the longer-term secondary prevention trials.

The EPAT Trial. The Estrogen and Prevention of Atherosclerosis Trial (EPAT) was a placebo-controlled, randomized, double-blind clinical trial in postmenopausal subjects without CHD but with LDL levels ≥ 130 mg/dl (N = 199). They were randomized to receive either placebo or oral 17β-estradiol (1 mg/day) plus lipid-lowering medication (if their LDL levels ≥ 160 mg/dl). After 2 years, carotid wall thickness was greater in the placebo group than in the active treatment group ($p = 0.045$). However, when the analysis was limited to women not on lipid-lowering therapy, the treatment effect was even more significant. In contrast, among women who were treated with lipid-lowering therapy, there was no difference in progression of carotid intima-media thickness between HRT and placebo women [34].

Table 1. Overview of Randomized Clinical Trials of Hormone Replacement Therapy*

Trial	N	Treatment†	Duration	Main Results of Treatment
Secondary Prevention				
HERS	2763	CEE + MPA	4.1 yr	No change in events
ERA	309	CEE; CEE + MPA	3.2 yr	No change in angiographically measured CAA
WEST	652	17β-estradiol	2.7 yr	No effect on rates of recurrent TIA/stroke
Primary Prevention				
PHOREA	321	17β-estradiol + gestodene 12 d/mo; 17β-estradiol + gestodene 12 d/3 mo	48 wk	No effect on carotid artery intima-media thickness (IMT)
EPAT	199	17β-estradiol + LLM (if needed)	2 yr	Small effect on carotid IMT; greater effect in LLM users

* See text for definitions of study acronyms.
† All treatments versus a placebo group.

CAA = coronary artery atherosclerosis; CEE = conjugated equine estrogens; LLM = lipid-lowering medications; MPA = medroxyprogesterone acetate; TIA = transient ischemic attack.

Ongoing Trials of HRT

The Women's Estrogen-progestin Lipid Lowering Hormone Atherosclerosis Regression Trial (WELL-HART) is studying the progression of coronary stenosis in women receiving oral estradiol with or without cyclic MPA. Subjects in WELL-HART also receive statin therapy if their LDL levels are ≥ 160 mg/dl. Angiographic changes in the coronary arteries after 3 years of HRT and/or vitamins C and E versus placebo are being evaluated in 400 postmenopausal women in the Women's Angiographic Vitamin and Estrogen (WAVE) trial. The Estrogen And Graft Atherosclerosis Research (EAGAR) study is studying whether estrogen will help maintain the patency of coronary artery bypass grafts in approximately 80 postmenopausal women who have recently undergone bypass surgery.

The Women's International Study of long Duration Oestrogen after the Menopause (WISDOM) and the WHI are two large primary prevention clinical trials currently underway in primarily healthy postmenopausal women. WISDOM is now recruiting a multinational cohort of approximately 34,000 women randomized to CEE (with or without MPA, depending on uterine status) versus placebo over 10 years. The WHI has several components, one of which is examining the effects of the same treatments used in HERS on the risk of CHD in 27,348 women over a mean of 8.5 years. The results of these trials will provide valuable insight into the effects of long-term HRT on the primary prevention of cardiovascular disease in postmenopausal women.

In summary, there is mounting evidence that HRT is not effective at slowing the clinical and anatomic progression of established atherosclerosis and may in fact be associated with an early increase in risk – possibly in a subgroup of women. However, the effects of HRT for primary prevention of CHD are not yet established, and recent clinical trial data suggest that estrogen may yet be effective in slowing progression in healthy women.

References

1. Grady D, Rubin SM, Petitti DB, et al. Hormone therapy to prevent disease and prolong life in postmenopausal women. Ann Intern Med 1992;117:1016-37.
2. Grodstein F, Stampfer MJ, Goldhaber SZ, et al. Prospective study of exogenous hormones and risk of pulmonary embolism in women. Lancet 1996;348:983-87.
3. Mendelsohn ME, Karas RH. The protective effects of estrogen on the cardiovascular system. N Engl J Med 1999;340:1801-11.
4. The Writing Group for the PEPI Trial. Effects of estrogen or estrogen/progestin regimens on heart disease risk factors in postmenopausal women. The Postmenopausal Estrogen/Progestin Interventions (PEPI) Trial. JAMA 1995;273:199-208.
5. Adams MR, Kaplan JR, Manuck SB, et al. Inhibition of coronary artery atherosclerosis by 17-beta estradiol in ovariectomized monkeys. Lack of an effect of added progesterone. Arteriosclerosis 1990;10:1051-57.
6. Hulley S, Grady D, Bush T, et al. Randomized trial of estrogen plus progestin for secondary prevention of coronary heart disease in postmenopausal women. JAMA 1998; 280:605-13.
7. Herrington DM, Reboussin DR, Brosnihan KB, et al. Effects of estrogen replacement on the progression of coronary-artery atherosclerosis. N Engl J Med 2000;343:522-29.
8. Grodstein F, Manson JE, Stampfer MJ. Postmenopausal hormones and recurrence of coronary events in the Nurses' Health Study (abstract). Circulation 1999;100:I-871.
9. Grodstein F, Manson JE, Colditz GA, et al. A prospective, observational study of postmenopausal hormone therapy and primary prevention of cardiovascular disease. Ann Intern Med 2000;33:933-41.
10. Wenger NK, Knatterud GL, Canner PL. Early risks of hormone therapy in patients with coronary heart disease (letter). JAMA 2000;284:41-3.
11. Heckbert SR, Weiss NS, Psaty BM. Hormone replacement therapy for secondary prevention of coronary heart disease (letter). JAMA 1999;281:795-96.
12. Daly E, Vessey MP, Hawkins MM, et al. Risk of venous thromboembolism in users of hormone replacement therapy. Lancet 1996;348:977-80.
13. Jick H, Derby LE, Myers MW, Vasilakis C, Newton KM. Risk of hospital admission for idiopathic venous thromboembolism among users of postmenopausal oestrogens. Lancet

1996;348:981-83.

14. Grady D, Wenger NK, Herrington D, et al. Postmenopausal hormone therapy increases risk for venous thromboembolic disease. The Heart and Estrogen/progestin Replacement Study. Ann Intern Med 2000;132:689-96.
15. Vandenbroucke JP, Koster T, Briet E, et al. Increased risk of venous thrombosis in oral contraceptive users who are carriers of the Factor V Leiden mutation. Lancet 1994;344: 1453-57.
16. Margaglione M, D'Andrea G, Giuliani N, et al. Inherited prothrombotic conditions and premature ischemic stroke. Sex differences in the association with Factor V Leiden. Arterioscler Thromb Vasc Biol 1999;19:1751-56.
17. Glueck CJ, Wang P, Fontaine RN, et al. Effect of exogenous estrogen on atherothrombotic vascular disease risk related to the presence or absence of the Factor V Leiden mutation. Am J Cardiol 1999;84:549-54.
18. Poort SR, Rosendaal FR, Reitsma PH, Bertina RM. A common genetic variation in the 3' untranslated region of the prothrombin gene is associated with elevated plasma prothrombin levels and increase in venous thrombosis. Blood 1996;88:3698-703.
19. Hillarp A, Zoller B, Svensson PJ, Dahlback B. The 20210A allele of the prothrombotic gene is a common risk factor among Swedish outpatients with verified deep vein thrombosis. Thromb Haemost 1997;78:990-92.
20. Leroyer C, Mercier B, Oger E, et al. Prevalence of 20210A allele of the prothrombin gene in venous thromboembolism patients. Thromb Haemost 1998;80:49-51.
21. Psaty BM, Smith NL, Lemaitre RN, et al. Hormone replacement therapy, prothrombotic mutations, and the risk of incident nonfatal myocardial infarction in postmenopausal women. JAMA 2001;285:906-13.
22. Ridker PM, Hennekens CH, Buring JE, Rifai N. C-reactive protein and other markers of inflammation in the prediction of cardiovascular disease in women. N Engl J Med 2000; 342:836-43.
23. Cushman M, Legault C, Barrett-Connor E, et al. Effect of postmenopausal hormones on inflammation-sensitive proteins. The Postmenopausal Estrogen/Progestin Interventions (PEPI) study. Circulation 1999;100:717-22.
24. Cushman M, Meilahn EN, Psaty BM, et al. Hormone replacement therapy, inflammation, and hemostasis in elderly women. Arterioscler Thromb Vasc Biol 1999;19:893-99.
25. Herrington DM, Brosnihan KB. Effects of estrogen vs droloxifene on adhesion molecules and cytokines in healthy postmenopausal women (abstract). J Am Coll Cardiol 1999;33 (Suppl A):318A.
26. Herrington DM, Vittinghoff E, Hunninghake D, et al. Effects of statin therapy on cardiovascular events and all-cause mortality in women in the Heart and Estrogen/progestin Replacement Study. Circulation 2000;102(Suppl II):II-837.
27. Austin MA, Hokanson JE, Edwards KL. Hypertriglyceridemia as a cardiovascular risk factor. Am J Cardiol 1998;81:7B-12B.
28. Wakatsuki A, Ikenoue N, Sagara Y. Estrogen-induced small low-density lipoprotein particles in postmenopausal women. Obstet Gynecol 1998;91:234-40.
29. Wakatsuki A, Ikenoue N, Okatani Y, Fukaya T. Estrogen-induced small low density lipoprotein particles may be atherogenic in postmenopausal women. J Am Coll Cardiol 2001;37:425-30.
30. Raal FJ, Pilcher GJ, Waisberg R, et al. Low-density lipoprotein cholesterol bulk is the pivotal determinant of atherosclerosis in familial hypercholesterolemia. Am J Cardiol

1999;83:1330-33.
31. Clarke S, Kelleher J, Lloyd-Jones H, et al. Transdermal hormone replacement therapy for secondary prevention of coronary artery disease in postmenopausal women (abstract). Eur Heart J 2000;21:212.
32. Viscoli CM, Brass LM, Kernan WN, Sarrel PM, Horwitz RI. Effect of estrogen replacement on risk of recurrent stroke and death in the Women's Estrogen for Stroke Trial (WEST) (abstract). Stroke 2001;32:329.
33. Angerer P, Stork S, Kothny W, Schmitt P, von Schacky C. Effect of oral postmenopausal hormone replacement on progression of atherosclerosis. A randomized, controlled trial. Arterioscler Thromb Vasc Biol 2001;21:262-68.
34. Hodis HN, Mack WJ, Lobo RA, et al. Estrogen in the prevention of atherosclerosis trial (abstract). Circulation 2000;102:II-837.

Recent Findings in Cardiovascular Disease

Rogerio A. Lobo

Introduction

Hormone replacement therapy (HRT) plays a major role in the health care of postmenopausal women. We know HRT effectively relieves vasomotor symptoms, the primary reason why most women initially seek treatment, but it also offers a number of other advantages. Studies have provided strong evidence that HRT protects against osteoporosis, and there is evidence that potential benefits exist for Alzheimer's disease, colon cancer, and depression.

One of the most encouraging connections implicated between HRT and female health is the role that HRT may play in the prevention of cardiovascular disease (CVD). Numerous studies have demonstrated that HRT may convey a protective effect in this regard; however, other findings suggest that HRT offers no such benefit.

Despite such conflicting findings, the fact remains that HRT is an important, and often necessary, component of a woman's overall health care. Providers of women's health care need to acknowledge that HRT is a very individualized form of treatment. For the patient who clearly needs HRT for relief of vasomotor symptoms and is satisfied with treatment, there is no reason for her to discontinue HRT; she may experience other health benefits, including the prevention of osteoporosis, cognitive benefits, and possibly the primary prevention of CVD.

Considering the enormous health risks posed by CVD, particularly following menopause, and that HRT may offer some beneficial effect in the primary prevention of CVD, it is not surprising that studies continue to examine the effects of HRT in CVD. This chapter reviews some of the novel and unique strategies that are being evaluated for a new approach to HRT and its role in CVD. The research behind these ideas were presented at the Fourth International Symposium on Women's Health and Menopause this past May.

A Work in Progress

Numerous studies over the past several years have analyzed the role of HRT in CVD. Although substantial evidence strongly suggests a cardioprotective effect of HRT, recent studies have not confirmed this. The article "Hormone Replacement and Cardiovascular Disease" provides an overview of the studies that have significantly influenced the way

HRT is viewed today in terms of its role in CVD. Results from observational studies such as the Framingham Heart Study and the Nurses' Health Study are presented, as well as findings from two recent clinical trials, the Heart and Estrogen/progestin Replacement Study and the Estrogen Replacement and Atherosclerosis Trial. With this background information, the author gives us an understanding of how different study designs and patient populations influence final outcomes, which consequently has led to the controversy surrounding the role of HRT in CVD. As Karen C. Johnson, MD, MPH, points out, more long-term research is needed, and several important trials in this area are ongoing.

LINKING NEW RESEARCH TO A NEW FORM OF HRT

Research focusing on potassium deficiency and the negative effects associated with the hormone aldosterone has yielded intriguing results that could have a significant influence on the development of a different type of HRT.

The importance of potassium maintenance, particularly as it relates to reducing the risk of CVD, is reviewed in the article "The Role of Potassium" by Peter R. Kowey, MD. As the author explains, potassium plays a significant role in the electrophysiologic properties of the heart. Studies have shown that when the body's stores of potassium are deficient, the risk of hypertension, stroke, congestive heart failure (CHF), and cardiac arrhythmias is substantially increased. Likewise, increased potassium intake has been linked with lowered blood pressure, a reduced risk of mortality associated with stroke, and a reduced risk of sudden cardiac death in patients with CHF.

The hormone aldosterone has also been implicated in the manifestation of CVD. The role of aldosterone in the pathophysiology of CHF, and how aldosterone-receptor inhibitors can counter its detrimental effects, are discussed in "Aldosterone-Receptor Blocking Agents" by Bertram Pitt, MD, FACC. This article reviews clinical trial data on the cardioprotective effects seen with antialdosterone treatment, focusing primarily on the aldosterone blocker spironolactone. As the author explains, treatment with aldosterone-receptor blockers is generally associated with an increased risk of excess potassium retention (hyperkalemia). However, the author points out that in a recent study, spironolactone was attributed with significantly reducing the risk of morbidity and death in patients with severe heart failure without leading to serious hyperkalemia.

These findings from two very different areas of research provide important data for the treatment of CVD. Specifically, these data are extremely important for the purpose of developing a new HRT with a new progestin. The progestins used in current HRT formulations can cause problems for many women. Many of the side effects associated with HRT are attributable to the specific progestin; consequently, women often discontinue therapy because of intolerable side effects. Research efforts to find alternatives to standard progestins have revealed a novel progestin with a profile almost identical to that of natural progesterone. As described in my contribution, "Progestogens: New Approaches," the novel progestin drospirenone is associated with a reduction in the incidence of some adverse effects associated with conventional progestins. Studies have shown that potassium excretion is not affected by this new progestin; furthermore, because it is related to spironolactone, drospirenone possesses some antialdosterone properties. As such, this new progestin could give us the opportunity to improve the side-effect profile of HRT as well as potentially aid in the prevention of CVD.

On behalf of the clinicians who contributed to this chapter, I hope you will find the articles herein both enlightening and encouraging. I believe that the research presented in these articles has set us on a course of better understanding the importance of potassium balance and aldosterone antagonism in CVD and potentially achieving certain advances in HRT.

HORMONE REPLACEMENT AND CARDIOVASCULAR DISEASE

Karen C. Johnson

Introduction

Coronary heart disease (CHD) is an important health problem in the United States, responsible for more than 503,000 deaths annually [1]. It has traditionally been underestimated in women, even though CHD is the single leading cause of death and a significant cause of morbidity in female patients. In fact, CHD is now estimated to account for more than 236,000 deaths among women each year, resulting in billions of dollars in health care expenditures [2]. Furthermore, it is estimated that 1 in 2 women will die of heart disease or stroke, compared with 1 in 25 who will eventually die of breast cancer [3]. Unfortunately, women are not aware of this overwhelming risk presented by CHD. In a recent national survey by the American Heart Association, only 34% of women spontaneously identified CHD as the leading cause of death in women [3].

Population-based studies indicate that postmenopausal women have a significantly higher risk of cardiovascular disease (CVD) than do premenopausal women, with this increased risk attributed to loss of the protective effect of endogenous estrogens at menopause [4]. Consequently, an important area of active research has centered on determining whether administration of postmenopausal estrogen replacement therapy (ERT) or hormone replacement therapy (HRT) is effective in the prevention of CHD in women. Although administration of ERT or HRT to postmenopausal women provides effective treatment for vasomotor symptoms and osteoporosis, controversy still exists over the possible health risks associated with its use.

Epidemiological studies on the effects of ERT and HRT on CVD in postmenopausal women have provided conflicting evidence regarding the possible cardioprotective effects of ERT and HRT. Cautious evaluation of these studies is necessary when interpreting their findings, with careful consideration given to the type of study and its design.

Scrutinizing Study Design

In a critical review of any study, attention to the associations and causal inferences derived is imperative. It is important to remember that an association between a risk factor and a disease does not necessarily imply causation. For example, associations may be artifactual (spurious) — that is, resulting from chance or bias. Associations may be indirect and confounding. Finally, associations may also be direct, causal, or etiologic. Study investigators observe associations and attempt to determine whether an association exists between an exposure (such as HRT) and a disease or prevention of a disease (such as CVD), and then derive inferences regarding possible causal relationships. The criteria for determining whether an association is causal in nature can be judged according to the following:

- the strength of the association between the exposure and the disease
- consistency of association
- temporal relationship between the exposure and the disease
- biologic plausibility
- presence of a dose-response relationship.

A study also should be examined based on whether it is experimental or observational in design. In an experimental study (i.e. a clinical or community trial), the investigator controls the assignment of participants to groups and randomization is a common method used to avoid selection bias. In an observational study (i.e. cohort, case-control, cross-sectional), the participants essentially self-select into groups. A randomized, controlled clinical trial design is considered the "gold standard" for detecting associations and making causal inferences.

Observational HRT Studies

A number of observational studies have examined the effects of HRT on CVD in women. Two well-known, large-scale observational studies that have evaluated hormone replacement therapy are the Framingham Heart Study and the Nurses' Health Study.

Framingham Heart Study

Initiated more than 50 years ago, the Framingham Heart Study has identified and evaluated numerous risk factors and characteristics of CVD in both men and women [5]. This long-term prospective cohort study has utilized biennial health examinations and questionnaires regarding participants' health to analyze the epidemiology of CVD. In 1985, an article was published based on data collected from the twelfth biennial exam (between 1970 and 1972) of postmenopausal women aged 50 to 83 who were taking HRT at the time of their eighth through twelfth biennial exam [6]. It should be noted that a woman was classified as an estrogen user if she had used estrogen at any one of these biennial exams, whether or not she was taking estrogen currently. All other women were classified as nonusers (which created the potential for misclassification bias regarding exposure to ERT).

Participants were followed for 8 years to ascertain the events associated with ERT use. Study endpoints included CHD (defined as angina, myocardial infarction [MI], coronary death, and sudden death), cerebrovascular disease (defined as stroke and transient ischemic attack), CVD (defined as CHD, cerebrovascular disease, intermittent claudication, or potential for congestive heart failure [CHF]), and death.

Examination of baseline characteristics showed that estrogen users on average were thinner, had higher levels of high-density lipoproteins (HDL), lower levels of low-density lipoproteins (LDL), and lower total cholesterol levels than nonusers. This profile suggested that the estrogen users might be healthier and have less CVD than nonusers. Despite this favorable profile, estrogen users had an increased risk of cerebrovascular disease, CHD, angina, and risk of death from CVD. Stratification by smoking status showed that these risks were higher in cigarette smokers, with one exception — estrogen users who were nonsmokers continued to have an increased risk of cerebrovascular disease compared with nonestrogen users who were also nonsmokers. The investigators concluded that no cardiovascular benefits from estrogen use were observed in this study cohort.

NURSES' HEALTH STUDY

The Nurses' Health Study, initiated in 1976, is another ongoing, observational prospective cohort study, to assess the development of chronic diseases in 121,964 nurses aged 30 to 55 [7,8]. Every 2 years, participants receive a follow-up questionnaire on diseases and health-related topics, including smoking, hormone use, and menopausal status. At the beginning of the trial, data on postmenopausal hormone use were gathered and women were classified as current users, past users, and nonusers. Information on the type and dose of estrogen was not collected, and women with prevalent CVD at baseline were excluded from the analysis. In 1978 and 1980, the follow-up surveys determined the incidence of CVD-related events, specifically the endpoints of nonfatal MI and fatal CHD [9].

The investigators noted important differences among participants upon analyses of the baseline characteristics. Women who had never used were more likely to smoke and had higher body mass indices compared with current or past users, which placed them at a higher risk for CVD. Compared with women who had never used hormones, current users were less likely to have nonfatal MI or nonfatal MI plus fatal CHD. The same findings were seen in past users compared with nonusers. The authors concluded that these data support the hypothesis that postmenopausal use of hormones reduces the risk of CHD.

Weighing Observational Outcomes

Many other observational studies have suggested that postmenopausal use of HRT reduces the risk of cardiovascular disease in women [10]. Furthermore, meta-analyses of these observational studies estimate the risk reduction of CHD with HRT use at 35% to 50% [11,12].

Although the results of observational studies have been widely used to recommend HRT to postmenopausal women for the prevention of CVD [13], some investigators have cautioned that methodological issues inherent in observational studies, such as increased potential for selection bias, may be present and affect the results [14]. For example, as was demonstrated in both the Framingham Heart Study and the Nurses' Health Study, postmenopausal HRT users demonstrated a better CHD risk profile than nonusers at baseline, which infers that the CHD risk reduction may have been due to a healthy lifestyle and not necessarily to HRT [15]. Only a randomized, controlled clinical trial can eliminate these baseline potential confounders, allowing for an inference that the treatment (HRT) caused the observed outcomes (decreased CHD events) [10].

Clinical Trials of HRT

One of the first controlled clinical trials of HRT in CVD was the Coronary Drug Project, which evaluated the effects of estrogen in men. More recently, data from the Heart and Estrogen/progestin Replacement Study and the Estrogen Replacement and Atherosclerosis Trial have provided additional insight into the associations between HRT and CVD in women.

CORONARY DRUG PROJECT

Based on the knowledge that there are gender differences in CVD, and that the risk of CVD is greater in postmenopausal women, investigators reasoned that estrogen must have a protective effect and therefore may have a similar effect in men. In 1965, the Coronary Drug Project was initiated to assess the effects of estrogen in men with known CVD [16]. This randomized, multicenter clinical trial compared conjugated equine estrogen 2.5 mg daily (n = 1,101) and 5 mg daily (n = 1,119) with placebo (n = 2,789) in men aged 30 to 64 years (mean age, 52 years) with electrocardiographically documented MI. The primary endpoint of the study was 5-year total death, with secondary endpoints of MI or a thromboembolic event.

In 1970, after a mean follow-up of 1.5 years, the 5-mg-per-day estrogen treatment arm was stopped early. Men in this treatment group had experienced a statistically significant increase in MI, MI plus coronary death, pulmonary embolism (PE), and PE plus deep venous thrombus compared with those in the placebo group [17]. In 1973, after a mean follow-up of 4.7 years, the 2.5-mg-per-day group was also discontinued because of adverse events and absence of benefit for total mortality [18]. Several theories have been postulated to explain these results, many focusing on the fact that the high doses of estrogen administered to men with known CVD could have led to adverse effects in the coagulation system, thus precipitating the observed events.

HEART AND ESTROGEN/PROGESTIN REPLACEMENT STUDY

Considering the need for more randomized clinical trials of postmenopausal hormone therapy in CVD, the Heart and Estrogen/progestin Replacement Study (HERS) was conducted to evaluate the efficacy and safety of estrogen combined with a progestin in preventing nonfatal MI and CHD death among postmenopausal women with established coronary artery disease [19]. This double-blind, controlled, secondary-prevention clinical trial included 2,763 women aged 44 to 79 who were randomized to receive daily doses of 0.625 mg conjugated equine estrogen (CEE) plus 2.5 mg medroxyprogesterone acetate (MPA; n = 1,380) or placebo (n = 1,383). Patients were followed for 4 years. The primary endpoint was occurrence of CHD events, defined as nonfatal MI or CHD death. Secondary outcomes included coronary revascularization, unstable angina, CHF, resuscitated cardiac arrest, stroke or TIA, and peripheral arterial disease.

Overall, there were no significant differences noted between the groups in the primary outcome of CHD events. The investigators noted that this lack of effect occurred even though HDL levels were higher and LDL levels were lower in the HRT group. When the primary outcome was analyzed by treatment group and year since randomization, a time trend was noted — an increased risk for CHD events in year 1 for women taking CEE/MPA changed to no association by year 2 and approached benefit by year 4.

The authors concluded that treatment with oral CEE plus MPA did not reduce the overall rate of CHD events in postmenopausal women with established coronary disease. Based on the findings of no overall cardiovascular benefit and a pattern of early increased risk of CHD events, they did not recommend starting HRT for the purpose of secondary prevention of CHD.

THE ESTROGEN REPLACEMENT AND ATHEROSCLEROSIS TRIAL

The Estrogen Replacement and Atherosclerosis (ERA) trial was conducted to gain a better understanding of the effects of estrogen on coronary atherosclerosis, and how progestin might modify these effects [20]. The ERA trial was similar to HERS, in that it was a secondary prevention clinical trial. All 309 postmenopausal women enrolled in the trial had established CVD — in this case, angiographically verified coronary artery disease. Participants were randomized to receive estrogen only (CEE 0.625 mg/day, n=100), estrogen plus progestin (CEE 0.625 mg/d plus MPA 2.5 mg/d, n=104), or placebo (n=105). Angiographic progression of coronary artery disease was the primary endpoint.

After a mean follow-up of 3 years, despite the fact that both of the groups receiving active hormone therapy had a statistically significant reduction in LDL and an increase in HDL compared with the placebo group, the mean minimal coronary artery diameters at follow-up were not different among the three groups. CHD event rates were essentially the same in all three groups, but it must be noted the study was not powered to detect this outcome. These findings led the investigators to conclude that postmenopausal HRT use does not affect the progression of coronary atherosclerosis in women with established disease. They recommended that women with existing CVD not use postmenopausal HRT with the expectation of obtaining any cardiovascular benefit.

Future Directions

Although the results of the Coronary Drug Project, HERS, and the ERA trial add important information to the current knowledge base regarding the effects of HRT on CVD, there are no definitive answers as of yet; thus, the need for long-term studies remains. Fortunately, other randomized trials of postmenopausal HRT are underway.

WOMEN'S HEALTH INITIATIVE

The Women's Health Initiative (WHI), which began enrollment in 1993, is a randomized, controlled, primary prevention clinical trial and observational study designed to examine the causes of disease, death, and bone fragility in postmenopausal women [21]. For the HRT study arm of WHI, 40 clinical centers recruited 27,348 women aged 50 to 79 who will be followed for an average of 9 years. Women with a uterus were randomized to received either estrogen plus progestin (CEE 0.625 mg/d plus MPA 2.5 mg/d) or placebo; women without a uterus were randomized to estrogen only (CEE 0.625 mg/d) or placebo. The primary and secondary outcomes of the trial are CHD events, osteoporotic fractures, and cancer (breast and colon).

The final results of the WHI study have not been published. However, in 2000, the WHI investigators reported to the participants that the 1-year follow-up data for the HRT clinical trial revealed the following: Women taking HRT had an increased risk of MI and stroke compared with women taking placebo. It was noted that this risk was of a similar magnitude to that seen in HERS. Furthermore, in June 2001, the WHI investigators again reported that the 3-year follow-up data revealed that women taking HRT continued to have an increased risk of MI and stroke compared with women taking placebo — a pattern inconsistent with the HERS data. The WHI follow-up continues.

Conclusion

Although many observational studies have found decreased rates of CHD in women using postmenopausal HRT, the consistency of evidence from randomized clinical trials in men and in women leads to speculation that the associations observed between HRT use and increased early CVD are causal in nature and occur relatively rapidly. Concern has also been voiced that observational studies may be influenced by bias, misclassification of either exposure or outcome status, or the inability to control for potential confounders.

There are biologically plausible reasons why HRT may be protective, such as beneficial effects on lipids and increased vasodilatation. However, there may be potentially unfavorable effects of HRT as well, such as increases in triglycerides; increases in certain coagulation factors, such as prothrombin fragment 1+2 (a marker for thrombin generation); increases in certain inflammatory markers, such as c-reactive protein; and increases in metalloproteinases, such as MMP-9, that may cause acute plaque rupture.

Clearly, questions still remain regarding the long-term effects of postmenopausal HRT on CVD. Only long-term clinical trials, such as the Women's Health Initiative, can provide more definitive answers.

References

1. US Department of Health and Human Services, Centers for Disease Control and Prevention. Chronic diseases and their risk factors: The nation's leading causes of death. National Center for Chronic Disease Prevention and Health Promotion 1999.
2. American Heart Association. Women, heart disease, and stroke statistics. American Heart Association 2000.
3. American Heart Association. Women, heart disease and stroke: Survey highlights and

comparison, 2000. American Heart Association 2001.
4. Barrett-Connor E. Sex differences in coronary heart disease: why are women so superior? The 1995 Ancel Keys lecture. Circulation 1997;95:252–64.
5. National Institutes of Health. The Framingham Heart Study. Available at: http://www.nhlbi.nih.gov/_about/framingham. Accessed June 21, 2001.
6. Wilson PW, Garrison RJ, Castelli WP. Postmenopausal estrogen use, cigarette smoking, and cardiovascular morbidity in women over 50: The Framingham Study. N Engl J Med 1985;313:1038-43.
7. Nurses' Health Study home page. Available at: http://www.channing.harvard.edu/nhs. Accessed June 21, 2001.
8. Belanger CF, Hennekens CH, Rosner B, Speizer FE. The Nurses' Health Study. Am J Nurs 1978;78:1039-40.
9. Stampfer MJ, Willett WC, Colditz GA, Rosner B, Speizer FE, Hennekens CH. A prospective study of postmenopausal estrogen therapy and coronary heart disease in U.S. women. N Engl J Med 1985;313:1044-49.
10. Petitti DB. Hormone replacement therapy and heart disease prevention: Experimentation trumps observation [commentary].JAMA1998;280:650-52.
11. Stampfer MJ, Colditz GA. Estrogen replacement therapy and coronary heart disease: A quantitative assessment of the epidemiologic evidence. Prev Med 1991;20:47-63.
12. Grady D, Rubin SM, Petitti DB, et al. Hormone therapy to prevent disease and prolong life in postmenopausal women. Ann Intern Med 1992;117:1016-37.
13. Sullivan JM. Estrogen replacement therapy. Circulation. 1996;94(11):2699-2702.
14. Rossouw JE. Estrogens for prevention of coronary heart disease: Putting the brakes on the bandwagon. Circulation 1996:94;2982-85.
15. Matthews KA, Kuller CN, Wing RR, Mailahan EN, Plantinga P. Prior to use of estrogen replacement therapy, are users healthier than nonusers? Am J Epidemiol 1996;143:971-78.
16. Coronary Drug Project Research Group. The Coronary Drug Project design, methods, and baseline results. Circulation 1973;47(Suppl.3):I1-I50.
17. Coronary Drug Project Research Group. The Coronary Drug Project: Initial findings leading to modification of its research protocol. JAMA 1970;214:1303-13.
18. Coronary Drug Project Research Group. The Coronary Drug Project: Findings leading to discontinuation of the 2.5-mg/day estrogen group. JAMA 1973;226:652-57.
19. Hulley S, Grady D, Bush T, et al for the Heart and Estrogen/progestin Replacement Study (HERS) Research Group. Randomized trial of estrogen plus progestin for secondary prevention of coronary heart disease in postmenopausal women. JAMA 1998;280:605-13.
20. Herrington DM, Reboussin DM, Brosnihan KB, et al. Effects of estrogen replacement on the progression of coronary-artery atherosclerosis. N Engl J Med 2000;343:522-29.
21. The Women's Health Initiative Study Group. Design of the Women's Health Initiative clinical trial and observational study. Control Clin Trials 1998;19:61-109.

THE ROLE OF POTASSIUM

Peter R. Kowey

Introduction

Potassium is one of the main blood minerals, or electrolytes, essential to both cellular and electrical function. Potassium is the primary positive ion, or cation, found in the cells, where more than 90% of the total body stores of potassium is contained. Along with sodium, potassium regulates the water balance and the acid-base balance in the blood and tissues, and plays a critical role in the transmission of electrical impulses in the heart. The active transport of potassium into and out of the cells is crucial to cardiovascular and nerve function. When potassium enters the cell, it instigates a sodium-potassium exchange across the cell membrane. In the nerve cells, this generates the electrical potential that allows the conduction of nerve impulses. When potassium leaves the cell, it restores repolarization to the cell, which allows the nerve impulse to progress. This electrical potential gradient helps generate muscle contractions and regulates the heartbeat. Normal serum potassium levels are between 3.6 and 5.0 mmol/L. If the level of total body potassium declines by just 1% (35 mmol), a serious imbalance in the intracellular and extracellular potassium results. This imbalance alters the electrophysiologic properties of the cell membrane and causes detrimental effects on impulse generation and conduction throughout the heart [1].

Studies that have examined potassium deficiency, also called hypokalemia, have established the importance of potassium maintenance in cardiovascular disease (CVD). Accumulating evidence suggests that increased potassium intake may be key in lowering blood pressure and reducing the risk of stroke, congestive heart failure (CHF), and cardiac arrhythmias. Considering that the risk of CVD is dramatically increased in postmenopausal women, understanding the role of potassium maintenance in CVD is vital to providing optimal treatment to this patient population.

Understanding Hypokalemia

Hypokalemia is perhaps the most common electrolyte abnormality found in clinical practice, exhibited in more than 20% of hospitalized patients [2]. In otherwise healthy people, hypokalemia is well tolerated; in patients with CVD, even mild or moderate hypokalemia increases the risks of morbidity and mortality [2]. Hypokalemia may be diagnosed when the serum potassium level falls below 3.6 mmol/L [3]. Symptoms may not be present, especially in mild cases (serum potassium, 3.0 to 3.5 mmol/L), however, in more severe hypokalemia, symptoms may include generalized muscle weakness, fatigue, and constipation [2,3]. Muscle necrosis can occur when serum potassium decreases to 2.5 mmol/L, and at 2.0 mmol/L, paralytic ileus may develop. In patients with cardiac ischemia, heart failure, or left ventricular hypertrophy, even mild to moderate hypokalemia increases the risk of cardiac arrhythmias [2].

Diuretic Use

Inadequate dietary potassium intake, high dietary sodium intake, and hypomagnesemia are among the causes of hypokalemia (Table 1). However, the most common cause of hypokalemia is diuretic therapy. Diuretics inhibit sodium reabsorption in the kidneys, thereby creating a favorable electrochemical gradient for potassium excretion [2,4]. A retrospective analysis of the Studies of Left Ventricular Dysfunction (SOLVD) project revealed compelling data regarding diuretic therapy [5]. Among those patients receiving diuretics, the relative risk of arrhythmic death was 37% higher compared with patients not using diuretics. However, the authors pointed out that the outcome for individuals receiving potassium-sparing diuretics was as favorable as that for patients not using diuretics. It is advised that patients requiring diuretic therapy receive potassium-sparing diuretics or the lowest effective dose of nonpotassium-sparing diuretics, along with additional potassium, either through potassium-rich foods or potassium supplements.

Protective Effects

A number of studies have demonstrated that potassium maintenance or supplementation is effective in reducing the risk of stroke, hypertension, CHF, and cardiac arrhythmias.

Stroke

Findings from a 12-year prospective study of 859 men and women aged 50 to 79 years showed that the risk of stroke-associated mortality was significantly lower among those with higher potassium intake [6]. The authors found that a 10-mmol increase in daily potassium intake was associated with a 40% reduction in the relative risk of stroke mortality. This protective effect of potassium was independent of other dietary variables, including caloric intake; levels of fat, protein, and fiber; and calcium, magnesium, and alcohol intake. It was also independent of other known cardiovascular risk factors, including age, sex, blood pressure, blood cholesterol level, obesity, fasting blood-glucose level, and cigarette smoking.

Hypertension

Increasing potassium intake also appears to have an antihypertensive effect, as several trials have shown. In the Nurses' Health Study, a potassium-rich diet was inversely associated with systolic and diastolic blood pressure [7]. The 52-center international INTERSALT study [8], which analyzed electrolytes and blood pressure, found that 24-hour urinary potassium excretion, 24-hour urinary sodium excretion, and the ratio of urinary sodium to potassium were independently related to blood pressure.

Table 1. Potential Causes of Hypokalemia [3]

Inadequate dietary potassium intake
Diuretic therapy
High dietary sodium intake
Hypomagnesemia
Prolonged diarrhea
Vomiting
Primary or secondary aldosteronism
Cushing's syndrome or disease
Large doses of corticosteroids
Ectopic coticotropinism
Bartter's syndrome
Liddle's syndrome
Urinary loss in CHF
Catecholamines
Others (excessive use of licorice, insulin, antibiotics)

Recommendations that potassium intake be increased for the prevention and treatment of hypertension were made following a recent meta-analysis of 33 randomized clinical trials of the effects of potassium supplementation on blood pressure [9]. The analysis found that potassium supplementation — the only difference between the intervention and control groups in all the studies — was related to a significant reduction in mean systolic and diastolic blood pressure (-4.4 mm Hg and -2.4 mm Hg, respectively; $P < 0.001$). This protective effect was greatest in patients with high sodium intake. From this analysis, it can be surmised that potassium deficiency may have a critical role in the development of hypertension.

CONGESTIVE HEART FAILURE

Patients with CHF commonly have hypokalemia brought about by the physiologic abnormalities related to CHF that predispose to the development of electrolyte disturbances. In the United Kingdom Heart Failure Evaluation and Assessment of Risk Trial, Nolan and colleagues found that low serum potassium levels were related to sudden cardiac death [10]. Similarly, Grobbee and Hoes noted that the risk of sudden cardiac death was twice as high in patients with hypertension who were taking nonpotassium-sparing diuretics compared with patients using potassium-sparing therapy [11].

These findings underscore the importance of maintaining potassium in CHF patients through the use of potassium-sparing diuretics, as well as potassium supplements. The use of angiotensin-converting enzyme (ACE) inhibitors has also been recommended for patients with CHF, as these drugs enhance potassium retention. However, prescribed dosages of ACE inhibitors are often insufficient to protect against potassium loss. As such, serum potassium levels in all patients with CHF should be closely monitored, regardless of therapy.

CARDIAC ARRHYTHMIAS

As described at the beginning of this article, potassium is crucial to the transmission of electrical impulses in the heart; even a small decrease in potassium can negatively effect the generation and conduction of these impulses. Although a direct link between hypokalemia and cardiac arrhythmias is not certain, evidence suggests that hypokalemia can trigger sustained ventricular tachycardia or ventricular fibrillation. Several studies have found that individuals who take diuretics without potassium supplementation have a much higher concentration of ventricular premature beats and a much higher complexity of ventricular premature depolarizations [1]. Patients with hypokalemia have a significantly increased likelihood of developing ventricular fibrillation during acute ischemic events compared with patients who had normal potassium levels [12].

Potassium and CVD Risk

To expand on the observations made to date regarding the association between hypokalemia and CVD, Kowey and colleagues conducted an in-depth, detailed analysis to evaluate the role of potassium deficiency as a risk factor for cardiovascular events [13].

The objectives of the study were to demonstrate a link between potassium replacement and cardiovascular events, and to detect the protective effects of potassium therapy among patients using nonpotassium-sparing diuretic medications. The group also wished to quantify the financial impact of potassium replacement, as these data should be available in a managed care patient population. Finally, the authors set out to create a foundation for a screening tool that can be used to identify at-risk patients within a managed care population as a basis for appropriate intervention. An analysis of hypokalemia as a mediator of adverse events is believed to be particularly important in this regard.

The study team analyzed 5 years of medical and pharmacy claims data for 4,909 members of a commercial health maintenance organization. Approximately 64% of this patient population was female, 14.5% had experienced a cardiovascular event, 17.2% had diabetes, 55.1% had hypertension, and 26.1% were 65 years of age or older. The presence of hypokalemia was approximated by use of nonpotassium-sparing diuretics without potassium replacement. Control of confounding variables, such as prior cardiovascular events, use of digoxin, and depression, revealed two types of effects: Patients at high risk for cardiovascular events were more likely to have received potassium replacement, and the risk of cardiovascular events was significantly reduced with potassium replacement among the study's subgroups (which included diabetes, hypertension, use of multiple diuretics, and age). From our cost calculations, we assumed that each patient would assume medical and pharmacy charges of $6,000 per cardiovascular event.

We then matched this patient population against selected outcome measures, which included CHF, intermediate coronary syndromes, left heart failure, malignant hypertensive heart disease with or without CHF, paroxysmal ventricular tachycardia, complete atrioventricular block, phlebitis and thrombophlebitis, cardiac arrest, unspecified heart failure, ventricular fibrillation, and heart failure. The variables used to predict cardiovascular events were age, gender, potassium use, digoxin use, prior cardiovascular events, prior hypertension, and prior diabetes, all of which were statistically significant ($P = 0.05$). The variables of depression, alcohol use, drug dependence, tobacco use, prior CHF, and prior obesity were not statistically significant.

The cardiovascular risk reduction for each subgroup was determined based on potassium replacement within 90 days of receiving a prescription for diuretics (Table 2). Potassium replacement was associated with a profound risk reduction of 31% in diabetic patients, and hypertensive patients experienced a risk reduction of 24%. The risk of cardiovascular events for patients receiving multiple diuretics also was dramatically reduced with potassium replacement; those receiving two diuretics had a 30% risk reduction; those given three diuretics had a 42% risk reduction; and those receiving four diuretics had a 51% risk reduction.

The benefits of potassium replacement were particularly noteworthy in older patients. In those aged 65 years and younger who received potassium supplementation during diuretic therapy, there was an 18% risk reduction. This became greater with advanced age: In patients aged 75 years and younger, the risk reduction was 33%; in those aged 85 years and younger, there was a 45% reduction in the risk of cardiovascular events when potassium supplementation was provided.

From this analysis of a large Medicare population, it can be concluded that the addition of potassium to diuretic therapy provides a definite beneficial effect in reducing the risk of cardiovascular events in several different subgroups of patients, particularly the elderly. Potassium supplementation is, in fact, being used in high-risk patient populations. Although there are high event rates in those populations, potassium is actually responsible for a reduced risk when compared within patient subgroups.

To prove not only the medical benefit but also the economic impact, Kowey and co-workers found that the cardiovascular risk reduction was associated with significant cost savings across all patient subgroups. These data show that omission of potassium replacement for patients who are receiving diuretics — in particular, patients who have heart disease, diabetes, or hypertension, and in the elderly — is inevitably associated with worse outcomes, and exerts a tremendous economic toll on our health care system.

Conclusion

Given the important role of potassium in the electrophysiologic properties of the heart, it is essential that the body's stores of potassium are maintained in patients at risk for or with CVD. Increasing the intake of potassium in patients with various cardiovascular conditions has proven extremely effective in reducing the risk of cardiovascular events. Potassium supplements and diets high in potassium have been shown to reduce the risk of stroke-associated mortality; both systolic and diastolic blood pressure can be lowered with increased potassium intake; and the risk of sudden cardiac death seen in patients with CHF can be reduced dramatically when potassium levels are maintained or additional potassium is taken. Patients with diabetes and the elderly can also derive significant benefit from potassium replacement, as can patients who are taking multiple diuretics, which are the primary cause of potassium loss.

Considering these benefits, it is imperative that potassium levels are maintained in postmenopausal women — a patient population that is at increased risk for CVD. Potassium levels should be monitored regularly, particularly in women who are taking nonpotassium-sparing diuretics, and potassium supplements should be administered when necessary to reduce the risk of cardiovascular events.

References

1. Podrid PJ. Potassium and ventricular arrhythmias. Am J Cardiol 1990;65:33E-44E.
2. Gennari FJ. Hypokalemia. N Engl J Med 1998;339:451-58.
3. Cohn JN, Kowey PR, Whelton PK, Prisant M. New guidelines for potassium replacement in clinical practice: A contemporary review by the National Council on Potassium in Clinical Practice. Arch Intern Med 2000;160:2429-36.
4. Tannen RL. Potassium disorders. In: Kokko JP, Tannen RL, editors. Fluids and electrolytes, 3rd ed. Philadelphia, Pa: WB Saunders, 1996: Chapter 3.
5. Cooper HA, Dries DL, Davis CE, Shen YL, Domanski MJ. Diuretics and risk of arrhythmic death in patients with left ventricular dysfunction. Circulation 1999;100:1311-15.
6. Khaw K-T, Barrett-Connor E. Dietary potassium and stroke-associated mortality: A 12-year prospective population study. N Engl J Med 1987;316:235-40.
7. Belanger CF, Hennekens CH, Rosner B, Speizer FE. The Nurses' Health Study. Am J Nurs 1978;78:1039-40.
8. INTERSALT Cooperative Research Group. INTERSALT: An international study of electrolyte excretion and blood pressure: Results for 24-hour urinary sodium and potassium excretion. BMJ 1988;297:319-28.

9. Whelton PK, He J, Cutler JA, et al. Effects of oral potassium on blood pressure: meta-analysis of randomized controlled clinical trials. JAMA 1997;277:1624-32.
10. Nolan J, Batin PD, Andrews R, et al. Prospective study of heart rate variability and mortality in chronic heart failure: Results of the United Kingdom heart failure evaluation and assessment of risk trial (UK-heart). Circulation 1998;98:1510-16.
11. Grobbee DE, Hoes AW. Non-potassium-sparing diuretics and risk of sudden cardiac death. J Hypertens 1995;13:1539-45.
12. Duke M. Thiazide-induced hypokalemia: Association with acute myocardial infarction and ventricular fibrillation. JAMA 1978;239(1)43-45.
13. Kowey PR. Unpublished data.

Aldosterone-Receptor Blocking Agents

Bertram Pitt

Introduction

Study findings pertaining to aldosterone-receptor blocking agents hold important implications in the care of patients with congestive heart failure (CHF). Such research is critical to the cardiovascular care of the postmenopausal population. Since its discovery in 1954, the hormone aldosterone has been a target for therapy in CHF because of its role in sodium retention and potassium excretion [1]. However, it is now clear that aldosterone is responsible for a wide array of adverse effects that contribute to the manifestation of CHF, including myocardial fibrosis, direct vascular damage, endothelial cell and baroreceptor dysfunction, and ventricular arrhythmias [2–6]. To control the production of aldosterone and thereby counter these effects, inhibition of angiotensin II, the peptide hormone responsible for the production and release of aldosterone, with an angiotensin-converting enzyme (ACE) inhibitor is standard treatment, based on the assumption that suppressing angiotensin II production will, in turn, suppress aldosterone production. However, increasing evidence suggests that ACE inhibitors cannot sustain suppression of aldosterone production [5,7-10], even when combined with an angiotensin-receptor blocking agent [11]. In the Randomized Evaluation of Strategies for Left Ventricular Dysfunction (RESOLVD) pilot study, the ACE inhibitor enalapril combined with the angiotensin receptor blocking agent candesartin in heart failure patients produced a transient reduction in serum aldosterone levels at 17 weeks. By 43 weeks, however, aldosterone levels had risen above control (Figure 1) [11].

As studies reveal more about the role of aldosterone in the pathophysiology of CHF, the importance of aldosteron- receptor blocking agents in treatment becomes increasingly apparent. One of the most recent studies evaluating the aldosterone antagonist spironolactone found that, when combined with standard therapy, it significantly reduced the risk of morbidity and mortality in patients with severe heart failure without leading to serious hyperkalemia [12]. This article reviews these findings and those of other studies that have underscored the importance of aldosterone in the manifestation of CHF and the effectiveness of aldosterone inhibition with aldosterone receptor blocking agents, particularly spironolactone. For postmenopausal women, whose risk of cardiovascular disease (CVD) is inherently increased, these findings hold important implications.

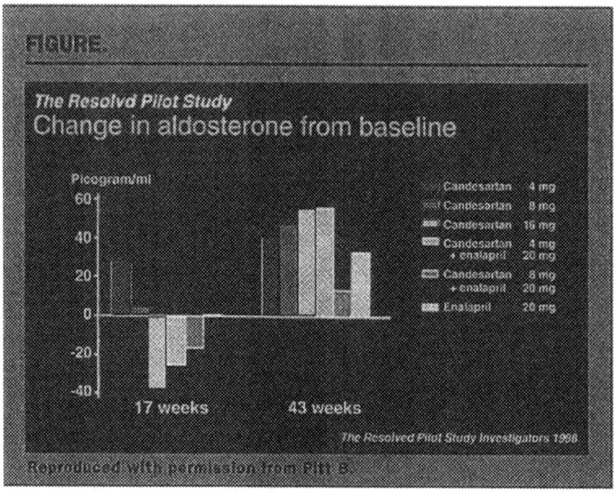

Figure 1. Change in Aldosterone From Baseline

A Study of Risk Reduction

The Randomized Aldactone Evaluation Study (RALES) tested the hypothesis that spironolactone combined with standard treatment would significantly reduce the risk of death from all causes in patients with severe CHF. This hypothesis was based on the results of an initial dose-finding study, which found spironolactone safe and effective in blocking the effects of aldosterone without causing serious hyperkalemia [13].

Patients were eligible for the double-blind study if they had symptomatic severe heart failure and systolic dysfunction (ejection fraction < 35%) and were receiving an ACE inhibitor and a loop diuretic. Digitalis, β-adrenergic blocking agents, potassium supplementation, and vasodilators were permitted, but treatment with potassium-sparing diuretics was not allowed. A total of 1,663 patients from 15 countries was included in the trial — 822 were randomized to 25 mg spironolactone daily and 841 patients were randomized to placebo.

In addition to the primary endpoint of death from any cause, secondary endpoints included death or hospitalization due to cardiac causes.

The 3-year trial was stopped prematurely after 2 years, when the planned interim analysis showed a significant benefit of spironolactone on the primary endpoint of death from all causes. At this point in the study, there were 386 deaths (46%) in the placebo group and 284 deaths (35%) in the spironolactone group. This represented a 30% reduction in the risk of death among spironolactone patients (relative risk of death 0.70; $P < 0.001$). Similar reductions were noted for risk of death from progressive heart failure, sudden death from cardiac causes, and hospitalization for cardiac causes.

These highly significant risk reductions with spironolactone were consistent across all subsets evaluated, and retrospective analyses found no differences in effectiveness related to sex, age, degree of heart failure, use of potassium supplements, and use of β blockers. The incidence of serious hyperkalemia was also minimal in both patient groups (1.7% for spironolactone, 1.2% for placebo). There were no significant adverse effects noted among women. Overall, spironolactone was well tolerated and the very low incidence of hyperkalemia emphasizes its safety in this group of severely ill patients.

The profound benefits seen with spironolactone in RALES suggest that the role of aldosterone receptor blockers extends beyond aversion of sodium retention and potassium loss. It is likely that these agents have a cardioprotective effect, with the ability to block many detrimental effects of aldosterone, including myocardial and past vascular fibrosis, diastolic dysfunction, free-radical production, and other adverse effects.

Role in CVD

Blocking Myocardial Fibrosis

Aldosterone plays a pivotal role in promoting myocardial fibrosis. It has been shown to cause increases in important signaling markers and pathways for vascular damage, which leads to microvascular damage, inflammation, and eventually fibrosis [14].

By reducing the vascular damage caused by aldosterone, aldosterone receptor blocking agents can effectively block myocardial fibrosis. Rocha and colleagues noted this in a study of stroke-prone, hypertensive rats treated with spironolactone [6]. Although spironolactone had no effect on blood pressure, histologic examination showed that it caused a marked reduction in urinary protein excretion and significantly less vascular damage in the brain, kidneys, and glomerulus compared with controls. These findings indicate a protective effect of spironolactone against the development of vascular damage in the absence of lowered blood pressure.

The effects of spironolactone in blocking myocardial fibrosis also have been demonstrated in a substudy of RALES, which examined serological markers of cardiac fibrosis in patients with CHF [15]. Specifically, three precursors of collagen formation were assessed: serum procollagen type I carboxy-terminal peptide (PICP), procollagen type I amino-terminal peptide (PINP), and procollagen type III amino-terminal peptide (PIIINP). High serum levels of these markers were associated with high rates of mortality and hospitalization, which continued to increase or remain the same in patients receiving placebo. In contrast, patients who received spironolactone showed a significant decrease in these serum markers. These changes in collagen formation suggest that a large part of the benefit of spironolactone in the RALES trial was due to blockade of aldosterone-stimulated collagen synthesis, which effectively blocked progressive myocardial fibrosis.

Improving Hypertension

In patients with hypertension, aldosterone-receptor blocking agents also have shown beneficial effects, including decreased blood pressure, improved diastolic dysfunction, and left ventricular hypertrophy (LVH).

Robledo and colleagues found that diastolic function improved by 37% in hypertensive patients receiving 100 mg/day spironolactone [16]. Patients with hypertension also exhibited LVH associated with increased urinary aldosterone levels. By blocking aldosterone, spironolactone causes a regression of LVH [17]. Furthermore, aldosterone-induced increases in intracellular calcium within the myocardium can be decreased with spironolactone [18]. These effects of spironolactone have important implications not only for hypertensive patients in general, but for postmenopausal women in particular.

Inhibiting Free-Radical Production

Evidence suggests that aldosterone may also contribute to the development of CHF and CVD as a free radical generator. Free radicals are extremely reactive chemical compounds that the body produces naturally during the metabolism of food. It is suspected that free radicals contribute to atherosclerosis and other diseases characterized by accumulation of insoluble fatty substances [19].

In a study of stroke-prone, hypertensive rats, Mathew and colleagues found that the hydroxyl radical inhibitor dimethylthiourea had no effect on blood pressure, yet significantly decreased tubular damage in the kidney caused by aldosterone [20]. The investigators reasoned, therefore, that the effects of aldosterone in CVD could be attributed in part to its role as a hydroxyl radical generator, and that the benefits of spironolactone could be a result of its action as a free-radical inhibitor.

In evaluating these roles of aldosterone and spironolactone, it is important to consider their association to nitric oxide (NO). Studies in rats and pigs have shown that long-term blockade of NO production using the NO antagonist N^{w}-nitro-L-arginine methyl ester (L-NAME) causes arterial hypertension, microvascular and perivascular fibrosis, and myocardial hypertrophy [21-27]. Upon further examination, Usui et al. found that blocking NO with L-NAME causes an increase in aldosterone synthesis [28]. Conversely, by increasing NO production in the adrenal gland, aldosterone production can be suppressed.

This effect of NO blockade can be seen in a study by Farquharson, which involved patients with heart failure who were maintained on an ACE inhibitor for 3 months followed by randomization to concomitant spironolactone treatment [29]. Patients receiving both agents showed significant improvement in endothelial-mediated vasodilation. These findings suggest that by blocking aldosterone, spironolactone decreases free-radical production, thereby increasing the net availability of NO.

Additional Benefits of Blocking Aldosterone

Improved Vascular Compliance

In a study of patients with heart failure, aldosterone was found to be correlated with large-vessel compliance [5]. The study evaluated the influence of aldosterone on arterial compliance in patients with mild to moderate heart failure who had been taking an ACE inhibitor, digoxin, furosemide, and aspirin for at least 3 months. Although angiotensin II was completely suppressed, aldosterone was not. The researchers noted that aldosterone escape was associated with decreased compliance of the aorta an its major side branches, which could lead to progressive heart failure.

This finding carries important implications for postmenopausal women, who have been shown to have a significant decrease in vascular compliance compared with younger women and with men. This change in vascular compliance is believed to contribute to hypertension, heart failure, and possibly myocardial infarction and sudden cardiac death. Considering these effects, the ability to block aldosterone could be extremely important to the cardiovascular health of postmenopausal women.

ENHANCED VARIABILITY

In patients with heart failure, hypertension, and postmyocardial infarction, it has been shown that heart rate variability, is a very powerful predictor of survival. Patients with a relative shift toward sympathetic tone have decreased survival, whereas those with increased vagal tone, or improved heart rate variability, have improved survival. Increased heart rate variability has been demonstrated in CHF patients treated with spironolactone. In a study by MacFadyen et al. [3], patients receiving spironolactone exhibited increased time-domain parameters of heart rate variability, despite concurrent ACE inhibitor treatment [3]. The most significant reductions occurred during the morning hours (6 AM-10 AM). In light of their findings, the researchers pointed out that residual aldosterone after ACE inhibitor treatment may play a role in arrhythmia and cardiac death. Thus, blocking aldosterone could effectively block these detrimental effects.

IMPROVED FIBRINOLYSIS

Blocking aldosterone could also have a favorable effect on fibrinolytic balance. Data suggest that angiotensin II impedes fibrinolysis by stimulating expression of plasminogen activator inhibitor-1 (PAI-1), which may promote the progression of vascular disease [30]. Elevated PAI-1 levels are associated with insulin resistance [31] and appear to be a risk factor for recurrent myocardial infarction [32].

In a study examining the interaction between the renin angiotensin system and fibrinolytic system, Brown et al. noted that aldosterone alone had very little effect on PAI-1 levels; however, when they combined angiotensin II and aldosterone, there was a significant additive effect levels of PAI-1 [33]. Additionally, they noted that blocking aldosterone decreased PAI-1.

Conclusion

As the role of aldosterone in the pathophysiology of CHF has become more clear, so has the role of aldosterone-receptor blocking agents in the treatment of CHF. Considering that aldosterone cannot be fully suppressed with ACE inhibitors or angiotensin receptor blocking agents, the use of aldosterone blockers such as spironolactone may be effective in treating or preventing CHF and other cardiovascular conditions. Aldosterone-receptor antagonists may have particular value in treating postmenopausal women who are at increased risk for hypertension and atherosclerosis.

Clinical trials have demonstrated repeatedly that aldosterone receptor blocking agents such as spironolactone express numerous cardioprotective effects. Most recently, the RALES trial found that, when combined with standard therapy, spironolactone effected a significant reduction in the risk of mortality and death in patients with severe heart failure, without causing serious hyperkalemia. Findings from these studies of aldosterone receptor blocking agents are important for CHF patients in general, and they hold enormous implications for postmenopausal women as well. Research is moving forward in evaluating a component of spironolactone in hormone replacement therapy, and it is hoped that it will provide additional benefit in the prevention and treatment of CVD in this high-risk population.

References

1. Soberman JE, Weber KT. Spironolactone in congestive heart failure. Curr Hypertens Rep 2000;2:451-56.
2. Barr CS, Lang CC, Hanson J, Arnott M, et al. Effects of adding spironolactone to an angiotensin-converting enzyme inhibitor in chronic congestive heart failure secondary to coronary artery disease. Am J Cardiol 1995;76:1259-65.
3. MacFadyen RJ, Barr CS, Struthers AD. Aldosterone blockade reduces vascular collagen turnover, improves heart rate variability and reduces early morning rise in heart failure in heart failure patients. Cardiovasc Res 1997;35:30-34.
4. Wang W. Chronic administration of aldosterone depresses baroreceptor reflex function in the dog. Hypertension 1994;24:571-75.
5. Duprez DA, De Buyzere ML, Rietzschel ER, et al. Inverse relationship between aldosterone and large artery compliance in chronically treated heart failure patients. Eur Heart J 1998 Sep;19(9):1371-76.
6. Rocha R, Chander PN, Khanna K, et al. Mineralocorticoid blockade reduces vascular injury in stroke-prone hypertensive rats. Hypertension 1998Jan;31(1Pt.2):451-58.
7. Borghi C, Boschi S, Ambrosioni E, et al. Evidence of a partial escape of renin-angiotensin-aldosterone blockade in patients with acute myocardial infarction treated with ACE inhibitors. J Clin Pharmacol 1993;33:40-45.
8. Cleland JGF, Dargie HJ, Hodsman GP, et al. Captopril in heart failure: A double blind controlled trial. Br Heart J 1984;52:530-35.
9. Biollaz J, Brunner HR, Gavras I, et al. Antihypertensive therapy with MK421: Angiotensin II-renin relationships to evaluate efficacy of converting enzyme blockade. J Cardiovasc Pharmacol 1982;4:966-72.
10. Staessen J, Lijnen P, Fagard R, et al. Rise in plasma concentration of aldosterone during long-term angiotensin II suppresion. J Endocrinol 1981;91:457-65.
11. McKelvie RS, Yusuf S, Pericak D, et al, for the RESOLVD Pilot Study Investigators. Comparison of candesartan, enalapril, and their combination in congestive heart failure: Randomized evaluation of strategies for left ventricular dysfunction (RESOLVD) pilot

study. Circulation 1999;100:1056-64.

12. Pitt B, Zannad F, Remme WJ, et al., for the Randomized Aldactone Evaluation Study Investigators. The effect of spironolactone on morbidity and mortality in patients with severe heart failure. N Engl J Med 1999;341:709-17.

13. Effectiveness of spironolactone added to an angiotensin-converting enzyme inhibitor and a loop diuretic for severe chronic congestive heart failure (the Randomized Aldactone Evaluation Study [RALES]). Am J Cardiol 1996;78:902-7.

14. Sun Y, Zhang J, Zhang JQ, Ramires FJ. Local angiotensin II and transforming growth factor-ß 1 in renal fibrosis of rats. Hypertension 2000;35:1078-884.

15. Zannad F, Alla F, Dousset B, et al, for the RALES Investigators. Limitation of excessive extracellular matrix turnover may contribute to survival benefit of spironolactone therapy in patients with congestive heart failure: Insights from the randomized aldactone evaluation study (RALES). Circulation 2000;102:2700-6.

16. Robledo GA. Role de la spironolactone dans le traîtement de l'hypertension arterille: Effets sur la function diastolique du ventricle gauche et sur la structure cardiaque. Réalités Cardiologiques 1996.

17. Hiltgen, et al. Régression sous spironolactone de l'hypertrophie ventriculaire gauche dans l'hypertension artérilles moderée: être echocardiographique de 125 cas. Réalités Cardiologiques 1995.

18. Benitah JP. Aldosterone upregulates calcium in adult rat myocite. Circ Res 1999;85:1139-45.

19. Barrett JR. Measuring the health effects of free radicals. NCRR Reporter Spring 1999. Available at: http://www.ncrr.nih.gov/newspub/apr99rpt/Radicals.htm. National Center for Research Resources page for the NCRR Reporter.

20. Mathew R, Fan NY, Yuan N, et al. Inhibition of NOS enhances pulmonary vascular changes in stroke-prone spontaneously hypertensive rats. Am J Physiol Lung Cell Mol Physiol 2000;278:L81-L89.

21. Ito A, Egashira K, Kadokami T, et al. Chronic inhibition of endothelium-derived nitric oxide synthesis causes coronary microvascular structural changes and hyperreactivity to serotonin in pigs. Circulation 1995;92:2636-44.

22. Numaguchi K, Egashira K, Takemoto M, et al. Chronic inhibition of nitric oxide synthesis causes pathologic coronary microvascular remodeling and myocardial fibrosis. Hypertension 1995;26(pt 1):957-62.

23. Kadokami T, Egashira K, Kuwata K, et al. Altered serotonin receptor subtypes contribute to microvascular hyperreactivity to serotonin in pigs with chronic inhibition of nitric oxide. Circulation 1996;94:182-89.

24. Arnal JF, Warin L, Michel JB. Determinants of aortic cyclic guanosine monophosphate in hypertension induced by chronic inhibition of nitric oxide synthase. J Clin Invest 1992; 90:647-52.

25. Baylis C, Mitruka B, Deng A. Chronic blockade of nitric oxide synthesis in the rat produces systemic hypertension and glomerular damage. J Clin Invest 1992;90:278-81.

26. Bank N, Aynedjian HS, Khan GA. Mechanism of vasoconstriction induced by chronic inhibition of nitric oxide in rats. Hypertension 1994;24:322-28.

27. Ribeiro MO, Antunes E, Nicci G, et al. Chronic inhibition of nitric oxide synthesis: A new

model of arterial hypertension. Hypertension 1992;20:298-303.

28. Usui M, Ichiki T, Katoh M, et al. Regulation of angiotensin II receptor expression by nitric oxide in rat adrenal gland. Hypertension 1998;32:527-33.

29. Farquharson CAJ, Struthers AD. Spironolactone increases nitric oxide bioactivity, improves endothelial vasodilator dysfunction, and suppresses vascular angiotension I/angiotension II conversion in patients with chronic heart failure. Circulation 2000;101 (6);594-97.

30. Vaughan DE, Lazos SA, Tong K. Angiotensin II regulates the expression of plasminogen activator inhibitor-1 in cultured endothelial cells. J Clin Invest 1995;95:995-1001.

31. Juhan-Vague I, Alessi MC. PAI-1, obesity, insulin resistance and risk of cardiovascular events. Thromb Haemost 1997;78:656-60.

32. Hamsten A, de Fairde U, Walldius G, et al. Plasminogen activator inhibitor in plasma: risk factor for recurrent myocardial infarction. Lancet 1987;2:3-9.

33. Brown NJ, Agirbasli MA, Williams GH, et al. Effect of activation and inhibition of the renin-angiotensin system on plasma PAI-1. Hypertension 1998;32:965-71.

PROGESTOGENS: NEW APPROACHES

Rogerio A. Lobo

Introduction

The benefits of hormone replacement therapy (HRT) are numerous: It provides relief of menopausal symptoms, reduces the risk of osteoporosis and accompanying fractures and may potentially aid in the prevention of various other illnesses, including Alzheimer's disease and cardiovascular disease (CVD) [1-4]. Despite the established and potential benefits of HRT, which have been shown to outweigh its possible risks, fewer than one-half of eligible women in the United States are currently using it [1,5]. Furthermore, only a fraction of current users will continue therapy for more than 2 years [6]. Part of the reason for this problem with discontinuation is the lack of consistency in the literature regarding risks and benefits. For example, the American Heart Association recently suggested in a position paper that there is no benefit to taking estrogen for secondary prevention of CVD and questioned whether there is any benefit to it in primary prevention [7].

A Significant Factor

In one study, the vast majority of former HRT users reported that their decision to stop HRT was linked to intolerable side effects, most notably bleeding (Figure 1) [1]. For women with a uterus, progestogens are a necessary component of HRT. They are known, however, to lead to somatic complaints, breast tenderness, and mood disturbances. They have also contributed to the uterine bleeding and cramps experienced by some postmenopausal women on HRT [8,9].

Evaluating the impact of HRT on quality of life, Tosteson et al noted that current HRT users had significantly better health-related quality of life compared with past users and those who had never used HRT. Nevertheless, nearly all current HRT users (95.5%) stated they would trade time to avoid the side effect of bleeding, and most would trade time to avoid breast tenderness (90.4%), weight gain (87.4%), and endometrial biopsy (82.7%) [10].

Drospirenone

Concerns about progestogen use include the complaints described above, as well as the potential attenuation of some benefits. These findings and the potential for alternative strategies have been reviewed elsewhere [11]. Among the efforts to develop alternatives to standard progestogen therapy is the evolution of newer progestogens that would more closely resemble the pharmacologic profile of natural progesterone. This has resulted in the novel progestogen drosperinone (DRSP), an analogue of 17α-spironolactone. Unlike other conventional progestins, all of which are derivatives of 17α-hydroxyprogesterone or 19-nortestosterone, DRSP possesses potent progestogenic, antiandrogenic, and antimineralocorticoid activity almost identical to that of natural progesterone [12,13]. With this unique profile, DRSP is consistently proven effective in improving tolerance and reducing the incidence of side effects seen with other progestins.

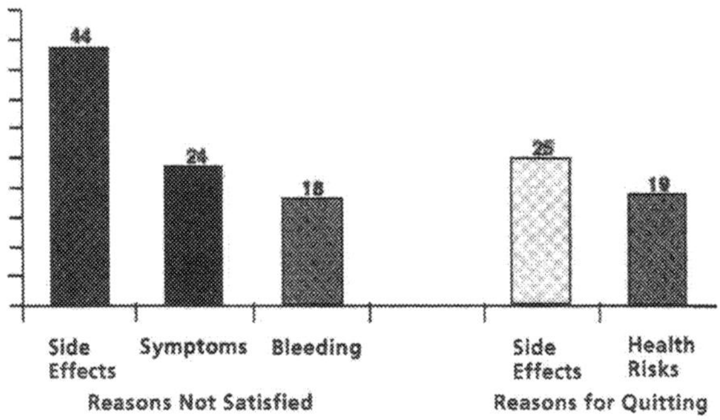

Figure 1. Former HRT Users — Reasons For Dissatisfaction

ANTIMINERALOCORTICOID ACTIVITY

Like natural progesterone, DRSP has affinity for both the progesterone and mineralocorticoid receptors, a characteristic that other progestins lack [14]. This antimineralocorticoid effect enables DRSP to counterbalance the sodium-retaining effects of ethinyl estradiol (EE) without affecting potassium excretion. This was demonstrated by Oelkers and colleagues in a trial of healthy young women who received a diet with controlled sodium (100 mmol/day) and potassium (60-70 mmol/day) from days 3 through 13 of their menstrual cycle [15]. From day 8 through 13, one-half of the women received 2 mg per day DRSP and one-half received placebo. A cumulative sodium excretion of 84 mmol per day was seen in the DRSP group, as well as a significant rise in plasma renin and aldosterone, compared with no change in the placebo group. By preventing sodium and water retention, DRSP not only reduces the likelihood of bloating and weight gain associated with EE but also offers the potential benefit of preventing increases in systolic and diastolic blood pressure [14].

The authors also noted no change in potassium excretion with DRSP, which was reaffirmed in a open-label study of women with normal renal function or mild or moderate renal impairment [15]. At steady-state DRSP treatment, all serum potassium concentrations were not significantly changed from baseline [16].

In a comparison trial of 3 mg DRSP combined with 15, 20, or 30 µg EE, Oelkers et al found that all three DRSP/EE regimens effected benefits on body weight compared with the control regimen of 150 µg levonorgestrel and 30 µg EE [17]. Improvements in high density lipoprotein (HDL) cholesterol and low density lipoprotein (LDL) cholesterol profiles were also noted; the opposite effect was seen with the control regimen (Figures 2A and 2B).

It has been surmised that 3 mg of DRSP is approximately equivalent to 25 mg of spironolactone.

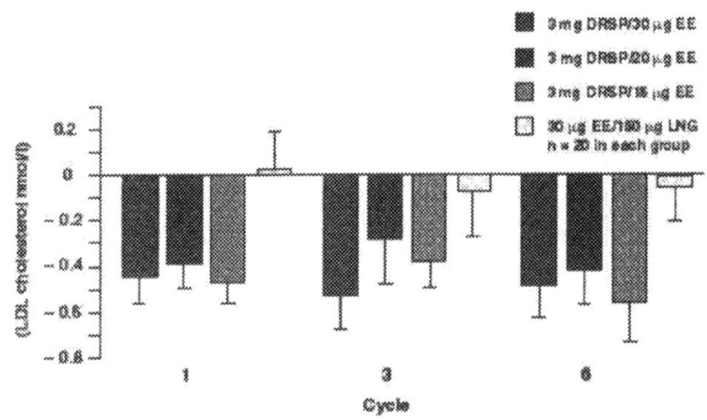

Figure 2A. Changes in LDL- Cholesterol [17]

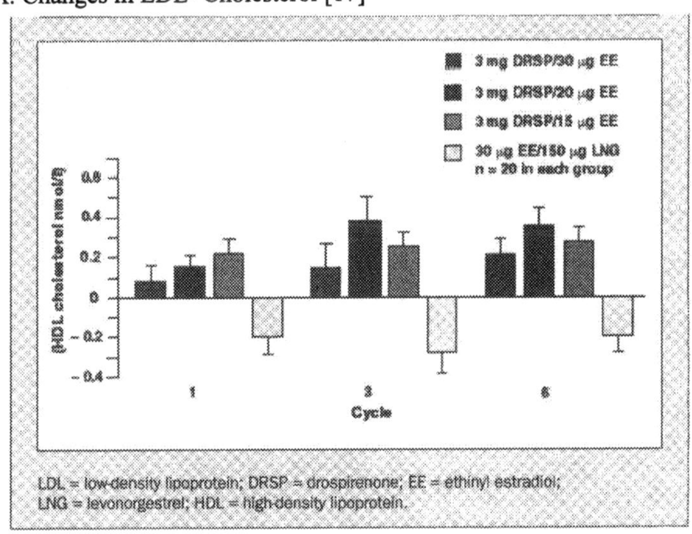

Figure 2B. Changes in HDL-Cholesterol [17}

ANTIANDROGENIC ACTIVITY

Studies of DRSP and progesterone have established that the antiandrogenic effects of DRSP are indeed potent [12–18], as much as 5 to 10 times greater than those of progesterone [19]. Although DRSP has very low affinity for the androgen receptor, it does not prevent binding of sex hormone binding globulins (SHBG) and androgens. Furthermore, DRSP does not counteract estrogen-induced increases in SHBG levels [20].

Other beneficial effects of the antiandrogenic activity of DRSP have been demonstrated in comparison trials of OC regimens combining DRSP and EE [21]. Two large, randomized, multicenter, open-label studies compared the contraceptive efficacy of 30 μg EE combined with either 3 mg DRSP or 150 μg desogestrel [21]. While both preparations exhibited effective contraception, the antimineralocorticoid and antiandrogenic benefits of the DRSP/EE combination were obvious when compared with the desogestrel/EE regimen. The antiandrogenic effects of DRSP resulted in improved skin appearance and reduced seborrhea, as well as good cycle control and improved mood.

In a follow-up study of this trial, participants reported that they felt worse after they stopped taking DRSP/EE regimens and resumed their conventional OC preparations.

SIDE EFFECTS

Studies to date have shown DRSP to have a favorable side-effect profile. A recent open-label study evaluating the safety of DRSP in 326 women reported that more than one-half (54%) of women had no intermenstrual bleeding during the 13-cycle study [22]. Of those who did, the majority (64%) experienced bleeding during only one or two pill cycles. These levels of breakthrough bleeding, spotting, and amenorrhea are similar to those of other low-dose OCs.

Discontinued study participation was noted in 6% of women and was due to adverse effects, including uncontrollable mood, headache, nausea, dysmenorrhea, intermenstrual bleeding, or depression. However, fewer than 2% cited each of these effects as their reason for discontinuation.

DRSP Use in HRT

The consistently positive findings in trials of DRSP used in OC preparations not only led to the development of a new OC, but also formed the rationale for analyzing the efficacy of this new progestin in HRT. Preliminary study results with four different doses of DRSP combined with 17β-estradiol in menopausal and postmenopausal women have proven extremely encouraging. All four DRSP regimens were effective as HRT and provided favorable side-effect profiles — specifically, prevention of hyperplasia, good cycle control, and decreases in blood pressure.

Prevention of Hyperplasia

A multicenter trial included 1,142 women ranging in age from 45 to 75 years who were given 1 mg 17β-estradiol alone or combined with daily doses of either 0.5, 1, 2, or 3 mg DRSP [22]. After 1 year, one case of endometrial hyperplasia was reported in the 0.5-mg DRSP group (n = 191), compared with 19 cases in the estradiol-only group (n = 197). There were no cases of hyperplasia found among women receiving 1, 2, or 3 mg DRSP.

Cycle Control

At study initiation, the investigators noted that maintenance of amenorrhea was highest in the estradiol-only group at 96.9%, with relatively good cycle control in all four DRSP groups: 78.3% in the 0.5-mg group, 79.4% in the 1-mg group, 71.6% in the 2-mg group, and 84.3% in the 3-mg group. However, as the study progressed, only negligible differences in cycle control were seen among all treatment groups after 6 months. By the study's end, at cycle 13, all four DRSP regimens were providing good cycle control in more than 80% of women, the highest percentage with 2-mg DRSP regimen at 88.2%. In contrast, 80.1% of women in the estradiol-only regimen had good cycle control, representing a decline of 17% from the start of the study.

Decreases in Blood Pressure

All four DRSP regimens also proved effective in maintaining or lowering blood pressure. Statistically significant decreases in systolic blood pressure from baseline were noted, with the greatest decreases seen in the 3-mg DRSP regimen ($P < 0.001$) and 1-mg DRSP regimens ($P = 0.002$).

Conclusion

The new progestin DRSP has afforded the opportunity to develop a new HRT with a favorable side-effect profile. With its antialdosterone activity, DRSP effects excretion of excess sodium and water while maintaining potassium levels, thereby resulting in decreased blood pressure as well as reduced bloating, weight gain, breast pain, and other symptoms of water retention. DRSP also has antiandrogenic activity, which has been shown to promote good cycle control, improved sense of well-being, and improved skin appearance. By reducing many of the side effects associated with the progestin component of HRT, the use of DRSP in a new HRT formulation could have the potential of leading to improved compliance and continued use.

References

1. The Gallup Organization, Inc. The 2000 Gallup Study of Women's Experiences with Hormone Replacement Therapy. Princeton, NJ: Multi-Sponsor Surveys, Inc. Conducted

for Berlex Laboratories, April 2000.

2. Purdie DW. Consequences of long-term hormone replacement therapy. Br Med Bull 2000; 56:809-23.
3. Yaffe K, Browner W, Cauley J, Launer L, Harris T. Association between bone mineral density and cognitive decline in older women. J Am Geriatr Soc 1999;47:1176-82.
4. Zweifel JE, O'Brien WH. A meta-analysis of the effect of hormone replacement therapy upon depressed mood. Psychoneuroendocrinology 1997;22:189-212.
5. Salamone LM, Pressman AR, Seeley DG, Cauley JA. Estrogen replacement therapy. A survey of older women's attitudes. Arch Intern Med 1996;156:1293-97.
6. Sarrel PM, Dobay B, Witta B. Estrogen and estrogen-androgen replacement in postmenopausal women dissatisfied with estrogen-only therapy. J Reprod Med 1998;43: 847-56.
7. Mosca L, Collins P, Herrington DM, et al. Hormone replacement therapy and cardiovascular disease: A statement for healthcare professionals from the American Heart Association. Circulation 2001;104:499-503.
8. Nerhood RC. Making a decision about ERT/HRT. Evidence to consider in initiating and continuing protective therapy. Postgrad Med 2001;109:167-70,173-74,178.
9. Achieving long-term continuance of menopausal ERT/HRT: Consensus opinion of the North American Menopause Society. NAMS Web site. Available at: http://www.menopause.org/consensus1.htm. Accessed June 4, 2001.
10. Tosteson AN, Gabriel SE, Kneeland TS, et al. Has the impact of hormone replacement therapy on health-related quality of life been undervalued? J Womens Health Gend Based Med 2000;9:119-30.
11. Lobo R, Kelsey J, Marcus R, editors. Menopause: Biology and pathobiology. Burlington, Mass: Academic Press, 2001.
12. Fuhrmann U, Krattenmacher R, Slater EP, Fritzemeier KH. The novel progestin drospirenone and its natural counterpart progesterone: Biochemical profile and antiandrogenic potential. Contraception 1996;54:243-51.
13. Oelkers W. Drospirenone — A new progestogen with antimineralocorticoid activity, resembling natural progesterone. Eur J Contracept Reprod Health Care 2000;5(Suppl.3): 17-24.
14. Drospirenone/ethinyl estradiol (Yasmin®): New oral contraceptive promises improved tolerance and less side effects. OBGYN.net Web site. Available at: http://www.obgyn.net/women/articles/MMC/MMC-yasmin.htm. Accessed June 1, 2001.
15. Oelkers W, Berger V, Bolik A, et al. Dihydrospirenone, a new progestogen with antimineralocorticoid activity: Effects on ovulation, electrolyte excretion, and the renin-aldosterone system in normal women. J Clin Endocrinol Metab 1991;73:837-42.
16. Data on file, Berlex Laboratories, Inc.
17. Oelkers W, Foidart JM, Dombrovicz N, Welter A, Heithecker R. Effects of a new oral contraceptive containing an antimineralocorticoid progestogen, drospirenone, on the renin-aldosterone system, body weight, blood pressure, glucose tolerance, and lipid metabolism. J Clin Endocrinol Metab 1995;80:1816-21.
18. Blode H, Wuttke W. Loock W, Roll G, Heithecker R. A 1-year pharmacokinetic investigation of a novel oral contraceptive containing drospirenone in healthy female

volunteers. Eur J Contracept Reprod Health Care 2000;5:256-64.

19. Fuhrmann U, Krattenmacher R, Slater EP, Fritzemeier KH. The novel progestin drospirenone and its natural counterpart progesterone: Biochemical profile and antiandrogenic potential. Contraception 1996;54:243-51.

20. Krattenmacher R. Drospirenone: Pharmacology and pharmacokinetics of a unique progestogen. Contraception 2000;62(1):29-38.

21. Foidart JM. The contraceptive profile of a new oral contraceptive with antimineralocorticoid and antiandrogenic effects. Eur J Contracept Reprod Health Care 2000;5(Suppl.3):25-33.

22. Data on file, Berlex

AROMATASE, NUCLEAR RECEPTORS, ADIPOSE TISSUE, AND BREAST CANCER

Evan R Simpson, Colin Clyne, Caroline Speed, and Gary Rubin

Introduction

Models of estrogen insufficiency have revealed new and often unexpected roles for estradiol in both females and males [1]. These models include natural mutations in humans of the aromatase gene, of which there are some ten cases known, of whom two are men, as well as one man with a mutation in the estrogen receptor (ER) α. They also include mice with targeted disruptions of the ERα and ERβ, the double ERα and β knockout [2-4], as well as the aromatase knockout (ArKO) mouse [5]. Some of these roles challenge the definition of the terms estrogen and androgen. For example the lipid and carbohydrate phenotype of estrogen insufficiency is nonsexually dimorphic and appears to apply equally to males and females [6,7], as does the bone phenotype of undermineralization and failure of epiphyseal closure. Even more dramatically, the role of estradiol in male germ cell development would indicate that at least in this local context estradiol would be more appropriately defined as an androgen [8]. The second important point is that in men and in postmenopausal women when the ovaries cease to produce estrogens, estradiol does not function as a circulating hormone. It is no longer an endocrine factor, instead estradiol is produced in a number of extragonadal sites and acts locally at these sites as a paracrine or even intracrine factor [9,10]. These sites include the mesenchymal cells of adipose tissue, osteoblasts and chondrocytes of bone, numerous sites in the brain, and also the Leydig cells and germ cells of the testes. Thus circulating levels of estrogens in postmenopausal women and in men do not drive estrogen action. Rather they are derived from the production of estrogen in extragonadal sites where it has acted locally and which then escapes local metabolism to re-enter the circulation. Thus circulating levels reflect rather than direct estrogen action in postmenopausal women and men.

Estrogens are synthesized from androgens and the enzyme responsible for this is called aromatase which is a member of the superfamily of genes known collectively as cytochrome P450. Aromatase belongs to family 19 hence its designation as CYP19. In humans aromatase is expressed in a number of tissue sites corresponding to the sites of estrogen biosynthesis. An important feature of this expression is that tissue-specific expression of aromatase is regulated by a number of upstream untranslated first exons which are spliced into the mature transcript in a tissue-specific fashion [11]. Thus expression in the gonads as well as in estrogen-synthesizing tumors is driven by a proximal promoter immediately upstream of the start of translation, promoter II. By contrast, expression in placenta is driven by a distal promoter, promoter I.1, whereas expression in mesenchymal cells of adipose tissue is driven by another distal promoter, promoter I.4. However in adipose tissue proximal to a breast tumor, promoter II is the dominant promoter utilized. Each of these promoters is regulated by a different cohort of signaling pathways and transcription factors. Thus estrogen biosynthesis is differentially regulated in the various tissue sites of expression. In gonads and in tumors, expression is regulated primarily by cyclic AMP. In the ovary the factor which drives cyclic AMP formation is FSH. In tumors it appears to be prostaglandin E2. In normal adipose mesenchymal cells, expression from promoter I.4 is driven primarily by Class 1 cytokines such as interleukin 6, interleukin 11, LIF, and oncostatin M via a Jak 1-Stat 3 pathway. TNFα also activates expression from promoter I.4 probably via a MAP kinase-AP1 pathway. The untranslated first exons downstream of these tissue-specific promoters are all spliced into a common 3'-splice junction upstream of the start of translation. Thus the coding region in each of the tissue-specific sites of expression is identical, and thus the aromatase protein in each of these sites is the same [11].

Breast Cancer

In studies conducted within the United States in which large numbers of women were given either tamoxifen or raloxifene [12], there was a substantial decrease in the incidence of invasive breast cancer in women of all ages regardless of whether they were pre- or postmenopausal. This implies that there is a source of estrogen in postmenopausal women which directs breast cancer development, in spite of the fact that the ovaries cease to make estrogens at the time of menopause. This source of estrogen appears to be aromatase expression either within the breast tumor itself, or within the mesenchymal cells of the breast surrounding the tumor. It has been shown that the levels of estradiol present in breast tumors are at least an order of magnitude greater than those present in the circulating plasma of postmenopausal women [13]. This can only be due to local estrogen biosynthesis. As an aside, this helps to account for the fact that HRT appears to present little increase in risk of breast cancer, at most 0.30-fold [14]. Even if HRT resulted in an increase in the circulating plasma estrogen levels of several fold, these levels would still be much lower than those present within the tumor due to local synthesis. This again illustrates the concept that was stated earlier, namely that circulating levels of estrogens in postmenopausal women are not the drivers of estrogen action, but rather reflect local production at extragonadal sites. We conclude therefore that local aromatase expression within the breast is the main source of estrogen implicated in breast cancer development in postmenopausal women.

Over the years [11] we have studied the regulation of aromatase expression in breast and have shown that in normal breast adipose mesenchymal tissue, aromatase expression is driven primarily by Class 1 cytokines and TNFα as mentioned previously. This is because the principal promoter utilized in this tissue is the distal promoter I.4 which responds to signaling pathways stimulated by these factors. However if a breast tumor is present, there is a switch in promoter utilization such that promoter II, the proximal promoter, is now the principle promoter utilized. The factor which is driving expression via promoter II appears to be prostaglandin E2 either produced by the epithelial cells of the tumor or else by macrophages recruited to the tumor site [15]. This results in a gradient of aromatase expression with highest levels within and proximal to the tumor, and decreasing with increased distance from the tumor.

As mentioned previously, if promoter II reporter gene constructs are transfected into ovarian granulosa cells, addition of forskolin, which stimulates adenylate cyclase, results in an increase in reporter gene expression. If the SF1 half site on promoter II is mutated, this results in a dramatic loss of reporter activity. When similar experiments were conducted in mouse 3T3L1 cells which are of adipose mesenchymal origin, a different result was observed. When the SF1 site was mutated, instead of a loss of reporter gene activity, in fact there was an increase in reporter gene activity. This suggests that in these adipose-derived fibroblasts there is a factor which is bound to the SF1 site under normal circumstances, and which represses aromatase expression. When the cells were co-transfected with an SF1 expression plasmid there was a large increase in reporter gene expression. Current efforts are directed towards cloning and characterizing this putative repressive protein present in adipose fibroblasts of breast. If this repressor protein turns out to be an orphan member of the nuclear receptor family, then in principle it might be possible to discover a ligand for this factor which increases its repressive activity. Since promoter II is not involved in aromatase expression in bone cells [16], such a ligand would prove to be a highly specific inhibitor of aromatase expression in breast tissue.

Although this putative repressor protein has yet to be characterized, there is another class of compounds which we have found to be potent inhibitors of aromatase expression in breast adipose cells, namely ligands for PPARγ and for RXR. PPARγ-RXR heterodimers are critical factors involved in adipocyte differentiation. Our studies have shown that in adipose tissue, aromatase is expressed primarily in the pre-adipocyte stromal mesenchymal cells rather than in mature adipocytes. Since factors which stimulate aromatase expression in these cells, namely Class 1 cytokines and TNFα are all inhibitors of adipocyte differentiation, then one might predict that stimulators of adipocyte differentiation would inhibit aromatase expression. Ligands for PPARγ such as troglitazone, rosiglitazone, and the putative natural ligand 15-deoxy-$\Delta^{12\text{-}14}$ - prostaglandin J2 are all powerful stimulators of adipocyte differentiation in model systems. We have examined the effect of these compounds on aromatase expression in breast adipose stromal cells and have found that as predicted, they are powerful inhibitors of aromatase expression in these cells [17]. The synthetic PPARγ ligands have found utility in the management of Type 2 insulin-resistant diabetes. Based on the above results, we suggest that they would also be potentially useful in breast cancer therapy.

Yet a third class of compounds with potential therapeutic value as breast cancer therapy are inhibitors of prostaglandin biosynthesis. A case-controlled study published some years ago indicated that daily use of nonsteroidal anti-inflammatory drugs such as ibuprofen reduced the incidence of breast tumors by up to 40% [18]. This is consistent with the observations described above that PGE2 is a powerful stimulator of aromatase expression in breast adipose tissue via promoter II. Moreover, expression of aromatase was correlated with COX-1 and COX-2 expression in human breast cancer and normal tissue specimens [19]. From these considerations it appears likely that prostaglandin synthesis inhibitors could prove to have utility in breast cancer therapy as tissue-specific inhibitors of aromatase, particularly as promoter II is not involved in aromatase expression in bone cells, as mentioned above.

Selective Aromatase Modulators

In conclusion therefore, we wish to introduce the concept of Selective Aromatase Modulators (SAMs). This concept is critically dependent on the fact that in postmenopausal women as in men, estradiol does not function as a circulating hormone but rather functions in a paracrine and intracrine fashion, namely it is produced locally in a number of extragonadal sites and acts within the same site to effect its biological activity. It is also dependent on the finding that tissue-specific expression of aromatase is dependent on tissue-specific promoters which are differentially regulated by a variety of stimulatory or inhibitory co-factors. Clearly if estradiol functioned primarily as a circulating hormone in postmenopausal women, these principles would not apply. As we proceed to analyze the specific co-activators and co-repressors of aromatase in the various tissue sites of expression, it should be possible to select targets for the development of drugs which will inhibit aromatase in a tissue-specific fashion. The first generation of SAMs might well be ligands of PPARγ and RXR or cyclooxygenase inhibitors, but we believe there are other possibilities waiting to be discovered.

As was stated previously, the problem with the Phase 3 inhibitors of aromatase activity is that they inhibit this activity globally, not only in the desired site but also in other sites such as bone and brain. While this may not be so critical in elderly women with advanced breast cancer, it becomes an issue when considering treatment of young women with early disease or even as chemoprevention. Thus we would anticipate that tissue-specific inhibitors of aromatase expression, i.e. SAMs, would find utility in breast cancer treatment, not only as a backup therapy, for example following tamoxifen breakthrough, but also as first-line therapy in their own right.

Acknowledgments

This work was supported by USPHS Grants # R-37 AG 08174 and , as well as by the Victorian Breast Cancer Research Consortium. Sue Elger provided skilled editorial assistance.

References

1. Grumbach MM, Auchus RJ. Estrogen: Consequences and implications of human mutations in synthesis and action. J Clin Endoc Metab 1999;85: 4677-94.
2. Lubahn DB, Moyes JS, Golding TS, Couse JF, Korach KS, Smithies O. Alteration

of function but not pre-natal sexual development after insertional disruption of the mouse estrogen receptor gene. Proc Natl Acad Sci USA 1993;90:11162-66.
3. Krege JH, Hodgin JB, Couse JF, et al. Generation and reproductive phenotypes of mice lacking estrogen receptor β. Proc Natl Acad Sci USA 1998;95:15677-82.
4. Couse JF, Hewitt SC, Bunch DO, et al. Postnatal sex reversal of the ovaries in mice lacking estrogen receptors alpha and beta. Science 1999;286:2328-31.
5. Fisher CR, Graves KH, Parlow AF, Simpson ER. Characterization of mice deficient in aromatase (ArKO) because of targetted disruption of the cyp19 gene. Proc Natl Acad Sci USA 1998;95:6965-70.
6. Jones MEE, Thorburn AW, Britt KL, et al. Aromatase-deficient (ArKO) mice have a phenotype of increased adiposity. Proc Natl Acad Sci USA 2000;97:12735-40.
7. Heine PA, Taylor JA, Iwamoto GA, Lubahn DB, Cooke PS. Increased adipose tissue in male and female estrogen receptor-α knockout mice. Proc Natl Acad Sci USA 2000;97:12729-34.
8. Robertson KM, O'Donnell L, Jones MEE, et al. Impairment of spermatogenesis in mice lacking a functional aromatase (cyp19) gene. Proc Natl Acad Sci USA 1999; 96:7986-91.
9. Labrie F, Belanger A, Cusan L, Gomez JL, Candas B. Physiological changes in dehydroepiandrosterone are not reflected by serum levels of active androgens and estrogens but of their metabolites:intracrinology. J Clin Endo Metab 1997;82:2403-9.
10. Simpson ER, Davis SR. Why do the clinical sequelae of estrogen deficiency affect women more frequently than men? J Clin Endo Metab 1998;83:2214.
11. Simpson ER, Zhao Y, Agarwal VR, et al. Aromatase in health and disease. Rec Prog Horm Res 1997;52:185-214.
12. Jordan VC. Targeted antiestrogens to prevent breast cancer. Trends Endocrinol Metab 1999;10:312-17.
13. Pasqualini JR, Chetrite G, Blacker C, et al. 1996. Concentrations of estrone, estradiol, and estrone sulfate and evaluation of sulfatose and aromatase activities in pre- and postmenopausal breast cancer patients. J Clin Endocrinol Metab 1996;81: 1460-64.
14. Collaborative Group on Hormonal Factors in Breast Cancer. Collaborative re-analysis of data from 51 epidemiological studies of 52,705 women with breast cancer and 108,441 women without breast cancer. Lancet 1997;350:1047-59.
15. Zhao Y, Agarwal VR, Mendelson CR, Simpson ER. Estrogen biosynthesis proximal to a breast tumor is stimulated by PGE2 via cyclic AMP, leading to activation of promoter II of the cyp19 gene. Endocrinology 1996;137:5739-42.
16. Shozu M, Simpson ER Aromatase expression of human osteoblast-like cells. Mol Cell Endocrinol 1998;139:117-29.
17. Rubin GL, Zhao Y, Kalus AM, Simpson ER. Peroxisome proliferator-activated receptor gamma ligands inhibit estrogen biosynthesis in human breast adipose tissue:possible implications for breast cancer therapy. Cancer Res 2000;60:1604-8.
18. Harris RE, Namboodiri KK, Farrar WB. Non-steroidal anti-inflammatory drugs and

breast cancer. Epidemiology 1996;7:203-5.
19. Brueggemeier RW, Quinn AL, Parrett ML, Joarder FS, Harris RE, Robertson FM. Correlation of aromatase and cycloxygenase gene expression in human breast cancer specimens. Cancer Lett 1999;140:27-35.

ENVIRONMENTAL FACTORS RELATED TO CANCERS IN POSTMENOPAUSAL WOMEN

Louise A. Brinton

Introduction

Cancer in women is a very serious public health concern, given that approximately 40% of American women will be diagnosed at some time in their life with a cancer other than a superficial skin cancer and 20% will die from cancer [1].

A number of challenges exist to identifying environmental factors related to female cancers. In approaching the prevention of cancers in women, special emphasis must be placed on understanding exposures which are unique to women and which merit special consideration, either because of changing prevalences or unique interactions with other risk factors. In addition, different cancer sites are affected divergently by various risk factors. Furthermore, for many identified risk factors our understanding of the associated biologic mechanisms is quite limited. Fortunately, recent studies have provided many new insights regarding possible effects of a variety of potential etiologic agents. These efforts have been greatly aided by technologic advances which have expanded our understanding of underlying biologic processes and the natural history of these lesions.

This presentation will focus on a number of possible etiologic agents for cancer among women which require special consideration. This includes effects of cigarette smoking, anthropometric measures, dietary factors, physical activity, iatrogenic agents (including effects of hormones and ovulation stimulating drugs), general environmental agents (including endocrine disruptors), occupational factors, and genetic susceptibility.

Cigarette Smoking

The effects of cigarette smoking on cancer risk in women are of obvious concern. The increasing prevalence of smoking in women has led to major increases in lung cancer incidence [2]. Of concern is that the risk of lung cancer associated with smoking may be greater in women than men for comparable amounts of smoking [3]. This suggests a possible hormonal etiology for lung cancer. Although cigarette smoking is best recognized for its effects on lung cancer risk, results are emerging that it may also affect the risk of several others cancers in women. The relationship with breast cancer has been well investigated, with results generally showing no overall association [4]. However, it has been suggested that results in some studies may have been obscured by the failure to account for passive smoking effects. Notably, in several recent studies, when active smokers have been compared to individuals unexposed to either active or passive smoking, an increased risk of breast cancer associated with active smoking has been observed [5,6]. At least one cancer, endometrial cancer, has been shown to be reduced among cigarette smokers [7-9]. Although several alternative biologic mechanisms have been proposed, including the alteration of the absorption, distribution or metabolism of hormones, the precise mode of action remains unclear.

Anthropometric Measures

There is clear evidence that body size has an effect on a number of cancers in women. The strongest associations have been observed for endometrial cancer, where obese women have been reported to be at a 4-5-fold increased risk compared to thin women [10]. Of note is that the distribution of body fat also appears to relate to risk [11]. Thus, women whose weight distributes abdominally have higher risks than those with fat that distributes peripherally, presumably due to unique endogenous hormonal profiles. Relationships with breast cancer are more difficult to interpret, given differing relationships depending on when the cancers are diagnosed. A consistent inverse relationship has been noted for premenopausal breast cancers [12]. Although it has been suggested that this may reflect greater difficulties in detecting tumors in heavier women, this does not appear to be the entire explanation. Also proposed as important is that obesity is associated with more anovulatory cycles and lower levels of progesterone. In contrast, for postmenopausal breast cancers, a direct relationship with obesity has been observed [12]. This is generally believed to be due to greater opportunity for conversion of precursors to estrone in peripheral fat tissue, leading to increased circulating estrogens and decreased serum hormone binding globulin levels.

Dietary Factors

The relationship of dietary factors to risk of cancer in women has long been of concern. For many years, it was hypothesized that dietary fat would have a major impact on breast cancer risk, based on animal data, international studies showing a correlation between per capita fat intake and breast cancer rates, temporal increases in breast cancer incidence paralleling higher rates of fat intake, and studies showing relatively rapid changes in breast cancer incidence when women migrated from low-incidence to high-incidence areas (presumably due to dietary changes). Analytic studies, however, have generally been unable to confirm much of an effect on breast cancer risk of dietary fat intake [13,14]. This may relate to the fact that most studies have been conducted in populations with homogenous diets, making it difficult to detect effects. In addition, the imprecision of dietary methodology tools is well recognized. Furthermore, most studies have focused on recent diet, while it may be adolescent diet that is more etiologically important.

In general, studies of the last decade have stressed the importance of considering the etiologic role of other dietary components for breast as well as other cancers. There is increasing evidence that various micronutrients might protect against various cancers. Ways in which foods are prepared have also become of concern, including potential effects of heterocyclic aromatic amines produced in meats cooked at high temperatures [15]. The effect of phytoestrogens on the risk of hormonally-related cancers has also been of intense recent interest [16]. Other examples of a broadening of nutritional assessment are studies which have suggested a possible effect of lactose intolerance on ovarian cancer risk [17] and of iron intake on colorectal cancer risk [18].

Despite abilities to relate most dietary constituents to breast cancer risk, alcohol consumption has been fairly consistently related [19]. Thus, in one meta-analysis, daily consumption of one alcoholic drink was associated with an 11 percent increase in breast cancer risk. The relationship is biologically plausible, given the recognized effects of alcohol on a variety of endogenous hormones. Of interest is that the effect of alcohol on breast cancer risk appears restricted to women with low levels of folate intake [20], supporting the notion that dietary relationships are complex and must consider many interrelated factors.

Physical Activity

The relationship of physical activity to risk of cancers in women has received recent widespread attention [21]. Although relationships with most cancer sites remain obscure, a potential effect is biologically plausible, through a number of proposed mechanisms. This includes the recognition that physical activity reduces body fat, which may affect hormonal conversion. Among individuals with intense activity, delay of menarche, amenorrhea, and anovulary cycles have been noted. Furthermore, reductions in luteal phase length and follicle stimulating hormone and progesterone levels have been recorded. Physical activity is also related to reduced insulin levels and altered response of the muscle to insulin. Furthermore, physical activity can lead to increased bowel motility, which has been proposed as a mediator for the effect on colorectal cancer risk [22].

Iatrogenic Agents

An important exposure among women is exogenous hormone use, including menopausal hormones. Although menopausal hormones are well recognized as increasing the risk of endometrial cancer, their relationship to breast cancer has been less well understood [23]. Results from a recent large meta-analysis support a modest increase with long-term use of estrogens [24]. However, estrogens are increasingly being prescribed in conjunction with progestins, given well-recognized benefits of this regimen against estrogen-induced endometrial hyperplasia and associated endometrial cancer [25]. Of concern is that progestins appear to have very different effects on endometrial than breast tissue. In endometrial tissue, progestogens counteract the epithelial proliferative effects of estrogens, but in breast tissue appear to act as mitogens, inducing cellular proliferation. This has led to the hypothesis that the combined therapy may be more hazardous to breast cancer risk than estrogens alone, a notion that has received some support from epidemiologic investigations [26-28].

In terms of cancer risk, there are a number of other concerns regarding possible iatrogenic agents, some of which have intensified over recent times. Ovulation stimulating drugs have been hypothesized to lead to a possible increase in the risk of ovarian cancer, although effects remain unresolved [29-31]. In addition, new hypotheses have arisen regarding other drugs, including tranquilizers, whose usage in women far exceeds that of men. Observations of an increase in ovarian cancer risk associated with these drugs merit further attention [32]. Fortunately, not all news about drugs is bad, with some medications having been linked with reductions in cancer risk. This includes possible reductions in colorectal and ovarian cancer with aspirin and other nonsteroidal anti-inflammatory drugs [33,34].

Environmental Agents

The effects of environmental agents have come under intense scrutiny, particularly given the widespread geographic variation in cancers, including a concentration of many cancers in highly industrialized areas [35]. For most cancers in women, there is little biologic evidence to support the notion that general environmental factors play a major etiologic role. However, recent observations have emphasized a possible etiologic role in various hormonally related cancers for a class of agents known as endocrine disruptors, including DDT, PCBs, and possibly some other chemicals. The relationship of these agents to cancer risk in women is currently unresolved, although certainly a topic of intense investigation [36-38].

Occupational Factors

In men, major etiologic clues regarding cancer have derived from studies of occupational exposures. However, in women, few occupational studies have been undertaken. This undoubtedly reflects the limited numbers of women that were actively employed in industrial occupations in past eras. However, given that increasing numbers of women are entering the workforce, studies are beginning to emerge suggesting that certain exposures merit attention, including possible effects of asbestos and metals on lung cancer risk [39,40], pharmaceutical and selected chemicals on breast cancer risk [41,42], and herbicides on ovarian cancer risk [43]. Although it may still be years before we are fully able to resolve effects in this country, research opportunities exist in many other countries where women have been actively employed for many years. A number of such investigations are currently underway, and results are awaited with great interest.

Genetic Susceptibility

This presentation would be remiss without reference to the revolution that has been made in identifying genetic determinants of risk. Foremost among the genetic advances are the identification of some major genes involved in the etiology of several cancers in women, including BRCA1 and BRCA2, the colorectal adenomatous polyposis gene (APC), and a variety of tumor suppressor genes (including p53). Although several of these genes are highly penetrant, i.e. individuals with the genes have a high likelihood of developing disease, it appears that the genes are relatively rare and explain only a relatively small proportion of cancer cases [44].

In addition to the identification of highly penetrant genes, advances have been made towards identifying a number of more common genetic polymorphisms involved in either carcinogen or hormone metabolism. Population studies evaluating the role of common polymorphisms are only beginning to emerge and it is unclear whether findings will have practical preventive implications. Nonetheless, it appears to be an exciting period of discovery and one that holds great promise for advancing our understanding of carcinogenic mechanisms. Particularly exciting are studies that attempt to integrate genetic markers with other identified disease risk factors, i.e. the assessment of gene-environment interactions. Some leads that have been pursued include interactive effects of cigarette smoking and N-acetyltransferase (NAT1 and NAT2) genotype on breast cancer risk [45,46], alcohol consumption and methylenetetrahydrofolate (MTHRF) genotype on colorectal cancer risk [47], and various reproductive and menstrual parameters and genes involved in hormone metabolism [48-49], including the cytochrome P450 P450c17α (CYP17) and catechol O-methyltransferase (COMT) enzymes, on risk of breast and endometrial cancers.

Future Research Directions

There are a number of research directions that may be useful in elucidating the causes of cancer in women. Given what we have learned about the etiology of cervical cancer from careful natural history studies, it would appear advantageous to use these as models for cancer sites where less is known about the progression of precursor conditions. Studies of factors involved in the progression of endometrial hyperplasias, benign ovarian tumors, proliferative breast diseases, and *in situ* cancers may be especially useful. Future studies may also benefit from careful assessments of the timing of exposures. Recent studies have clarified that weight gain late in life appears to be most predictive of breast cancer risk [50], but the timing of other exposures remains less clear, including dietary patterns and physical activity. The adolescent period has come under scrutiny as a possible window of opportunity, although the challenges in how to accurately measure such exposures for cancers that generally occur late in life are obvious [51]. Even more challenging is how to account for pre- and postnatal exposures, which have recently been postulated to also affect some cancers, including breast cancer [52,53]. Research has obviously greatly benefitted from the careful integration of molecular markers into epidemiologic studies, allowing more precise assessment of exposures as well as definition of disease subtypes. Nonetheless, descriptive studies should also not be overlooked, as they also can provide important clues regarding the etiology of diseases. In particular, most cancers in women show tremendous geographic variation, oftentimes as much as a 5-10-fold difference in incidence and/or mortality across countries. These studies may be especially useful in clarifying effects of dietary or genetic factors.

References

1. Devesa SS. Cancers in women. In: Goldman MB, Hatch MC, editors. Women and health. San Diego: Academic Press, 2000: 863-70.
2. Wu AH. Epidemiology of lung cancer in women. In: Goldman MB, Hatch MC, editors. Women and Health. San Diego: Academic Press, 2000: 949-61.
3. Zang EA, Wynder EL. Differences in lung cancer risk between men and women, examination of the evidence. J Natl Cancer Inst 1996;88:183-92.
4. Baron JA, Newcomb PA, Longnecker MP, et al. Cigarette smoking and breast cancer. Cancer Epidemiol Biomarker Prev 1996;5:399-403.
5. Lash TL, Aschengrau A. Active and passive cigarette smoking and the occurrence of breast cancer. Am J Epidemiol 1999;149:5-12.
6. Morabia A, Bernstein M, Heritier S, Khatchatrian N. Relation of breast cancer with passive and active exposure to tobacco smoke. Am J Epidemiol 1996;143:918-28.
7. Brinton LA, Barrett RJ, Berman ML, Mortel R, Twiggs LB, Wilbanks GD. Cigarette smoking and the risk of endometrial cancer. Am J Epidemiol 1993;137:281-91.
8. Parazzini F, La Vecchia C, Negri E, Moroni S, Chatenoud L. Smoking and risk of endometrial cancer: Results from an Italian case-control study. Gynecol Oncol 1995;56: 195-99.
9. Weiderpass E, Baron JA. Cigarette smoking, alcohol consumption and endometrial cancer risk: A population-based study in Sweden. Cancer Causes Control 2001;12:239-47.
10. Shoff SM, Newcomb PA. Diabetes, body size, and risk of endometrial cancer. Am J Epidemiol 1998;148:234-40.
11. Swanson CA, Potischman N, Wilbanks GD, et al. Relation of endometrial cancer risk to past and contemporary body size and body fat distribution. Cancer Epidemiol Biomarkers Prev 1993:2:321-27.
12. Van den Brandt PA, Spiegelman D, Yaun SS, et al. Pooled analysis of prospective cohort studies on height, weight, and breast cancer risk. Am J Epidemiol 2000;152:514-27.
13. Howe GR, Hirohata T, Hislop TG, et al. Dietary factors and risk of breast cancer: Combined analysis of 12 case-control studies. J Natl Cancer Inst 1990;82:561-69.
14. Hunter DJ, Spiegelman D, Adami H-O, et al. Cohort studies of fat intake and the risk of breast cancer—a pooled analysis. N Engl J Med 1996;334:358-61.
15. Zheng W, Gustafson DR, Sinha R, et al. Well-done meat intake and risk of breast cancer. J Natl Cancer Inst 1998;90:1724-29.
16. Davis SR, Dalais FS, Simpson ER, Murkies AL. Phytoestrogens in health and disease. Recent Prog Horm Res 1999;54:185-210.
17. Cramer DW, Harlow BL, Eillett WC, et al. Galactose consumption and metabolism in relation to the risk of ovarian cancer. Lancet 1989;2:66-71.
18. Wurzelmann JI, Silver A, Schreinemachers DM, Sandler RS, Everson RB. Iron intake and the risk of colorectal cancer. Cancer Epidemiol Biomarkers Prev 1996;5:503-7.
19. Longnecker MP. Alcoholic beverage consumption in relation to risk of breast cancer: meta-analysis and review. Cancer Causes Control 1994;5:73-82.
20. Zhang S, Hunter DJ, Hankinson SE, et al. A prospective study of folate intake and the risk of breast cancer. JAMA 1999;281:1632-37.
21. Friedenreich CM. Physical activity and cancer prevention: From observational to intervention research. Cancer Epidemiol Biomarkers Prev 2001;10:287-301.
22. Peters HP, De Vries WR, Vanberge-Henegouwen GP, Akkarmans LM. Potential benefits

and hazards of physical activity and exercise on the gastrointestinal tract. Gut 2001;48: 435-39.
23. Pike MC, Ross RK. Progestins and menopause: Epidemiologic studies of risks of endometrial and breast cancer. Steroids 2000;65:659-64.
24. Collaborative Group on Hormonal Factors in Breast Cancer. Breast cancer and hormonal contraceptives: Collaborative reanalysis of individual data on 53,297 women with breast cancer and 100,239 women without breast cancer from 54 epidemiological studies. Lancet 1996;347:1713-27.
25. Key TJA, Pike MC. The role of oestrogens and progestagens in the epidemiology and prevention of breast cancer. Eur J Cancer Clin Oncol 1988;24:29-43.
26. Colditz GA, Hankinson SE, Hunter DJ, et al. The use of estrogens and progestins and the risk of breast cancer in postmenopausal women. N Engl J Med 1995;332:1589-93.
27. Schairer C, Lubin J, Troisi R, Sturgeon S, Brinton L, Hoover R. Menopausal estrogen and estrogen-progestin replacement therapy and breast cancer risk. JAMA 2000;283:485-91.
28. Ross RK, Paganini-Hill A, Wan PC, Pike MC. Effect of hormone replacement therapy on breast cancer risk: Estrogen versus estrogen plus progestin. J Natl Cancer Inst 2000;92: 328-32.
29. Rossing MA, Daling JR, Weiss NS, Moore DE, Self SG. Ovarian tumors in a cohort of infertile women. N Engl J Med 1994;331:771-76.
30. Venn A, Watson L, Lumley J, et al. Breast and ovarian cancer incidence after infertility and in vitro fertilisation. Lancet 1995;346:995-1000.
31. Whittemore AS, Harris R, Itnyre J, the Collaborative Ovarian Cancer Group. Characteristics relating to ovarian cancer risk: Collaborative analysis of 12 US case-control studies. Am J Epidemiol 1992;136:1184-1203.
32. Harlow BL, Cramer DW, Baron JA, Titus-Ernstoff L, Greenberg ER. Psychotropic medication use and risk of epithelial ovarian. Cancer Epidemiol Biomarkers Prev 1998;7: 697-702.
33. Berkel HJ, Holcombe RF, Middlebrooks M, Kannan K. Nonsteroidal antiinflammatory drugs and colorectal cancer. Epidemiol Rev 1996;18:205-17.
34. Cramer DW, Harlow BL, Titus-Ernstoff L, Bohlke K, Welch WR, Greenberg ER. Over-the-counter analgesics and risk of ovarian cancer. Lancet 1998;351:104-7.
35. Sturgeon SR, Schairer C, Gail M, McAdams M, Brinton LA, Hoover Rn. Geographic variation in mortality from breast cancer among white women in the United States. J Natl Cancer Inst 1995;87:1846-52.
36. Woolf MS, Toniolo PG, Lee EW, et al. Blood levels of organochlorine residues and risk of breast cancer. J Natl Cancer Inst 1993;85:648-52.
37. Hoyer AP, Grandjean P, Jorgensen T, Brock JW, Hartvig HB. Organochlorine exposure and risk of breast cancer. Lancet 1998;352: 816-20.
38. Helzlsouer KJ, Alberg AJ, Huang H-Y, et al. Serum concentrations of organochlorine compounds and the subsequent development of breast cancer. Cancer Epidemiol Biomarkers Prev 1999;8:525-32.
39. Brownson RC, Alavanja MCR, Chang JC. Occupational risk factors for lung cancer among nonsmoking women, a case-control study in Missouri (United States). Cancer Causes Control 1993;4:449-54.
40. Wu-Williams AH, Xu ZY, Blot WJ, et al. Occupation and lung cancer risk among women in northern China. Am J Ind Med 1993;24:67-79.
41. Blair A, Hartge P, Stewart PA, McAdams M, Lubin J. Mortality and cancer incidence of

aircraft maintenance workers exposed to trichloroethlene and other organic solvents and chemicals: Extended follow-up. Occup Environ Med J 1998;55:161-71.
42. Goldberg MS, Labreche F. Occupational risk factors for female breast cancer: A review. J Occup Environ Med 1996;53:145-56.
43. Donna A, Crosignani P, Robutti F, et al. Triazine herbicides and ovarian epithelial neoplasms. Scand J Work Environ Health 1989;15:47-53.
44. Streuwing JP, Hartge P, Wacholder S, et al. The risk of cancer associated with mutations of BRCA1 and BRCA2 among Ashkenazi Jews. N Engl J Med 1997;336:1401-8.
45. Ambrosone CB, Freudenheim JL, Graham S, et al. Cigarette smoking, N-acetyltransferase 2 genetic polymorphisms, and breast cancer risk. JAMA 1996;276:1494-1501.
46. Zheng W, Deitz AC, Campbell DR, et al. N-acetyltransferase 1 genetic polymorphism, cigarette smoking, well-done meat intake, and breast cancer risk. Cancer Epidemiol Biomarkers Prev 1999;8:233-39.
47. Ma J, Stampfer MJ, Giovannucci E, et al. Methylenetetrahydrofolate reductase polymorphism, dietary interactions, and risk of colorectal cancer. Cancer Res 1997;57:1098-1102.
48. Huang CS, Chern HD, Chang KJ, Cheng CW, Hus SM, Shen CY. Breast cancer risk associated with genotype polymorphisms of the estrogen-metabolizing genes CYP17, CYP1A1, and COMT: A multigenic study on cancer susceptibility. Cancer Res 1999;59: 4870-75.
49. Haiman CA, Hankinson SE, Colditz GA, Hunter DJ, De Vivo I. A polymorphism in CYP17 and endometrial cancer risk. Cancer Res 2001;61:3955-60.
50. Ballard-Barbash R. Anthropometry and breast cancer. Body size—a moving target. Cancer 1994;74:1090-1100.
51. Coliditz GA, Frazier AL. Models of breast cancer show that risk is set by events of early life: Prevention efforts must shift focus. Cancer Epidemiol Biomarkers Prev 1995;4:567-71.
52. Hilakivi-Clarke L, Clarke R, Lippman ME. Perinatal factors increase breast cancer risk. Breast Cancer Res Treat 1994;31:273-84.
53. Trichopoulos D. Is breast cancer initiated in utero? Epidemiology 1990;1:95-96.

GROWTH FACTORS AND CANCER – THE ROLE OF INSULIN-LIKE GROWTH FACTORS

Herbert Yu

Introduction

A large group of growth factors with important biological functions have been identified and characterized. Many of the growth factors regulate fundamental cellular activities, such as cell proliferation, differentiation, transformation, and programmed cell death. These cellular activities are not only crucial for normal cell function, but also involved in the process of many diseases. Growth factors have been found to play pivotal roles in cancer development and progression. Evidence suggests that insulin-like growth factors (IGFs) are especially important in this aspect [1,2]. The importance of IGFs in cancer is not only because they have profound impacts on cell proliferation and apoptosis, but also because they are influenced by our lifestyles. In this presentation, findings of the effect of IGFs on cancer from laboratory experiments and epidemiological studies are briefly reviewed. Based on the findings and other evidence, a new hypothesis is proposed that explains the possible role of IGFs in linking our lifestyles, high-energy diet, and low physical activity, to insulin resistance, diabetes, and increased risk of several common cancers in Western societies.

Insulin-Like Growth Factors (IGFs)

Insulin-like growth factors include two members, IGF-I and IGF-II. The two molecules are small polypeptides with single chain structure and substantial homology to each other [3]. Functionally, IGFs exert insulin-like anabolic action on carbohydrate and protein metabolism. In addition to the acute action, IGFs also have long-term effects on cell proliferation, differentiation, and apoptosis [4]. The effect of IGFs on cell activities is regulated by a large group of molecules, including growth hormone, steroid hormones, and other growth factors. The action of IGFs is mediated by a specific receptor called the IGF-I receptor (IGF-IR), which is a cell membrane receptor with tyrosine kinase activity.

Binding of IGFs to IGF-IR activates the enzyme which triggers two signal transduction pathways [5]. One is the MAP kinase-involved signal transduction pathway which is responsible for the mitogenic action of IGFs; the other pathway involves PI-3 kinase which mediates the anti-apoptotic effect of IGFs.

The IGF-I receptor has a similar structure to the insulin receptor, both of which are tetramers with two identical α chains and two identical β chains. Both IGFs and insulin are able to interact with these receptors. The two receptors are able to form a hybrid receptor which consists of half of the insulin receptor and half of the IGF-I receptor [5]. The hybrid receptor mediates the effect of IGFs [6]. The presence of the receptor may be the key linking Western lifestyle, i.e. high-energy diet and low physical activity, to high risk of several cancers and other health problems.

The interaction between IGFs and the IGF-I receptor is regulated by a group of IGF binding proteins. There are six specific IGF binding proteins, named IGFBP-1 through IGFBP-6 [7]. IGFBPs have both IGF-dependent and IGF-independent actions. With regard to IGF-dependent action, IGFBPs regulate the interaction between IGFs and IGF-IR, protect IGFs from degradation, and transport IGFs to local tissue. The effect of IGFBPs can result in either suppression of IGF actions by blocking the interaction between IGFs and IGF-IR or potentiation of IGF actions by increasing their bioavailability in target tissues. The dual regulatory effect of IGFBPs on IGFs is mainly determined by the molecular structure of the IGF binding proteins. IGFBPs undergo substantial post-translational modification, including phosphorylation and proteolysis. There exist a large group of IGFBP proteases which can indirectly regulate the action of IGFs. A lot of antiproliferative molecules exert their actions through interacting with IGFBPs to antagonize the mitogenic action of IGFs.

IGFs and Cancer

A large body of evidence has indicated that IGFs play an important role in cancer development and progression. Laboratory experiments show that both IGF-I and IGF-II are strong mitogens for a wide variety of cancer cells [1,8]. The mitogenic effect of IGFs is mediated mainly by cyclin D1 which is a regulatory subunit of cyclin-dependent kinase (CDK) [9]. Binding of cyclin D1 to CDKs activates the kinase which accelerates cell cycle from G1 to S phases. Studies have shown cyclin D1 is over-expressed in many types of cancer and that the effect of cyclin D1 can be suppressed by tumor suppressor gene products [10].

In addition to mitogenic stimulation, IGFs also suppress cell apoptotic pathway to enhance their effect on cell proliferation. IGFs inhibit Bax expression and stimulate the expression of Bcl proteins to increase Bax/Bcl heterodimer which inhibits the initiation of the apoptotic pathway [11]. The IGF-I receptor is also involved in cell transformation induced by tumor virus and oncogene products [12].

Besides their independent effects on cell proliferation and apoptosis, IGFs also interact with a large number of molecules involved in cancer development or progression. IGFs have synergistic interaction with other mitogenic molecules, such as EGF and estrogens [13,14]. IGFs mediate the mitogenic effects of tumor viruses and stimulate the expression of VEGF to enhance angiogenesis [15,16]. IGFs also antagonize the effect of antiproliferative molecules, including TGF-β, vitamin D, and retinoic acid [17,18], and counteract the action of tumor suppressor gene products, such as p53, WT1, PTEN, and BRCA1 [19-22].

Findings from epidemiological studies further support the involvement of IGFs in cancer. Two case-control studies nested from two large prospective cohorts show that high levels of IGF-I in plasma are associated with increased risk of colorectal cancer both in men and women [23,24]. Women with high IGF-I have a 2-fold increase in colorectal cancer risk compared to those with low IGF-I. There is also an inverse association between IGFBP-3 and colorectal cancer; high IGFBP-3 is associated with low risk of colorectal cancer. The important feature of these studies is that the blood samples used for IGF test were collected before the diagnosis of the disease. Therefore, the level of IGF-I is less likely to be affected the disease status.

The relationship between circulating IGF-I and breast cancer was examined in two nested case-control study [25,26]. The study found that plasma levels of IGF-I were associated with breast cancer risk. Women with high IGF-I had 2- to 3-fold increase in breast cancer risk compared to those with low IGF-I. This association, however, was seen only among premenopausal women. No association was found in postmenopausal women. In these studies, no significant association was found for IGFBP-3. The possible link between IGF-I and breast cancer risk has also been observed in a number of case-control studies, including our own studies [27-31]. One of our studies suggests that free IGF-I is more strongly associated with breast cancer risk than total IGF-I [30]. Functionally, free IGF-I is more biologically active than bound IGF-I because free IGF-I can freely cross blood vessel and directly interact with its receptor. Our study also found high plasma levels of IGF-I to be associated with increased risk of breast cancer in Chinese women [31]. Similar to the findings in Caucasians, this association was more evident in premenopausal women. In contrast to the findings in Caucasians, our study found a strong positive association between IGFBP-3 and breast cancer risk; high IGFBP-3 was associated with increased risk of breast cancer. The reason for the inconsistent finding of IGFBP-3 in relation to breast cancer risk remains to be determined.

In addition to colorectal cancer and breast cancer, epidemiological studies also found high circulating IGF-I to be associated with increased risk of prostate and lung cancers [32,33]. Overall, most human studies have demonstrated that IGF-I is associated with the risk of several common cancers in Western societies. However, the association between IGFBP-3 and cancer risk has not been found consistently in epidemiological studies. This inconsistency may support the findings of laboratory experiments which suggest IGFBP-3 having dual regulatory effect on IGF action. In addition, the inconsistency may also indicate the effect of our lifestyle on the IGF binding protein or as a whole on the IGF family.

IGFs and Lifestyle

Lifestyle factors, especially diet, have a significant impact on IGF-I levels in the circulation. Studies have showed that children suffering from malnutrition have significantly low levels of serum IGF-I and that the level could be restored back to normal in response to improvement in nutrition [34]. Similar results are also found in animal experiments. Circulating levels of IGF-I were declined in mice when the animals were put on diet, either restriction on total energy intake or protein intake. Lifting the restriction could restore normal IGF-I concentration in the circulation of the animals. Moreover, It has been shown in animal experiments that restriction on total energy intake slows down tumor growth and reduces the risk of developing new tumors [35]. This inhibitory effect of energy restriction on tumor growth is correlated with IGF-I concentrations in the circulation [36]. Finally, IGF-I administration can abolish the inhibitory effect of energy restriction on tumor growth [37].

Dietary habit and lifestyle are substantially different between Caucasians and Chinese women. To assess the impact of diet and lifestyle on IGF, we made a preliminary comparison on circulating levels of IGF-I between the two populations. The results of our comparison indicate that plasma levels of IGF-I are 20-40% higher in Caucasian women from the Nurses' Health Study [25] than in Chinese women from our study [31].

All these observations lead to the speculation that IGF may link certain lifestyles to cancer risk [2]. High-energy diet increases the expression of IGF-I which results in high IGF activity. High IGF activity subsequently stimulates cell proliferation and suppresses apoptosis. High proliferating cells tend to suffer extensive oxidative stress due to the large consumption of energy to maintain the activity of cell replication. Oxidative stress is an endogenous source of DNA damage and is associated with cancer risk. Low cell death rate is also in favor of cancer development because it allows vulnerable and unhealthy cells to survive, which increases their chance for transformation. With the combination of high cell proliferation and low apoptosis, it is conceivable that cancer risk can be elevated. However, this initial speculation may underestimate the importance of IGF in cancer. Based on emerging evidence, the IGF family may have a much more profound impact on our health.

It is known that Western lifestyle characterized by high-energy diet and low physical activity is associated with, in addition to cancer, several other health problems, including overweight, obesity, insulin resistance, and diabetes. These health problems are also associated with cancer risk. Furthermore, animal experiments and human studies demonstrate that reducing energy intake and increasing physical activity can reduce cancer risk and improve the condition of insulin resistance and diabetes. Despite the recognition of all the associations, the underlying mechanism remains unknown. Since these conditions and lifestyle factors are highly interrelated to one another, dissecting the relationships to evaluate the effect of each individual condition or factor on cancer risk is difficult.

New Hypothesis

Based on the improvement in our understanding of IGF, insulin and their receptors, it is now possible for us to propose a new hypothesis that may explain all the associations under one biological mechanism. The main issue regarding Western lifestyle is high-energy diet and low physical activity. The combination of the two creates a fundamental problem, positive energy imbalance. This problem is featured by (a) a huge surplus and (b) a sustained imbalance. These conditions impose a huge pressure on our energy metabolism system in terms of balancing energy intake and expenditure. Increasing energy storage and accelerating expenditure are the only ways to remove excess energy. Insulin and IGFs are the systems in our body dealing with energy homeostasis. The insulin system is mainly responsible for energy distribution and storage, and the IGF system takes care of energy expenditure through increasing the number of cells. The two systems work coordinately to maintain energy homeostasis.

The effect of insulin and IGF-I is mediated through their receptors, and besides the insulin receptor and IGF-I receptor, there exists another receptor, the insulin/IGF-I hybrid receptor. This hybrid receptor has higher binding affinity to IGF-I and mainly mediates the effect of IGF-I. Formation of the hybrid receptor is a dynamic process depending upon the balance of energy intake and expenditure. Features of the hybrid receptor suggest that this receptor may play a critical role in the development of health problems related to positive energy imbalance. Positive energy imbalance creates a pressure on energy metabolism. Initially, this pressure is handled mainly by the insulin system. To maintain energy homeostasis, most excess energy is stored by the insulin-dominant energy metabolism. Because of this, overweight and obesity are developed as the first sign of the problem. As the problem prolongs, the energy metabolism system undergoes changes to adjust for the mounting pressure of energy imbalance. The system gradually shifts from the insulin-dominant energy metabolism to the IGF-dominant energy metabolism. From the energy homeostatic point of view, the change increases the efficiency of the system to remove excess energy, but however, this shift also creates problems, which are insulin resistance and high cell growth rate.

Although long-term positive energy imbalance could cause increases in IGF-I expression and IGF-IR activity, these changes are relatively minor compared to the overall IGF activity. The major change could be the formation of the insulin/IGF-I receptor. The increase in the presence of this receptor will result in two bad consequences. First, the number of insulin receptors is reduced and/or the function of insulin receptors is adversely affected due to the formation and/or presence of the hybrid receptor. Second, the effect of IGF-I is dramatically amplified by the receptor. All these lead to insulin resistance and high cell proliferation. Insulin resistance is characterized by hyperinsulinemia and dyslipidemias that are further linked to hypertension, type 2 diabetes, and all kinds of cardiovascular disorders. High cell proliferation accompanied by low apoptosis increases cancer risk.

Evidence also suggests that these changes are reversible at an early stage. Energy restriction could reduce the pressure of positive energy imbalance, lowering the effect of IGFs. Physical exercise also helps to lower the pressure by stimulating energy expenditure. Energy consumption by the muscle requires insulin to store energy, which stimulates the presence of insulin receptor and reduces the hybrid receptor. Lowering the level of the hybrid receptor and increasing insulin receptors could reverse the condition of insulin resistance and diminish the effect of IGFs. All these changes will help to reduce cancer risk and to improve the condition of insulin resistance.

In summary, IGFs have direct impacts on cancer through their mitogenic and anti-apoptotic effects on cells. IGFs also have synergistic interaction with other mitogenic and carcinogenic molecules and antagonize the effect of antiproliferative molecules and tumor suppressor gene products. The expression and action of IGFs are affected by our lifestyle factors, and therefore, IGFs may link our lifestyle to cancer risk. Potentially, IGFs and their receptors can be used as biomarkers for disease prevention and risk assessment.

References

1. Macaulay VM. Insulin-like growth factors and cancer. Br J Cancer 1992;65:311-20.
2. Yu H, Rohan T. Role of the insulin-like growth factor family in cancer development and progression. J Natl Cancer Inst 2000;92:1472-89.
3. Sara VR, Hall K. Insulin-like growth factors and their binding proteins. Physiol Rev 1990; 70:591-614.
4. Jones JI, Clemmons DR. Insulin-like growth factors and their binding proteins: Biological actions. Endocr Rev 1995;16:3-34.
5. LeRoith D, Werner H, Beitner-Johnson D, Roberts CT. Molecular and cellular aspects of the insulin-like growth factor I receptor. Endocr Rev 1995;16:143-613.
6. Seely BL, Reichart DR, Takata Y, Yip C, Olefsky JM. A functional assessment of insulin/insulin-like growth factor-I hybrid receptors. Endocrinology 1995;136:635-41.
7. Kelley KM, Oh Y, Gargosky SE, et al. Insulin-like growth factor-binding proteins (IGFBPs) and their regulatory dynamics. Int J Biochem Cell Biol 1996;28:619-37.
8. Toretsky A, Helman LJ. Involvement of IGF-II in human cancer. J Endocrinol 1996;149: 367-72.
9. Furlanetto RW, Harwell SE, Frick KK. Insulin-like growth factor-I induces cyclin-D1 expression in MG63 human osteosarcoma cells in vitro. Mol Endocrinol 1994;8:510-17.
10. Weinstein IB. Disorders in cell circuitry during multistage carcinogenesis: The role of homeostasis. Carcinogenesis 2000;21:857-64.
11. Minshall C, Arkins S, Straza J, et al. IL-4 and insulin-like growth factor-I inhibit the decline in Bcl-2 and promote the survival of IL-3-deprived myeloid progenitors. J Immunol 1997;159:1225-32.
12. Sepp-Lorenzino L. Structure and function of the insulin-like growth factor I receptor. Breast Cancer Res Treat 1998;47:235-53.
13. Hembree JR, Agarwal C, Eckert RL. Epidermal growth factor suppresses insulin-like growth factor binding protein 3 levels in human papilomavirus type 16-immortalized cervical epithelial cells and thereby potentiates the effects of insulin-like growth factor 1. Cancer Res 1994;54:3160-66.
14. Ruan W, Catanese V, Wieczorek R, Feldman M, Kleinberg DL. Estrodiol enhances the stimulatory effect of insulin-like growth factor-I (IGF-I) on mammary development and growth hormone-induced IGF-I messenger ribonucleic acid. Endocrinology 1995;136: 1296-1302.
15. Kim SO, Park JG, Lee YI. Increased expression of the insulin-like growth factor I (IGF-I) receptor gene in hepatocellular carcinoma cell lines: implications of IGF-I receptor gene activation by hepatitis B virus X gene product. Cancer Res 1996;56:3831-36.
16. Bermont L, Lamielle F, Fauconnet S, Esumi H, Weisz A, Adessi GL. Regulation of vascular endothelial growth factor expression by insulin-like growth factor expression in endometrial adenocarcinoma cells. Int J Cancer 2000;85:117-23.
17. Gucev ZS, Oh Y, Kelley KM, Rosenfeld RG. Insulin-like growth factor binding protein 3 mediates retinoic acid- and transforming growth factor b2-induced growth inhibition in human breast cancer cells. Cancer Res 1996;56:1545-50.
18. Huynh H, Pollak M, Zhang JC. Regulation of insulin-like growth factor (IGF) II and IGF binding protein 3 autocrine loop in human PC-3 prostate cancer cells by vitamin D metabolite 1, 25 (OH) 2D3 and its analog EB1089. Int J Oncol 1998;13:137-43.
19. Buckbinder L, Talbott R, Velasco-Miguel S, et al. Induction of the growth inhibitor IGF-

binding protein 3 by p53. Nature 1995;377:646-49.
20. Werner H, Rauscher FJ 3rd, Sukhatme VP, Drummond IA, Roberts CT Jr, LeRoith D. Transcriptional repression of the insulin-like growth factor I receptor (IGF-I-R) gene by the tumor suppressor WT1 involves binding to sequences both upstream and downstream of the IGF-I-R gene transcription start site. J Biol Chem 1994;269:12577-82.
21. Wick W, Furnari FB, Naumann U, Cavenee WK, Weller M. PTEN gene transfer in human malignant glioma: sensitization to irradiation and CD95L-induced apoptosis. Oncogene 1999;18:3936-43.
22. Maor SB, Abramovitch S, Erdos MR, Brody LC, Werner H. BRCA1 suppresses insulin-like growth factor-I receptor promoter activity: Potential interaction between BRCA1 and Sp1. Mol Genet Metab 2000;69:130-36.
23. Ma J, Pollak MN, Giovannucci E, et al. Prospective study of colorectal cancer risk in men and plasma levels of insulin-like growth factor (IGF)-1 and IGF-binding protein-3. J Natl Cancer Inst 1999;91:620-25.
24. Giovannucci E, Pollak MN, Platz EA, et al. A prospective study of plasma insulin-like growth factor-1 and binding protein-3 and risk of colorectal neoplasia in women. Cancer Epidemiol Biomarkers Prev 2000;9:345-49.
25. Hankinson SE, Willett WC, Colditz GA, et al. Circulating concentrations of insulin-like growth factor-1 and risk of breast cancer. Lancet 1998;351:1393-96.
26. Toniolo P, Bruning PF, Akhmedkhanov A, et al. Serum insulin-like growth factor-I and breast cancer. Int J Cancer 2000;88:828-32.
27. Bruning PF, van Doorn J, Bonfrèr MG, et al. Insulin-like growth-factor binding protein 3 is decreased in early-stage operable pre-menopausal breast cancer. Int J Cancer 1995;62: 266-70.
28. Bohlke K, Cramer DW, Trichopoulos D, Mantzoros CS. Insulin-like growth factor-1 in relation to premenopausal ductal carcinoma in situ of the breast. Epidemiol 1998;9:570-73.
29. Agurs-Collins T, Adams-Campbell L, Kim KS, Cullen KJ. Insulin-like growth factor-1 and breast cancer risk in postmenopausal African-American women. Cancer Detect Prev 2000; 24:199-206.
30. Li BDL, Khosravi MJ, Berkel HJ, et al. Free insulin-like growth factor-I and breast cancer risk. Int J Cancer 2001;91:736-39.
31. Yu H, Jin F, Li B, Shu XO, Dia Q, Berkel H, Zheng W. Insulin-like growth factors and breast cancer risk in Chinese women (abstract). Am J Epidemiol 2001;153(Suppl.):S108.
32. Chan JM, Stampfer MJ, Giovannucci E, et al. Plasma insulin-like growth factor-1 and prostate cancer risk: a prospective study. Science 1998;279:563-66.
33. Yu H, Spitz MR, Mistry J, Gu J, Hong Wk, Wu X. Plasma levels of insulin-like growth factor-1 and lung cancer risk: a case-control study. J Natl Cancer Inst 1999;91:151-56.
34. Thissen JP, Ketelslegers JM, Underwood LE. Nutritional regulation of the insulin-like growth factors. Endocr Rev 1994;15:80-163.
35. Kritchevsky D. Caloric restriction and experimental carcinogenesis. Adv Exp Med Biol 1992;322:134-41.
36. Mukherjee P, Sotnikov AV, Mangian HJ, Zhou JR, Visek WJ, Clinton SK. Energy intake and prostate tumor growth, angiogenesis, and vascular endothelial growth factor expression. J Natl Cancer Inst 1999;91:512-23.
37. Dunn SE, Kari FW, French J, et al. Dietary restriction reduces insulin-like growth factor I levels, which modulates apoptosis, cell proliferation, and tumor progression in p53-deficient mice. Cancer Res 1997;57:4667-72.

Postmenopausal Hormone Use and Endometrial Cancer: Reassessment of the Epidemiological Data

Gijs A. van Unnik, Curt W. Burger, and Peter Kenemans

Introduction

Cancer of the uterine corpus is the most common pelvic malignancy in women today. As estimated by the American Cancer Society, it accounted for around 36,000 new cases in the United States in 2000, thus affecting 1 in 38 women in their lifetime. More than 95% of these cancers are endometrial carcinomas. Even among Western industrialized countries, annual incidence rates vary substantially, from 10 per 100,000 in Spain to 25 per 100,000 in the U.S.A. The incidence increases steadily with age before reaching a peak between 70 and 74 years [1]. Incidence rates have declined since the early seventies, parallelling the popularity of unopposed estrogen replacement therapy [2].

Female Sex Hormones and Cancer Risk

A well-documented effect of estrogens on the endometrium is an increase in mitotic activity, leading to proliferation and growth of occult, pre-existing tumors [3]. In addition, estrogens by inducing incessant mitoses, could increase the risk of DNA damage to occur, that is not adequately repaired. Estrogens thus could possibly also lead to the development of a new endometrial carcinoma [4]. Progestagens, however, reverse the proliferating endometrium into a mere secretory, nonmitotic state. This counteraction of progestins on the estrogen-primed endometrium is the result of various mechanisms, including reduction in nuclear estrogen receptors, suppression of DNA synthesis, and reduction of the availability of estrogens by stimulating the conversion of potent estradiol (E2) into the weaker estrone (E3), and its sulfate [4,5]. Consequently, conditions accompanied by a shift in the estrogen/progestin balance towards a predominance of estrogens potentially increase endometrial cancer risk, whereas a predominance of progestin could have a protective effect.

It is therefore not surprising that important risk factors for endometrial cancer involve any excessive or prolonged E2 exposure, and/or a relatively short exposure to progestagens: obesity, nulliparity, early menarche, late menopause, Stein-Leventhal syndrome, and theca-granulosa cell tumors [6-10]. Hypertension and diabetes mellitus are also positively associated with endometrial cancer risk, but this might merely be the result of a higher prevalence of these disease entities in older, obese women [11].

Hormonal subfertility is often characterized by anovulation or infrequent ovulations (resulting in a prolonged follicular phase) or an insufficient functioning of the corpus luteum (resulting in a progesterone deficiency). Thus, it was no surprise to find subfertility to be associated with an elevated risk of endometrial cancer [12]. An increased risk was not only found for subfertility *per se*, but also for the use of fertility drugs. However, the number of reports on this matter is small and their outcomes are susceptible to confounding effects, such as nulliparity and low use of oral contraception (OC) [13-15], and therefore inconclusive [12].

In addition to endogenous estrogens, exogenous estrogens have been related with endometrial cancer too. In the late sixties, interest had already been aroused in this matter, but at that time no definite conclusions were drawn [16]. In 1975, two case-control studies were published reporting a significant increase in relative risk (RR) of endometrial cancer in women who ever used unopposed estrogen replacement therapy (ERT), when compared to never-users [17,18]. In the years that followed, many case-control and cohortstudies confirmed this increase in risk, which turned out to be higher with longer duration of use [19]. Not only ERT, but also sequential OC use, i.e. estrogen alone followed by progestagen, seemed to be associated with an increased risk of endometrial cancer [20,21]. (Interestingly, this association was not found for combined OC, which is consistently associated with a substantial reduction of endometrial cancer risk. [22-25].)

In this review we will focus on the effect of different hormone replacement therapy (HRT) regimens on endometrial cancer risk. As will be discussed, addition of a progestagen leads to a much lower risk than supplementation with estrogens alone. However, the exact scheme by which progestagens are being administered (sequentially or continuously, more than 10 days per cycle or less than 10 days per cycle, monthly or long-cycle) and probably also the type of progestagen, have substantial impact on the ultimate endometrial effect. In this respect, we will address the results of the most relevant studies and some promising new HRT schemes will be discussed. Finally, we will discuss the data available for HRT use in women who have been treated for endometrial cancer.

ERT and Endometrial Cancer

There is a large body of evidence showing a consistent, positive association between ERT use and endometrial cancer risk, both for current and for previous use. Table 1 summarizes the 15 most recent case-control and cohort studies [26-40]. In 1995, Grady et al. published a meta-analysis [41] that analyzed 30 studies with adequate controls and risk estimates including 4 studies from Table 1 [28-31]. This analysis resulted in a relative risk (RR) estimation of 2.3 (95% confidence interval (CI): 2.1-2.5) for ever-users of ERT compared with never-users [41]. In this meta-analysis, the RR was higher with longer duration of exposure, increasing approximately 1.0 for each year of use, up to 9.5 (95% CI: 7.4-12.3) for more than 10 years of treatment. The large cohort study by Paganini-Hill et al. even reports a RR of 20 (95% CI: 7.2-54) for more than 15 years of ERT [26].

Studies addressing the effect of different dosages of estrogens used fail to show a

Table 1. Case-control Studies and Cohort Studies on HRT and Endometrial Cancer

Case-control studies	Cases Patients / controls	ERT (previous use) RR (95% CI)	ERT (long-term use) RR (95% CI)	Dose used (mg) of ERT RR (95% CI)	ERT (current use) RR (95% CI)	HRT (SC[b]/ CC[c]) RR (95% CI)
Rubin 1990[28]	196/986	1.9 (1.3-2.8)	6y[a]: 3.5 (1.7-7.4)	0.625: 1.2 (0.5-2.7)1.25: 3.8 (1.7-8.5)		
Voigt 1991[29]	158/182	3.1 (1.6-5.8)	3y[a]: 5.7 (2.5-12.8)			1.3 (0.6-2.8)
Brinton 1993[30]	300/207	3.0 (1.7-5.1)	10y[a]: 16.1 (5.1-50.5)	0.3: 2.8 (0.4-19) 0.625: 4.0 (1.6-9.9) 1.25: 2.8 (0.9-8.6)		1.8 (0.6-4.9)
Jick 1993[31]	172/1720		5y[a]: 22.0 (6.5-74.1)	0.3: 4.3 (1.2-16) 0.625: 7.1 (2.8-17.6) 1.25: 8.4 (2.0-36.5)	6.5 (3.1-13.3)	1.9 (0.9-3.8)
Pike 1997[32]	833/791		1-5y[a]: 2.2 (1.9-2.5)		2.2 (p<0.0001)	1-5y[a]: SC: 1.1 (0.8-1.4) CC: 1.1 (0.8-1.4)
Beresford 1997[33]	832/1114				4.0 (3.1-5.1)	1.4 (1.0-1.9)
Weiderpass 1999[35]	789/3368		oral E3, 1-5y[a]: 3.0 (2.0-4.4) vaginal E3, 1-5y[a]: 1.2 (0.9-1.7)			
Weiderpass 1999[36]	687/3270		<5y[a]: 2.2 (1.1-4.6) >5y[a]: 6.6 (3.6-12.0) >10y[a]: 9.2 (4.4-19.4)			SC: <5y[a]: 1.5 (1.0-2.2) >5y[a]: 2.9 (1.8-4.6) CC: >5y[a]: 0.2 (0.1-0.8)
Parslov 2000[37]	237/538					1-5y[a]: 3.1 (1.4-7.0) >5y[a]: 2.8 (0.7-11.6)
Jain 2000[38]	512/513		<3y[a]: 1.3 (0.8-2.2) >3y[a]: 4.2 (2.2-7.7)		2.2 (1.5-3.4)	SC: <3y[a]: 0.6 (0.3-1.1) >3y[a]: 1.5 (0.9-2.4) CC: 1.5 (0.7-3.4)
Hill 2000[39]	969/1325					SC: 0.4 (0.2-1.1) CC: 0.6 (0.3-1.3)

Table 1 Continued. Case-control Studies and Cohort Studies on HRT and Endometrial Cancer

Cohort Studies	Cohort / patients					
Paganini-Hill 1989[26]	5160/50	10 (n.r.)[d]	15y[a]: 20 (7.2-54)	0.625: 15 (n.r.)[d] 1.25: 11 (n.r.)[d]	25 (9.2-69)	
Persson 1989[27]	23244/74	1.4 (1.1-1.9)	>6y[a]: 1.8 (1.1-3.2)			0.9 (0.4-2.0)
Persson 1999[34]	8438/66		>6y[a]: 4.2 (2.1-8.4)		<6y*: 0.9 (0.3-2.5)	<6y[a]: 1.1 (0.4-3.1) >6y[a]: 1.4 (0.6-3.3)
Pukkala 2001[40]	15956cy[e] / 78549cy[e]					1 mnth[f]: 1.3 (1.1-1.6) 3 mnth[f]: 2.0 (1.6-2.6)

a. Years of use; b. continuously combined; c. sequentially combined; d. not reported;
e. cycles; f. monthly

significant dose-related increase of endometrial cancer risk [26,28,30,31]. This lack of association was also found in four older studies not listed in Table 1 [42-45] and also in the meta-analysis by Grady et al [41]. Apparently, in the genesis of endometrial carcinoma, duration of estrogen exposure is more important than dose. However, we should take into account, that the absence of an obvious dose-effect might be due to a lack of power, since confidence intervals are wide in all studies cited. Moreover, in the CHART study, a 2-year randomized trial, biopsies showed significantly higher rates of hyperplastic endometrial changes with higher dosages of estrogens (1, 2.5, 5, and 10 μg of ethinyl estradiol, respectively) [46].

Whether (unopposed) estrogens are administered on a continuous or interrupted basis (with a stop week every cycle), it does not have any effect on endometrial cancer risk: similar risks for both regimens were reported in various studies [41,44,45].

Persistence of Effect

There is strong evidence to show that endometrial cancer risk related to ERT use remains increased for many years after discontinuation of therapy. Table 2 shows the results of 6 case-control studies, 1 cohort study and 1 meta-analysis, all finding a persistently increased endometrial cancer risk up to 15 years after cessation of ERT [26,32,41,43,45,47-49].

Table 2. Relative Risk of Developing Endometrial Cancer after Discontinuation of Therapy Compared with Never Users

	Design	Years after stopping ERT	RR (95% CI)
Mack 1976 [47]	case-control	> 2 years	3.4 (1.3-8.6)
Weiss 1979 [43]	case-control	3-7 years	3.8 (1.5-9.5)
Buring 1986 [45]	case-control	> 5 years	4.5 (1.1-19)
Levi 1993 [48]	case-control	> 10 years	2.3 (1.2-4.5)
Green 1996 [49]	case-control	> 8 years	1.6 (1.1-2.3)
Pike 1997 [32]	case-control	> 10 years	1.6 (1.0-2.5)
Paganini-Hill 1989 [26]	cohort	> 15 years	5.8 (2.0-17)
Grady 1995 [41]	meta-analysis	> 5 years	2.3 (1.8-3.1)

ERT and Endometrial Cancer Mortality

The overall prognosis of endometrial cancer is good, with a 5-year survival rate of 73% [11], since most patients present with early stage disease. Most of the times, the typical symptoms (abnormal bleeding and vaginal discharge) are easily recognized leading to little delay by patient or doctor. Moreover, women using ERT tend to be monitored on a regular basis possibly even resulting in the disease to be diagnosed in a presymptomatic stage. This means that the increased cancer risks mentioned earlier apply in particular to morbidity due to endometrial cancer, rather than to mortality. Mortality rates of endometrial cancer among ERT users are estimated to be not significantly different from those of never-users: RR 2.7 (95% CI: 0.9-8.0) [41]. An additional explanation for the difference in morbidity and mortality rates lies in the fact that hormone-induced carcinomas of the endometrium seem actually biologically different from "spontaneous" endometrial carcinomas [50,51]. In 1983, Bokhman postulated the existence of two different pathogenic types of endometrial carcinoma [52]. The first type (endometrioid carcinoma, type I carcinoma) arises from hyperplastic precursors in a relatively hyperestrogenic state. In general, these are well-differentiated tumors being sensitive to progestational therapy. The second type (serous carcinoma, type II carcinoma) develops and grows largely unrelated to estrogens and it tends to lack responsiveness to progestagens [11]. Estrogen therapy may primarily promote growth of type I carcinomas thus only leading to a very modest increase in endometrial cancer mortality, if any increase at all. This view is supported by data from large cohort studies finding no increased mortality due to (endometrial) cancer for ERT users [53,54].

HRT and Endometrial Cancer

Progestagens are able to prevent the development of endometrial hyperplasia and carcinoma [55]. In the early eighties, it became routine to prescribe combined estrogen-progestagen replacement therapy (hormone replacement therapy, HRT) to nonhysterectomized women leading to a considerable decline in endometrial cancer incidence [2]. However, the question whether the increase in risk of endometrial cancer associated with ERT is totally eliminated by adding a progestagen, cannot be answered unequivocally. Available data on this matter lack uniformity and case-control studies and cohort studies show conflicting results.

Sequential Combined HRT and Endometrial Cancer

In relation to endometrial carcinoma, the regimen studied most thoroughly of adding a progestagen is the sequentially combined scheme (scHRT). This type of HRT is not found to increase endometrial cancer risk significantly in most case-control studies (Table 1). Statistical significance was found only for long-term use and in only two studies, namely those of Beresford et al. [33] and Weiderpass et al. [36]. The cohort studies in Table 1 (cohort studies are often considered to be methodologically superior to case-control studies) found no significant difference in risk between scHRT-users and non-users [27,34]. The 1995 meta-analysis by Grady et al. [41] came up with a significant RR of 1.8 (95% CI, 1.1-3.1) based on three case-control studies [29-31] and 0.4 (95% CI, 0.2-0.6) based on three cohort studies [27,56,57].

When considering the magnitude of risk in scHRT users, an essential issue is the number of days a progestagen is administered each month. Maximal progestational effects in endometrial specimens in terms of reduction of DNA synthesis have been shown to occur after administration of progestagens for at least six days [58]. It has also been found that the number of mitoses are not reduced until after nine days of progestagen therapy [59].

Epidemiological data are in line with these findings. Three case-control studies compared the RR of endometrial cancer for women using HRT with addition of a progestagen for fewer than 10 days per cycle with the RR for women using a regimen with a progestagen added for 10 days or more [29,33,32]. All three studies found higher risks among long-term HRT users being administered progestagen 10 days or less each cycle, although only in the study by Pike et al. this increase was statistically significant [32]. None of the studies found an increase in risk for use with a progestagen for 10 days or more each cycle. The relatively large differences in RRs between these methodologically comparable studies may be due to confounding factors: in the study by Beresford et al. [33], subjects had a significantly higher body mass index and they had used (sequential) OCs preceding HRT for a significantly shorter period of time than controls did. Both factors are well known to increase endometrial cancer risk [10,11].

Continuous Combined HRT and Endometrial Cancer

Continuous combined HRT (ccHRT) has been introduced in order to overcome the scheduled withdrawal bleedings associated with scHRT regimens [60]. The main drawback of ccHRT, however, is the occurrence of unscheduled bleeding episodes in about 40% of women during the first six months of treatment [61]. This can possibly lead to patients' discontinuation of therapy [62-64], although others found adherence during the first year of therapy to be higher among women prescribed ccHRT than scHRT [65]. Spotting while on ccHRT seems to occur less frequently in older women and in women, who are postmenopausal for a longer period of time [61].

Regimens with continuous addition of a progestagen appear to be safe with respect to the endometrium, though the number of studies on this matter is limited. The first endometrial cancers in ccHRT users were reported by Comerci et al. [66] and Beresford et al. [33], but numbers were too small for RRs to be calculated. Since then, four case-control studies have been published investigating the impact of ccHRT on endometrial cancer risk (see Table 1) [32,36,38,39]. The only study [36] finding a significant association reported a reduced RR of 0.2 (95% CI, 0.1-0.8) for more than 5 years of ccHRT use. The other studies showed either an insignificantly positive association between ccHRT use and cancer risk [32,38] or an insignificantly negative one [39]. Obviously, these reports have contradictory results, probably due to limited follow-up and confounding factors that are inherent in case-control studies, like selection bias and recall bias.

Alternative HRT Regimens

Despite well-documented advantages of both short-term and long-term HRT, HRT uptake and continuation rate are generally poor [67]. Often the reason women discontinue hormone supplementation is the return of vaginal bleeding [68]. Therefore, quarterly (3-monthly) regimens have been developed, in which a progestagen is added for 10 to 14 days every 12 weeks, thus minimizing the frequency of bleeding episodes and other progestagen-related side effects. Studies on this matter claim good endometrial response [69] and high continuation rates [70], and women were reported to prefer the quarterly regimen by nearly four to one [71]. However, the one study that evaluated the endometrial effects in a randomized trial with sufficient follow-up (4 years) found a significantly higher incidence of endometrial neoplastic changes (simple and complex hyperplasia, atypia, and cancer) in women receiving progestagens on a 3-monthly basis compared to those on a monthly regimen: annual incidence was 5.6% versus 1%, respectively ($p = 0.003$) [72]. Studies on long-cycle HRT and endometrial cancer are sparse. In 2001, Pukkala et al. [40] evaluated the association between long-cycle HRT and endometrial cancer. They studied a cohort of 15,956 women exposed to a 3-monthly regimen versus 78,549 women exposed to a conventional scHRT scheme. The standardized incidence rates for endometrial cancer were 2.0 (95% CI, 1.6-2.6) and 1.3 (95% CI, 1.1-1.6) respectively [40].

Recently, a new regimen has been introduced, the so-called interrupted progestin HRT, in which estrogen is administered continuously and progestagen (norgestimate) is given in a 3-days on, 3-days off pulsed fashion [73,74]. This regimen would allow stimulation of estrogen and progestagen receptors in target tissues during the (short) estrogen-only periods thus preventing the substantial down-regulation of both types of receptors one sees in conventional HRT regimens [75]. Consequently, lower doses progestagens would ultimately be required to be sufficiently effective in inducing anti-proliferative changes in the endometrium. Preliminary results of phase III trials show good symptom control and low bleeding rates. In dose-finding studies, a daily dose of 1 mg estradiol and 90 μg norgestimate was shown to be well tolerated and to offer endometrial protection [76]. Theoretically, this seems a promising new way of hormone supplementation, but more clinical studies are required to reliably establish its actual efficacy and safety.

HRT in Women Treated for Endometrial Cancer

Although endometrial cancer primarily affects postmenopausal women, in 20-25% of patients the disease develops before the onset of menopause [11]. Since its therapy routinely includes bilateral ovariectomy, the option to start with hormonal supplementation can be of great importance to the individual patient. Most gynecologists are reluctant to prescribe HRT in endometrial cancer patients, but there are no data available showing any increase in recurrence rate for women using HRT. Table 3 summarizes the results of four case-control studies suggesting that HRT use in women treated for endometrial cancer has no unfavorable effect on their prognosis [77-80]; two studies even found a significantly longer disease-free interval among HRT users [77,80]. We should keep in mind, however, that these are all retrospective studies. Although at least three studies appear to have adequately matched the controls for stage of the disease and risk factors for recurrence, it is possible that HRT was predominantly prescribed to women who had a predetermined more favorable prognosis for some other reason (selection bias).

Obviously, there is a strong need for randomized trials on HRT use in endometrial cancer patients [81]. At present, one such a study is ongoing, conducted by the GOG group, having included two-third of the number of patients needed. Furthermore, the EORTC

Gynecological Oncology Group is preparing a prospective study on this subject which is due to start recruiting patients by the end of 2001.

Table 3. Relative Risk of Recurrent Disease for Women Treated for Endometrial Cancer Using/not Using ERT or HRT

	Recurrence for ERT/HRT users	Recurrence for nonusers	P value	Remarks
Creasman 1986 [77]	1/47 (2.1%)	26/174 (14.9%)	< 0.05	- only stage I disease - only ERT use; 72% vaginally, 28% orally (and vaginally)
Lee 1990 [78]	0/44 (0%)	8/99 (8.1%)	NS	- only stage I disease - ERT (66%) and HRT use (34%); only orally
Chapman 1996 [79]	2/62 (3.2%)	6/61 (9.8%)	NS	- stage I (91%) and stage II (9%) disease - nonusers more often stage IC and II (p=0.04) - ERT (47%) and HRT use (53%); 97% orally
Suriano 2001 [80]	2/75 (2.7%)	11/75 (14.7%)	0.006	- stage I, II and III disease - ERT (51%) and HRT use (49%), only orally - preoperative HRT use: 49% resp. 17%

Conclusion

After decades of ERT and HRT use by millions of peri- and postmenopausal women, the effect of hormonal supplementation on endometrial cancer risk still remains subject to debate. There are three major reasons for this lack of conclusive data. First, most studies are case-control or cohort studies and like any observational study, these are susceptible to bias. It takes an enormous effort and a long period of time to conduct a randomized trial with sufficient power and follow-up to demonstrate the very modest changes in endometrial cancer risk that are expected to apply for HRT users. In 1998, recruitment was completed for the Women's Health Initiative (WHI), a large, randomized, primary prevention trial (27,000 women in the HRT arm, follow-up 9 years) on benefits and risks of hormonal supplementation. This trial may offer us more conclusive answers regarding HRT in relation with endometrial cancer.

Second, during the course of time, regimens have changed substantially. Since it became obvious that ERT use leads to an increased endometrial cancer risk, progestagens have been added: initially sequentially, later also continuously. In addition, the type and dose of estrogens and progestagens administered have varied greatly too, and they still do. Third, not only regimens, but also women are different. Risk modifiers, such as age, weight, parity, former OC use, and smoking may all have their consequences on the HRT- mediated cancer risk.

Despite the fact that more data are needed to elucidate all aspects of endometrial cancer risk in HRT users, it seems very unlikely that hormonal supplementation has deleterious effects on the chance of developing this disease provided that one sticks to a few basic principles. If the uterus is present, addition of a progestagen is obligatory, at least for 10 days per month. With respect to the endometrium, ccHRT might be slightly preferable to scHRT, though this is not a foregone conclusion yet. Long-cycle therapy offers less endometrial protection than conventional monthly regimens. New schemes of supplementation, like interrupted progestin HRT, are promising indeed, but results of more studies are needed to evaluate its effects on the endometrium and on other organs definitively.

In the decision to start with HRT, a woman and her doctor have to take many aspects into account. When HRT is prescribed for a relatively short period of time (for the treatment of climacteric complaints), one has little reason to worry about risk of endometrial cancer (or breast cancer), since short-term use has never been associated with an increased risk.

When HRT is administered for a longer period of time, however, with the aim to prevent diseases later in life (such as osteoporosis), pros and cons have to weighed up carefully. This is not an easy thing to do. Whereas the effectiveness of HRT in the prevention of osteoporosis is well established [82,83], data to show that HRT prevents Alzheimer's disease [84,85] and colon carcinoma [86,87] are much less consistent. While observational studies have demonstrated a large reduction in risk of cardiovascular diseases in HRT users [88,89], recent randomized, secondary prevention trials [90,91,92] raised doubts.

Not only inconsistencies exist in studies on the (presumed) advantages of HRT, the extent of risks of HRT also have been insufficiently elucidated, including stroke [93] and breast cancer [94]. Here again, data from randomized trials are urgently needed to provide insight in the ultimate effects of HRT. For the time being, we must make shift with what we have and treat our patients based on their individual needs and their individual risk profile. This also counts for patients who have been treated for endometrial cancer, though some reservedness in prescribing HRT in this particular group of patients is probably indicated, until results of randomized trials on this matter have proved otherwise.

References

1. Ball HG, Elkadry EA. Endometrial cancer: Current concepts and management. Surg Oncol Clin North Am 1998;7:271-84.
2. Ziel HK, Finkle WD, Greenland S. Decline in incidence of endometrial cancer following increase in prescriptions for opposed conjugated estrogens in a prepaid health plan. Gynecol Oncol 1998;68:253-55.
3. Key TJ. Hormones and cancer in humans. Mutat Res 1995;333:59-67.
4. Kenemans P, van Unnik GA. Postmenopausal sex hormones and cancer of the endometrium and breast. J Br Meno Soc 2000;6(Suppl.3):4-9.

5. Emons G, Fleckenstein G, Hinney B, Huschmand A, Heyl W. Hormonal interactions in endometrial cancer. Endocr Relat Cancer 2000;7:227-42.
6. Wynder EL, Escher GC, Mantel N. An epidemiological investigation of cancer of the endometrium. Cancer 1966;19:489-520.
7. Gusberg SB, Kardon P. Proliferative endometrial response to theca-granulosa cell tumors. Am J Obstet Gynecol 1971;111:633-43.
8. MacMahon B. Risk factors for endometrial cancer. Gynecol Oncol 1974;2:122-29.
9. Jafari K, Javaheri G, Ruiz G. Endometrial adenocarcinoma and the Stein-Leventhal syndrome. Obstet Gynecol 1978;51:97-100.
10. Pettersson B, Adami HO, Bergstrom R, Johansson ED. Menstruation span--a time-limited risk factor for endometrial carcinoma. Acta Obstet Gynecol Scand 1986;65:247-55.
11. Creasman WT. Endometrial cancer: incidence, prognostic factors, diagnosis, and treatment. Sem Oncol1997;24:S1.
12. Klip H, Burger CW, Kenemans P, van Leeuwen FE. Cancer risk associated with subfertility and ovulation induction: a review. Cancer Causes Control 2000;11:319-44.
13. Venn A, Watson L, Lumley J, Giles G, King C, Healy D. Breast and ovarian cancer incidence after infertility and in vitro fertilisation. Lancet 1995;346:995-1000.
14. Modan B, Ron E, Lerner-Geva L, et al. Cancer incidence in a cohort of infertile women. Am J Epidemiol 1998;147:1038-42.
15. Venn A, Watson L, Bruinsma F, Giles G, Healy D. Risk of cancer after use of fertility drugs with in-vitro fertilisation [In Process Citation]. Lancet 1999;354:1586-90.
16. Acken HS, Jr. Estrogen replacement therapy. Obstet Gynecol 1969;34:46-49.
17. Smith DC, Prentice R, Thompson DJ, Herrmann WL. Association of exogenous estrogen and endometrial carcinoma. N Engl J Med 1975;293:1164-67.
18. Ziel HK, Finkle WD. Increased risk of endometrial carcinoma among users of conjugated estrogens. N Engl J Med 1975;293:1167-70.
19. Burger CW, Kenemans P. Postmenopausal hormone replacement therapy and cancer of the female genital tract and breast. Curr Opin Obstet Gynecol 1998;10:41-45.
20. Henderson BE, Casagrande JT, Pike MC, Mack T, Rosario I, Duke A. The epidemiology of endometrial cancer in young women. Br J Cancer 1983;47:749-56.
21. Weiss NS, Sayvetz TA. Incidence of endometrial cancer in relation to the use of oral contraceptives. N Engl J Med 1980;302:551-54.
22. Kaufman DW, Shapiro S, Slone D, et al. Decreased risk of endometrial cancer among oral-contraceptive users. N Engl J Med 1980;303:1045-47.
23. Hulka BS, Chambless LE, Kaufman DG, Fowler WC, Jr., Greenberg BG. Protection against endometrial carcinoma by combination-product oral contraceptives. JAMA 1982; 247:475-77.
24. Oral contraceptive use and the risk of endometrial cancer. The Centers for Disease Control Cancer and Steroid Hormone Study. JAMA 1983;249:1600-1604.
25. Rosenblatt KA, Thomas DB. Hormonal content of combined oral contraceptives in relation to the reduced risk of endometrial carcinoma. The WHO Collaborative Study of Neoplasia and Steroid Contraceptives. Int J Cancer 1991;49:870-74.
26. Paganini-Hill A, Ross RK, Henderson BE. Endometrial cancer and patterns of use of oestrogen replacement therapy: a cohort study. Br J Cancer 1989;59:445-47.
27. Persson I, Adami HO, Bergkvist L, et al. Risk of endometrial cancer after treatment with oestrogens alone or in conjunction with progestogens: results of a prospective study. Br Med J 1989;298:147-51.

28. Rubin GL, Peterson HB, Lee NC, Maes EF, Wingo PA, Becker S. Estrogen replacement therapy and the risk of endometrial cancer: remaining controversies. Am J Obstet Gynecol 1990;162:148-54.
29. Voigt LF, Weiss NS, Chu J, Daling JR, McKnight B, van Belle G. Progestagen supplementation of exogenous oestrogens and risk of endometrial cancer. Lancet 1991; 338:274-77.
30. Brinton LA, Hoover RN. Estrogen replacement therapy and endometrial cancer risk: unresolved issues. The Endometrial Cancer Collaborative Group. Obstet Gynecol 1993;81: 265-71.
31. Jick SS, Walker AM, Jick H. Estrogens, progesterone, and endometrial cancer. Epidemiology 1993;4:20-24.
32. Pike MC, Peters RK, Cozen W, et al. Estrogen-progestin replacement therapy and endometrial cancer [see comments]. J Natl Cancer Inst 1997;89:1110-16.
33. Beresford SA, Weiss NS, Voigt LF, McKnight B. Risk of endometrial cancer in relation to use of oestrogen combined with cyclic progestagen therapy in postmenopausal women. Lancet 1997;349:458-61.
34. Persson I, Weiderpass E, Bergkvist L, Bergstrom R, Schairer C. Risks of breast and endometrial cancer after estrogen and estrogen- progestin replacement. Cancer Causes Control 1999;10:253-60.
35. Weiderpass E, Baron JA, Adami HO, et al. Low-potency oestrogen and risk of endometrial cancer: a case-control study. Lancet 1999;353:1824-28.
36. Weiderpass E, Adami HO, Baron JA, et al. Risk of endometrial cancer following estrogen replacement with and without progestins. J Natl Cancer Inst 1999;91:1131-37.
37. Parslov M, Lidegaard O, Klintorp S, et al. Risk factors among young women with endometrial cancer: A Danish case- control study. Am J Obstet Gynecol 2000;182:23-29.
38. Jain MG, Rohan TE, Howe GR. Hormone replacement therapy and endometrial cancer in Ontario, Canada. J Clin Epidemiol 2000;53:385-91.
39. Hill DA, Weiss NS, Beresford SA, et al. Continuous combined hormone replacement therapy and risk of endometrial cancer. Am J Obstet Gynecol 2000;183:1456-61.
40. Pukkala E, Tulenheimo-Silfvast A, Leminen A. Incidence of cancer among women using long versus monthly cycle hormonal replacement therapy, Finland 1994-1997. Cancer Causes Control 2001;12:111-15.
41. Grady D, Gebretsadik T, Kerlikowske K, Ernster V, Petitti D. Hormone replacement therapy and endometrial cancer risk: a meta- analysis. Obstet Gynecol 1995;85:304-13.
42. Gray LA, Sr., Christopherson WM, Hoover RN. Estrogens and endometrial carcinoma. Obstet Gynecol 1977;49:385-89.
43. Weiss NS, Szekely DR, English DR, Schweid AI. Endometrial cancer in relation to patterns of menopausal estrogen use. JAMA 1979;242:261-64.
44. Hulka BS, Kaufman DG, Fowler WC, Jr., Grimson RC, Greenberg BG. Predominance of early endometrial cancers after long-term estrogen use. JAMA 1980;244:2419-22.
45. Buring JE, Bain CJ, Ehrmann RL. Conjugated estrogen use and risk of endometrial cancer. Am J Epidemiol 1986;124:434-41.
46. Speroff L, Rowan J, Symons J, Genant H, Wilborn W. The comparative effect on bone density, endometrium, and lipids of continuous hormones as replacement therapy (CHART study). A randomized controlled trial. JAMA 1996;276:1397-403.
47. Mack TM, Pike MC, Henderson BE, et al. Estrogens and endometrial cancer in a retirement community. N Engl J Med 1976;294:1262-67.

48. Levi F, La Vecchia C, Gulie C, Franceschi S, Negri E. Oestrogen replacement treatment and the risk of endometrial cancer: an assessment of the role of covariates. Eur J Cancer 1993;29A:1445-49.
49. Green PK, Weiss NS, McKnight B, Voigt LF, Beresford SA. Risk of endometrial cancer following cessation of menopausal hormone use (Washington, United States). Cancer Causes Control 1996;7:575-80.
50. Sherman ME, Sturgeon S, Brinton LA, et al. Risk factors and hormone levels in patients with serous and endometrioid uterine carcinomas. Mod Pathol 1997;10:963-68.
51. Sherman ME. Theories of endometrial carcinogenesis: A multidisciplinary approach. Mod.Pathol. 2000;13:295-308.
52. Bokhman JV. Two pathogenetic types of endometrial carcinoma. Gynecol Oncol 1983;15: 10-17.
53. Henderson BE, Paganini-Hill A, Ross RK. Decreased mortality in users of estrogen replacement therapy. Arch Intern Med 1991;151:75-78.
54. Schairer C, Adami HO, Hoover R, Persson I. Cause-specific mortality in women receiving hormone replacement therapy. Epidemiology 1997;8:59-65.
55. Lobo RA. The role of progestins in hormone replacement therapy. Am J Obstet Gynecol 1992;166:1997-2004.
56. Hammond CB, Jelovsek FR, Lee KL, Creasman WT, Parker RT. Effects of long-term estrogen replacement therapy. II. Neoplasia. Am J Obstet Gynecol 1979;133:537-47.
57. Gambrell RD, Jr., Massey FM, Castaneda TA, Ugenas AJ, Ricci CA, Wright JM. Use of the progestogen challenge test to reduce the risk of endometrial cancer. Obstet Gynecol 1980;55:732-38.
58. Whitehead MI, Townsend PT, Pryse-Davies J, Ryder TA, King RJ. Effects of estrogens and progestins on the biochemistry and morphology of the postmenopausal endometrium. N Engl J Med 1981;305:1599-605.
59. Moyer DL, de Lignieres B, Driguez P, Pez JP. Prevention of endometrial hyperplasia by progesterone during long-term estradiol replacement: influence of bleeding pattern and secretory changes. Fertil Steril 1993;59:992-97.
60. Staland B. Continuous treatment with natural oestrogens and progestogens. A method to avoid endometrial stimulation. Maturitas 1981;3:145-56.
61. Spencer CP, Cooper AJ, Whitehead MI. Management of abnormal bleeding in women receiving hormone replacement therapy. Br Med J 1997;315:37-42.
62. Mattsson LA, Cullberg G, Samsioe G. Evaluation of a continuous oestrogen-progestogen regimen for climacteric complaints. Maturitas 1982;4:95-102.
63. Magos AL, Brincat M, Studd JW, Wardle P, Schlesinger P, O'Dowd T. Amenorrhea and endometrial atrophy with continuous oral estrogen and progestogen therapy in postmenopausal women. Obstet Gynecol 1985;65:496-99.
64. Doren M, Schneider HP. The impact of different HRT regimens on compliance. Int J Fertil Menopausal Stud 1996;41:29-39.
65. Hill DA, Weiss NS, LaCroix AZ. Adherence to postmenopausal hormone therapy during the year after the initial prescription: A population-based study. Am J Obstet Gynecol 2000;182:270-76.
66. Comerci JT, Jr., Fields AL, Runowicz CD, Goldberg GL. Continuous low-dose combined hormone replacement therapy and the risk of endometrial cancer. Gynecol Oncol 1997; 64:425-30.
67. Kenemans P, van Unnik GA, Mijatovic V, van der Mooren MJ. Perspectives in hormone

replacement therapy. Maturitas 2001;38(Suppl.1):S41-S48.
68. Wren BG, Brown L. Compliance with hormonal replacement therapy. Maturitas 1991;13: 17-21.
69. Boerrigter PJ, van de Weijer PH, Baak JP, Fox H, Haspels AA, Kenemans. Endometrial response in estrogen replacement therapy quarterly combined with a progestogen. Maturitas 1996;24:63-71.
70. Hirvonen E, Salmi T, Puolakka J, et al. Can progestin be limited to every third month only in postmenopausal women taking estrogen? Maturitas 1995;21:39-44.
71. Ettinger B, Selby J, Citron JT, et al. Cyclic hormone replacement therapy using quarterly progestin. Obstet Gynecol 1994;83:693-700.
72. Bjarnason K, Cerin A, Lindgren R, Weber T. Adverse endometrial effects during long cycle hormone replacement therapy. Scandinavian Long Cycle Study Group. Maturitas 1999;32:161-70.
73. Casper RF. Estrogen with interrupted progestin HRT: A review of experimental and clinical studies. Maturitas 2000;34:97-108.
74. Rozenberg S. Clinical evidence supporting the rationale for constant oestrogen, intermittent progestogen hormone replacement therapy. Eur J Obstet Gynecol Reprod Biol 2001;94:86-91.
75. Moutsatsou P, Sekeris CE. Estrogen and progesterone receptors in the endometrium. Ann NY Acad Sci 1997;816:99-115.
76. Corson SL, Richart RM, Caubel P, Lim P. Effect of a unique constant-estrogen, pulsed-progestin hormone replacement therapy containing 17beta-estradiol and norgestimate on endometrial histology. Int J Fertil Womens Med 1999;44:279-85.
77. Creasman WT, Henderson D, Hinshaw W, Clarke-Pearson DL. Estrogen replacement therapy in the patient treated for endometrial cancer. Obstet Gynecol 1986;67:326-30.
78. Lee RB, Burke TW, Park RC. Estrogen replacement therapy following treatment for stage I endometrial carcinoma. Gynecol Oncol 1990;36:189-91.
79. Chapman JA, DiSaia PJ, Osann K, Roth PD, Gillotte DL, Berman ML. Estrogen replacement in surgical stage I and II endometrial cancer survivors. Am J Obstet Gynecol 1996;175:1195-200.
80. Suriano KA, McHale M, McLaren CE, Li KT, Re A, DiSaia PJ. Estrogen replacement therapy in endometrial cancer patients: a matched control study. Obstet Gynecol 2001;97: 555-60.
81. Burger CW, van Leeuwen F, Scheele F, Kenemans P. Hormone replacement therapy in women treated for gynaecological malignancy. Maturitas 1999;32:69-76.
82. Naessen T, Persson I, Adami HO, Bergstrom R, Bergkvist L. Hormone replacement therapy and the risk for first hip fracture. A prospective, population-based cohort study. Ann Intern Med 1990;113:95-103.
83. Cauley JA, Seeley DG, Ensrud K, Ettinger B, Black D, Cummings SR. Estrogen replacement therapy and fractures in older women. Study of Osteoporotic Fractures Research Group. Ann Intern Med 1995;122:9-16.
84. Baldereschi M, Di CA, Lepore V, et al. Estrogen-replacement therapy and Alzheimer's disease in the Italian Longitudinal Study on Aging. Neurology 1998;50:996-1002.
85. Brenner DE, Kukull WA, Stergachis A, et al. Postmenopausal estrogen replacement therapy and the risk of Alzheimer's disease: A population-based case-control study. Am J Epidemiol 1994;140:262-67.
86. Newcomb PA, Storer BE. Postmenopausal hormone use and risk of large-bowel cancer.

J Natl Cancer Inst 1995;87:1067-71.
87. MacLennan SC, MacLennan AH, Ryan P. Colorectal cancer and oestrogen replacement therapy. A meta-analysis of epidemiological studies. Med J Aust 1995;162:491-93.
88. Grady D, Rubin SM, Petitti DB, et al. Hormone therapy to prevent disease and prolong life in postmenopausal women [see comments]. Ann Intern Med 1992;117:1016-37.
89. Stampfer MJ, Colditz GA. Estrogen replacement therapy and coronary heart disease: a quantitative assessment of the epidemiologic evidence. Prev Med 1991;20:47-63.
90. Hulley S, Grady D, Bush T, et al. Randomized trial of estrogen plus progestin for secondary prevention of coronary heart disease in postmenopausal women. Heart and Estrogen/progestin Replacement Study (HERS) Research Group. JAMA 1998;280:605-13.
91. Herrington DM, Reboussin DM, Brosnihan KB, et al. Effects of estrogen replacement on the progression of coronary-artery atherosclerosis. N Engl J Med 2000;343:522-29.
92. Angerer P, Stork S, Kothny W, Schmitt P, von Schacky C. Effect of oral postmenopausal hormone replacement on progression of atherosclerosis: Arandomized, controlled trial. Arterioscler Tromb Vasc Biol 2001;21:262-68.
93. Paganini-Hill A. Hormone replacement therapy and stroke: Risk, protection or no effect? Maturitas 2001;38:243-61.
94. Kenemans P, van Unnik GA, Taets van Amerongen AHM, Scheele F. Hormone replacement treatment options and the breast. Adv Obstet Gynecol 2000;52:255-65.

Hormone Replacement Therapy and Breast Cancer: Still More Questions Than Answers

Susan Love

The Old Paradigm: Gasoline to the Fire

Estrogen replacement therapy (ERT) and hormone replacement therapy (HRT) have been suspected of increasing breast cancer risk for decades. Despite many observational studies the topic is still unsettled [1].

The old paradigm based on observational data was that ERT/HRT is good for symptom relief, and prevention of cardiovascular disease, osteoporosis, and Alzheimer's disease. On the other hand it is strongly believed that ERT/HRT is a cause or at least a promoter of breast cancer. Based largely on work in cell lines the common thinking was that "estrogen was to breast cancer as gasoline was to a fire." Recent randomized controlled data has called into question the cardiac benefits of ERT/HRT [2]. As a result, we now are demanding data to prove the reduction in fractures and Alzheimer's disease that has been attributed to ERT/HRT based on observational data. By the same token the data linking breast cancer and estrogen is also largely observational and needs to be reexamined.

Observational Data

Epidemiological studies have demonstrated a correlation between endogenous levels of estrogen, progesterone, and testosterone and breast cancer [3]. It has been consistently shown that the duration of reproductive levels of hormones correlates directly with the risk for breast cancer. That is the younger a woman is when she undergoes menarche and the older she is at menopause or the more menstruating years that she has, the higher her risk for breast cancer [4]. In addition early bilateral oophorectomy significantly reduces the risk of subsequent breast cancer, even in women who carry mutations in BRCA1 or 2 [5]. More direct evidence comes from the Study for Osteoporotic Fractures (SOF) where 97 women with breast cancer were matched with 244 controls without breast cancer. All the women were white, postmenopausal, and not on hormones. They found that estradiol levels were 30% higher and testosterone levels were 28% higher in cases than controls. Both the highest bioavailable estrogen and testosterone quartiles had 3.6 times the risk of breast cancer than those in the lowest quartiles [6].

There are several surrogate markers for endogenous hormone levels that have also been examined in observational studies. For example pregnancy increases the risk of breast cancer at the time of the pregnancy and to a lesser extent for the three subsequent years [7]. This is apart from the fact that an early pregnancy will ultimately decrease the risk of breast cancer. Bone density which is a surrogate marker for estrogen and testosterone levels has been shown to directly relate to breast cancer risk. Both the Framingham Study and SOF demonstrated that the higher the bone density the higher the risk of breast cancer [8,9]. Mammographic density has been shown to be one of the strongest indicators of breast cancer risk [10]. It appears to be related to both estrogen and progesterone levels increasing significantly in 30% of women on HRT [11] and decreasing when women take tamoxifen [12]. Finally postmenopausal obesity, a presumed marker for increased aromatase conversion of testosterone and androstenedione to estrogen, correlates with an increase risk of breast cancer [13].

Exogenous hormones have also been shown in observational studies to increase breast cancer risk. Oral contraceptives demonstrate a slight increase in breast cancer risk in current users [14]. This disappears soon after stopping the drugs. Diethylstilbesterol (DES) has been shown to increase breast cancer risk in the women who took it during pregnancy to prevent miscarriage [15]. On the other side, the SERMs tamoxifen and raloxifene have both been shown to decrease breast cancer risk, presumably by blocking the estrogen receptor [16,17]. This mechanism has received support with the MORE trial observation that only women with high estradiol levels benefit from raloxifene's breast cancer risk reduction [18]. Many observational studies have examined the relationship between ERT/HRT and breast cancer. Examining just the meta-analyses (Table 1) we find that any use versus never use of hormones postmenopausally has a small effect. The major effect is in the current users who have taken ERT/HRT for over ten years. Here the increased risk is a consistent 20-30%.

Table 1. Meta-Analysis of HRT and Breast Cancer Risk

Reference	No. of studies	Any use RR	Duration of current use
Dupont and Page 1991 [19]	28	1.07	
Steinberg et al. 1991 [20]	16	1.0	> 15 yrs 1.30 (1.20-1.60)
Grady and Ernster 1991 [21]	10	1.0	> 10 yrs 1.23 (1.04-1.51)
Sillero-Arenas et al 1992 [22]	37	1.06 (1.00-1.12)	> 8 yrs 1.20
Colditz 1993 [23]	31	1.40 (1.20-1.63) Current users	> 10 yrs 1.23 (1.08-1.49)
Oxford 1997 [24]	51	2.3% Current users	> 5 yrs 1.35 (1.21-1.49)

Biases in Observational Data

In fact for every 1,000 women who begin to take postmenopausal hormones at age 50 and who take them for ten years there are six excess cases of breast cancer; if they take them for fifteen years the increase is 12 excess cases. But these observational studies do not take into consideration several biases that slip into the analysis. Women who take ERT/HRT are followed every six months by their gynecologists. This means they are more likely to have regular breast exams and mammograms than women who do not take ERT/HRT. This might bias the studies to find more cancers in the women taking hormones. In addition most if not all of these studies lump together natural and surgical menopause as if they were the same. It is now recognized that the ovaries of natural menopausal women continue to produce estrone, testosterone, androstenedione well into their eighties albeit at lower levels than premenopausally [25]. And these lower levels are significant biologically. Ettinger recently showed that women with as low as 5 picograms of endogenous estrogen have significantly fewer hip fractures than women with less than that amount [26]. Women generally have their ovaries out when they are premenopausal and therefore may actually have a lower risk for breast cancer than the women who are naturally menopausal. Women who are surgically menopausal are more likely to take ERT than HRT. If progestins are important than these studies will underestimate the breast cancer risk. Most of these studies lump together all doses and durations of hormones making it hard to distinguish individual effects. Several recent studies (Table 2) have demonstrated the problem with lumping all regimens together. All have consistently shown that taking estrogen alone increases the risk of breast cancer by about 1-3% a year while adding a progestin (usually Provera) increases this to 5-9 %/year [27-29]. Estrogen and progestins appear to act synergistically on the breast. Since 60% of women taking hormones long term have had a surgical menopause and are taking ERT the large meta-analysis which lump ERT and HRT together are undoubtedly underestimating the breast cancer risk.

Table 2. Breast Cancer Risk in ERT Versus HRT

	ERT	HRT
Nurse's Health Study [27]	3.3%/year	9%/year
Schairer [28]	1%/year	8%/year
Ross [29]	6%/5 years	24%/5 years

Finally there is the issue of combinations of different regimens over time. It is only as the baby boomers age that we will have women who have taken oral contraceptives (OCPs) for extended periods of time and then followed them with ERT/HRT. In one provocative observational study Brinton et al. demonstrated another synergistic effect. Although women who had taken OCPs or HRT alone had not increased risk of subsequent breast cancer, those women who had taken OCPs for over ten years and then taken HRT for over three years had a 3.2 times increased risk of breast cancer [30]. We need to be careful about looking at postmenopausal hormones in isolation without considering the whole hormonal history of the woman.

Finally we have the fact that estrogen receptor (ER) positive cancers are treated by blocking or removing endogenous estrogen whether by oophorectomy or zoladex in the premenopausal woman [31] or by tamoxifen [32] or aromatase [33] inhibition in the postmenopausal woman.

The Paradox

All of these observations can be woven together into a coherent hypothesis suggesting that estrogen and progesterone either cause or promote breast cancer. The problem is that there are a few observations which would contradict this pat approach, and herein lies the paradox. In premenopausal women pregnancy increases the risk of breast cancer [34] but women who get breast cancer while pregnant have the same prognosis as women who are not pregnant, stage for stage [35]. In addition in the admittedly small, uncontrolled, observational studies of women who get pregnant after a diagnosis and treatment for breast cancer there is no change in prognosis [36]. Clearly the high levels of estrogen and progesterone during pregnancy are not "gasoline to the fire."

In postmenopausal women we see a parallel paradox. ERT/HRT appear to increase the risk of breast cancer over time but women who get breast cancer while on ERT/HRT have a slightly better prognosis than women who were not taking ERT/HRT when diagnosed [37]. And again in small, uncontrolled studies women with breast cancer who take ERT/HRT do not appear to fare any worse than women who do not take it [38]. Again the gasoline is not igniting this fire.

A recent study (Table 3) by O'Meara [39] bears further scrutiny. The HRT users had a decrease in recurrence and breast cancer mortality when compared to the nonusers. This could be because they are screened more or it could be a biological effect. More intriguing is the fact that the women on HRT had an increase in contralateral cancers when compared to the nonusers. It should be noted this is a relatively small study and uncontrolled but the findings parallel the paradox that we are describing: reproductive hormones appear to have a role in initiating breast cancer but do not have a subsequent effect. Is it possible that they are flipping a switch that once on stays on?

Table 3. Women Who Are on HRT when Diagnosed with Breast Cancer

	HRT user	Nonusers	RR
Recurrence	17/1000	30/1000	0.50 (0.30-0.85)
Breast cancer mortality	5/1000	15/1000	0.34 (0.13-0.91)
Overall morality	16/1000	30/1000	0.48 (0.29-0.78)
Contralateral cancers	12/1000	8/1000	1.42 (0.69-2.95)

While this is an interesting idea, it leaves out many more aspects of this paradox. For example, tamoxifen, initially thought to be an estrogenic blocker has now been rechristened a selective estrogen receptor modulator. In premenopausal women it increases their serum estrogen levels significantly and yet still reduces recurrences and second cancers. After five years, tamoxifen appears to stimulate breast cancers causing and slight increase in recurrences and second cancers [40]. And finally and most intriguing of all, its benefits persist at least 15 years after stopping its use [41].

Another example of the paradoxical effects of estrogen in breast cancer development revolves around atypical hyperplasia. This proliferative lesion is 95% ER positive and yet giving ERT/HRT does not seem to stimulate it [42]. On the other hand tamoxifen given to women with atypical ductal hyperplasia reduces the subsequent risk of breast cancer by 86% [16].

Genetic breast cancer adds to the muddle. In women who are carriers of BRCA1 pregnancy increases the risk [43] and oophorectomy decreases the risk [5] but tamoxifen has no effect [44]. Most cancers that develop in this subgroup are ER negative and may be independent from hormones from the beginning but then why would oophorectomy have a protective effect.

New Hypotheses?

Obviously we do not have the right hypothesis to understand these relationships. A brief glance at some of the recent biological findings suggest the complexities we have been overlooking. There are at least two estrogen receptors, alpha and beta [45]. These have different effects and are present in different organs. In addition the relationship between progesterone and estrogen is variable and organ specific. In the uterus progesterone blocks the proliferative effects of estrogen while in the breast they are synergistic [46]. In addition there are coactivators and corepressors of the ER which can determine the end effect of stimulation [47]. Finally there is some evidence that breast tissue in breast cancer patients responds differently to estrogen then normal breast tissue [48].

Could the problem be that it is the local levels of hormones that are important? Breast tissue is known to contain aromatase and therefore is capable of producing its own estrogen [49]. In addition studies of nipple aspirate fluid by Petrakis have demonstrated that the levels of estrogen and progesterone in the breast duct fluid do not correlate with those in the blood [50]. Does the breast tissue have its own microenvironment that is related to but not reflective of that of the blood? The data relating breast cancer prognosis to the time of surgery would suggest that the hormonal milieu at a point of time is important [51]. A recent report from Nandi showed that it not only matters when but also how much and how long. He showed that short-term exposure to pregnancy levels of estrogen was protective for breast cancer in rats [52].

We've obviously outgrown the simplistic hypothesis that the relationship of estrogen to breast cancer is like gasoline to a fire. Yet the correct hypothesis still eludes us. At this point all we can do is keep rearranging the pieces of the puzzle until a new paradigm emerges which ties them all together. Until then all we can do is admit that the relationship between estrogen and breast cancer is a paradox.

References

1. Bush TL, Whiteman M, Flaws JA. Hormone replacement therapy and breast cancer: A qualitative review. Obstet Gynecol 2001;98:498-508.
2. Hulley S, Grady D, Bush TL, et al. Randomized trial of estrogen plus progestin for the secondary prevention of coronary heart disease in postmenopausal women. JAMA 1998; 280:605-13.
3. Toniolo PG, Levitz M, Zeleniuch-Jacquotte A, et al. A prospective study of endogenous estrogens and breast cancer in potmenopausal women. J Natl Cancer Inst 1995;87:190-97.
4. Pike MC, Krailo MD, Henderson BE, Casagrande JT, Hoel DG. "Hormonal" risk factors, "breast tissue age" and the age-incidence of breast cancer. Nature 1983;303:767-70.
5. Rebbeck TR, Levin AM, Eisen A, et al Breast cancer risk after bilateral prophylactic oophorectomy in BRCA1 mutation carriers. J Natl Cancer Inst 1999;91(17);1475-79.
6. Cauley JA, et al. Elevated serum estradiol and testosterone concentrations are associated with a high risk for breast cancer. Ann Intern Med 1999;130:270-77.
7. Lambe M, Hsieh C, Trichopoulos D, et al. Transient increase in risk of breast cancer after giving birth. N Engl J Med 1994;331:5-9.
8. Cauley J, Lucas F, Kuller L, et al. Bone mineral density and the risk of breast cancer in older women. The study of osteoporotic fractures. JAMA1996;276:1404-8.
9. Zhang Y, Kiel D, Kreger B, et al. Bone mass and the risk of breast cancer among postmenopausal women. N Engl J Med 1997;336:611-17.
10. Verbeek ALM, Hendricks, JHCL, Peeters PHM, Sturmans F. Mammographic breast pattern and the risk of breast cancer. Lancet 1984;1:591-93.
11. Stomper PC, Van Voorhis BJ, Ravnikar VA, Meyer JE. Mammographic changes associated with postmenopausal hormone replacement therapy: A longitudinal study. Radiology 1990;174:487-90.
12. Atkinson C, Warren R, Bingham SA, Day NE. Mammographic patterns as a predictive biomarker of breast cancer risk: effect of tamoxifen. Can Epid Bio Prev 1999;8:863-66.
13. Huang Z, Hankinson SE, Colditz GA, et al. Dual effects of weight and weight gain on breast cancer risk. JAMA 1997;278:1407-11.
14. Collaborative Group on Hormonal Factors in Breast Cancer. Breast cancer and hormonal contraceptives: Collaborative reanalysis of individual data on 53,297 women with breast cancer and 100,239 women without breast cancer from 54 epidemiological studies. Lancet 1996;347:1713-27.
15. Titus-Ernstoff L, Hatch EE, Hoover RN, et al. Long-term cancer risk in women given diethylstilbestrol (DES) during pregnancy. Br J Cancer 2001;84:126-33.
16. Fisher B, Constantino JP, Wickerham DL, et al. Tamoxifen for prevention of breast cancer: Report of the National Surgical Adjuvant Breast and Bowel Project P1 Study. J Natl Cancer Inst. 1998;90:1371-88.
17. Cummings SR, Eckert S, Krueger KA, et al. The effect of raloxifene on risk of breast cancer in postmenopausal women: Results from the MORE trial. JAMA 1999;281:2189-97.
18. Cummings SR, et al. Estradiol level in postmenopausal women may indicate who benefits most from treatment to reduce risk of breast cancer. Annual Meeting of the American

Society for Bone and Mineral Research, Toronto Sept 11, 2000.
19. Dupont WD, Page DL. Menopausal estrogen replacement therapy and breast cancer. Arch InternMed 1991;151:67-72.
20. Steinberg KK, Thacker SB, Smith SJ, et al. A meta-analysis of the effect of estrogen replacement therapy on the risk of breast cancer. JAMA 1991;262(15):1985-90.
21. Grady D, Ernster V. Invited commentary: Does hormone replacement therapy cause breast cancer? Am J Epidemiol 1991;134:1396-1400.
22. Sillero-Arenas M, Delgado-Rodriguez M, Rodigues-Canteras R, Bueno-Cavanillas A, Galvez-Vargas R. Menopausal hormone replacement therapy and breast cancer: A meta-analysis. Obstet Gynecol 1992;79:286-94.
23. Colditz GA, Egan KM, Stampfer MJ. Hormone replacement therapy and risk of breast cancer: Results from epidemiologic studies. Am J Obstet Gynecol 1993;168:1473-80.
24. Collaborative Group on Hormonal Factors in Breast Cancer. Breast cancer and hormone replacement therapy: Collaborative reanalysis from SI epidemiological studies of 52705 women with breast cancer and 108411 women without breast cancer. Lancet 1997;350; 1047-1060.
25. Slujimer AV, Heineman MJ, DeJong FH, Evers JL. Endocrine activity of the postmenopausal ovary. Horm Res 1995;72:631.
26. Ettinger B, Pressman A, Sklarin P, Bauer DC, Cauley JA, Cummings SR. Associations between low levels of serum estradiol, bone density and fractures among elderly women: The study of osteoporotic fractures. J Clin Endocrinol Metab 1998;83:2239-43.
27. Colditz GA, Hankinson SE, Hunter DJ, et al The use of estrogens and progestins and the risk of breast cancer in postmenopausal women. N Engl J Med 1995;332:1589-93.
28. Schairer C, Lubin J, Troisi R, Sturgeon S, Brinton L, Hoover R. Menopausal estrogen and estrogen-progestin replacement therapy and breast cancer risk. JAMA;283:485-91.
29. Ross RK, Paganini-Hill A, Wan PC, Pike MC. Effect of hormone replacement therapy on breast cancer risk:estrogen versus estrogen plus progestin. J Natl Cancer Inst 2000;92:328-32.
30. Brinton LA, Brogan DR, Coates RJ, et al. Breast cancer risk among women under 55 years of age by joint usage of oral contraceptives and hormone replacement therapy. Menopause 1998;5:145-51.
31. Early Breast Cancer Trialists' Collaborative Group. Systemic treatment of early breast cancer by hormonal, cytotoxic, or immune therapy. Lancet 1992;339:1-15.
32. Klijn JG, Blamey RW, Boccardo F, et al. Combined tamoxifen and luteinizing hormone-releasing hormone (LHRH) agonist versus LHRH agonist alone in premenopausal advanced breast cancer: a meta-analysis of four randomized trials. J Clin Oncol 2001;19: 343-53.
33. Kuerer HM, Buzdar AU, Singletary SE. Biological basis and evolving role of aromatase inhibitors in the management of invasive carcinoma of the breast. J Surg Oncol 2001;77: 139-47.
34. Beral V, Reeves G. Childbearing, oral contraceptive use, and breast cancer. Lancet 1993; 341:1102.
35. Lethaby AE, O'Neill MA, Mason KE, et al. Overall survival from breast cancer in women pregnant or lactating at or after diagnosis. Int J Cancer 1996;67:751-55.
36. Gelber S, Coates AS, Goldhirsch A, et al. Effect of pregnancy on overall survival after the diagnosis of early-stage breast cancer. J Clin Oncol 19:1671-75.
37. Bergkvist L, Adami HO, Persson I, et al Prognosis after breast cancer diagnosis in owmen

exposed to estrogen and estrogen-progestin replacement therapy. Am J Epi 1980;130:221-27.
38. Col NF, Hirota LK, Orr RK, Erban JK, Wong JB, Lau J. Hormone replacement therapy after breast cancer: a systemic review and quantitative assessment of risk. J Clin Oncol 2001;19:2357-63.
39. O'Meara ES, Rossing MA, Daling JR, Elmore JG, Barlow WE, Weiss NS. Hormone replacement therapy after a diagnosis of breast cancer in relation to recurrence and mortality. J Natl Cancer Inst 2001;93:754-62.
40. Fisher B, Dignam J, Bryant J, et al. Five versus more than five years of tamoxifen therapy for breast cancer patients with negative lymph nodes and estrogen receptor-positive tumors. J Natl Cancer Inst 1996;88:1529-42.
41. Early Breast Cancer Trialists' Collaborative Group. Tamoxifen for early breast cancer: An overview of the randomized trials. Lancet 1998;351:1451-67.
42. Byrne C, Connolly JL, Colditz GA, Schnitt SJ. Biopsy confirmed benign breast disease postmenopausal use of exogenous female hormones and breast cancer risk. Cancer 2000; 89:2046-52.
43. Jernstrom H, Lerman C, Ghadirian P, et al. Pregnancy and risk of early breast cancer in carriers of BRCA1 and BRCA2. Lancet 1999;354:1846-50.
44. King, MC, Wieand S, Hale K, et al. Tamoxifen and breast cancer incidence among women with inherited mutations in BRCA1 and BRCA2: National Surgical Adjuvant Breast and Bowel Project (NSABP-P1)Breast Cancer Prevention Trial. JAMA 2001;286:2251-56.
45. Kuiper GG, Enmark E, Pelto-Huikko M, Nillson S, Gutafsson JA. Cloning of a novel receptor expressed in rat prostate and ovary. Proc Natl Acad Sci 1996;93:5925-30.
46. Horwitz KB, Sartorius CA, Hovland AR, et al. Surprises with anti porgestins: Novel mechanisms of progesterone receptor action. Ciba Foundation Symposium1995;191:235-49; (discussion) 250-53.
47. McKenna NJ, O'Malley BW. An issue of tissues: Divining the split personalities of selective estrogen receptor modulators. Nat Med 2000;6:960-62.
48. Chetrite GS, Cortes-Prieto J, Phillippe JC, et al. Comparison of estrogen concentrations, estrone sulfatase and aromatase activities in normal, and in cancerous, human breast tissues. J Steroid Biochem Mol Biol 2000;72:23-27.
49. Bhatnagar AS, Brodie AM, Long BJ, Evans DB, Miller WR. Intracellular aromatase and its relevance to the pharmacological efficacy of aromatase inhibitors. J Steroid Biochem Mol Biol 2001;76:199-202.
50. Petrakis NL, Wrensch MR, Ernster VL, et al. Influence of pregnancy and lactation on serum and breast fluid estrogen levels: Implications for breast cancer risk. In J Cancer 1987:40(5):587-91.
51. Veronesi U, Luini A, Mariani L, et al. Effect of menstrual phase on surgical treatment of breast cancer. Lancet 1994;343:1545-47.
52. Rajkumar L, Guzman RC, Yang J, Thordarson G, Talamantes F, Nandi S. Short-term exposure to pregnancy levels of estrogen prevents mammary carcinogenesis. Proc Natl Acad Sci 2001;98(20):11755-59.

HORMONAL APPROACH TO BREAST CANCER PREVENTION AND TREATMENT

Jose Russo and Irma H. Russo

Introduction

Epidemiological and clinical data have provided enough information for characterizing the profile of the woman at risk of developing sporadic breast cancer, which constitutes greater than 95% of all cancers diagnosed worldwide [1]. These data highlight the importance of events influenced by ovarian function in relation to age and parity history, such as the increased risk associated with early menarche, i.e. before age 12, nulliparity, late first full-term pregnancy, and late menopause [2-6]. Variations in this relationship among ovarian, age, and reproductive factors that result in protection are late menarche, early single or multiple parity [7], and early menopause [2-6]. Therefore, it can be concluded that these conditions represent the ideal goal to be achieved for protecting the population at large. Our work has been designed largely to clarify the ultimate mechanisms that mediate the protective effect of early pregnancy. Towards this purpose we have analyzed the development of the breast under the influence of endocrinological events occurring at various times during the lifespan of a woman [8-11]. These studies, in correlation with the pathogenesis of breast cancer [11,12], and comparative analyses of experimental *in vivo* and *in vitro* models [13-29], led us to conclude that the key element in the protection of the breast from cancer initiation was the differentiation of this organ induced by pregnancy "before" the mammary parenchyma was affected by a known or still unknown carcinogenic stimulus [30-33]. These findings have led us to postulate that one or more full-term pregnancies at an early age induce differentiation of the breast with the consequent "genomic changes" or "signature" that would ultimately be the responsible for the reduced lifetime breast cancer risk. This postulate is supported in great part by our studies of the 7,12-dimethylbenz (a) anthracene (DMBA)-induced carcinogenesis rodent model [34-39]. A full-term pregnancy induces in the rat complete differentiation of the mammary gland, which then becomes resistant to the carcinogenic effect of DMBA [8,11,13-16,39]. The protection conferred by pregnancy can be reproduced in virgin rats by the administration of human chorionic gonadotropin (hCG) for 21 days before exposure to the carcinogen [40-45]. This hormone, that induces mammary differentiation similar to that elicited by full-term pregnancy, also inhibits tumor progression [40,43]. Both pregnancy- and hCG-induced differentiation encompass progressive lobular development, which is accompanied of morphological and functional changes that result in activation of a variety of genes, namely those controlling programmed cell death and DNA repair [41,43,46,47]. A delay in establishing this "signature," such as might occur with late pregnancy, would alter the pattern of gene activation during early gland development and differentiation. These alterations might in turn affect gland involution, leading to an increase in the lifetime risk of developing breast cancer. This postulate is supported by the progressively increased breast cancer risk observed when childbearing is delayed beyond age 25 [6,7], inasmuch as the risk becomes greater than that of nulliparous women when the first full-term pregnancy occurs after 35 years of age [2-7,48]. In late parous women, in whom the span between menarche and the first pregnancy, a period identified as the "susceptibility window," had been lengthened by two- to three-fold over its length in early parous women, the breast have had greater chances of undergoing genomic damage caused by any given carcinogenic agent, such as radiation [49-52], environmental carcinogens [53], and/or hormonal imbalances [30,43]. An exception to this rule are women that are carriers of the BRCA1 or BRCA2 mutations, who are not protected by an early first full-term pregnancy [54,55]. Our work indicates that genetic predisposition is associated with an altered pattern of breast development and differentiation [56]. It is reasonable to postulate that the observed alterations in the developmental pattern of the breast may be associated with changes in the pathways of programmed cell death and DNA repair. Another important element in the equation that can affect the "signature" imprinted by early full-term pregnancy is the presence of common genetic polymorphisms [57] that have been identified to modify the pathways through which estrogens and environmental carcinogens are metabolized in the epithelium and/or the stroma of the breast at various stages of differentiation.

Role of Gland Differentiation in Breast Cancer Prevention

Our laboratory has demonstrated that in the rat model of DMBA-induced mammary carcinogenesis, maximal cancer incidence occurs when the carcinogen is administered to young virgin rats, but the same carcinogen fails to induce tumors when given to rats after a full-term pregnancy [8,25,29]. The high cancer incidence developed by young virgin rats is the result of the binding of DMBA to the DNA of rapidly dividing cells lining the mammary ducts, namely the terminal end buds (TEBs) [14,15,34-36,58]. This is followed by fixation of transformation, formation of polar metabolites, and deficient DNA repair [14,15], that leads to the development of intraductal proliferations (IDPs) and carcinomas *in situ* (CIS) in these structures. There are close similarities between the pathogenesis of these tumors and the disease spontaneously developed in women, in whom the least differentiated structure equivalent to the TEB is the lobule type 1 (Lob 1), or terminal ductal lobular unit (TDLU) identified in the breast of postpubertal nulliparous women, that is also the origin of ductal carcinomas [10,11]. These structures exhibit high rate of cell proliferation, or Ki67 index, and contain a high percentage of estrogen receptor (ER) alpha and progesterone receptor (PgR) positive cells [21,24,59]. Lob 1 progressively differentiate into Lob 2, and Lob 3, which by the last trimester of pregnancy reach the final stage of secretory Lob 4 [10]. The percentage of both proliferating and steroid receptor positive cells decreases progressively as the lobules mature [21]. After weaning, all the secretory units of the breast regress, progressively reverting in time to Lob 3 and Lob 2 [10]. The comparison between the architecture of the breast of nulliparous and parous women revealed that the breast of the former contained almost exclusively Lob1 throughout the lifespan of the individual. The breast of early parous women, instead, contained predominantly the more differentiated Lob 3 during the reproductive years, but they regressed to Lob 1 after menopause [10,24]. Even though during the postmenopausal years the breast of both parous and nulliparous women contained preponderantly Lob 1, nulliparous women are at higher risk of developing breast cancer [10,30]. Since ductal breast cancer originates in Lob 1 (TDLU) [11,12], the epidemiological observation that nulliparous women exhibit a higher incidence of breast cancer than parous women [3,4] indicates that Lob 1 in these two groups of women might be biologically different, or exhibit different susceptibility to carcinogenesis [16-18]. *In vitro* studies have demonstrated that each specific lobule type differs in biological behavior. Lob 1 and Lob 2 grow faster and have higher DNA labeling index, and a shorter doubling time than Lob 3 [60]. Cells obtained from Lob 1 and Lob 2 express *in vitro* phenotypes indicative of neoplastic transformation when treated with chemical carcinogens, whereas cells obtained from Lob 3 do not manifest those changes [16,17].

Comparison of Gene Expression Between Lob 1 of Nulliparous and Lob 3 of Parous Premenopausal Women

Studies performed in our laboratory using the RNA obtained by laser capture microdissection (LCM) of Lob 1 of three nulliparous and Lob 3 of three parous premenopausal women. The RNA was hybridized to cDNA filter arrays containing 1,176 human genes (Clontech Human Cancer 1.2 array). Lob 3 of parous women exhibited 82 genes differentially overexpressed or downregulated when compared with those expressed in Lob 1. It is of interest to note that a G/T mismatch-specific thymine DNA glycosylase [61] was overexpressed 4 fold in Lob 3, confirming previous data indicating that DNA repair is associated with the process of lobular differentiation [47]. Other genes that were also upregulated in Lob 3, and confirmed by semi-quantitative RT-PCR, were the BRCA1 associated protein, DNA excision repair protein, Endonuclease II homolog 1, DNA repair protein RAD 54, Rad 50 and DNA repair protein XRCC1, all genes known to regulate the synthesis of protein in DNA repair [62]. The insulin-like growth factor binding protein-3 [IGFBP-3], whose levels are developmentally regulated and influenced by a number of hormonal stimuli both *in vitro* and *in vivo* [63-65], was also significantly overexpressed in Lob 3. Of relevance is the observation that TP53 may regulate apoptosis in tumor cells via transactivation of the IGFBP-3 gene [65]. The expression of cytoskeletal proteins such as cytokeratins 18, 19, and 8, that are overexpressed in tumor cells [66], did not differ between Lob 1 and Lob 3. These preliminary data strongly suggest that new clusters of genes are expressed during the process of differentiation from Lob 1 to Lob 3, genes that will give us the specific signature of the fully differentiated breast.

USE OF HUMAN CHORIONIC GONADOTROPIN (HCG) IN THE PREVENTION AND THERAPY OF BREAST CANCER-PRECLINICAL STUDIES.

We have initiated research with the purpose of clarifying the mechanisms through which full-term pregnancy prevents the initiation of DMBA-induced rat mammary cancer led to the novel discoveries that the placental hormone hCG exerted similar protective effect [40,41,43]. Additional studies revealed that this hormone induced differentiation of the mammary gland and early activation of genes controlling programmed cell death, apoptosis, and differentiation [43,46]. The observations that treatment of tumor-bearing rats with recombinant hCG (r-hCG) induced regression of the cancerous lesions opened a new avenue for the utilization of this hormone in cancer therapy [67]. The following three systems derived from this model are being investigated in this project: the role of hCG in the prevention and therapy of DMBA-induced rat mammary cancer [40,41,43], *in vitro* effect of hCG on human breast epithelial cell gene expression [43,44], and clinical trials for testing the therapeutic effect of recombinant hCG on primary and metastatic breast cancer [67]. Recombinant hCG exerts an inhibitory effect on tumor progression through a dual mechanism, one mediated by ovarian stimulation in intact animals and the other independent of the ovary, as demonstrated by treatment of ovariectomized (OVX) rats supplemented with estrogen and progesterone, in which r-hCG significantly reduces the percentage of invasive adenocarcinomas. These preclinical data indicated that r-hCG is a a preventive and tumoristatic agent in mammary cancer, and served as the basis for developing a double-blind, placebo-controlled study. The aim of this study was to investigate the effect of r-hCG on tumor cell proliferation in postmenopausal patients with breast cancer. Twenty two postmenopausal women with primary operable breast cancer (T1–T3) received on alternate days for 2 weeks intramuscular injections of either r-hCG (500 μg); (n = 20) or placebo (n = 5). Core biopsies were collected on day 0 and surgery (mastectomy or lumpectomy) was performed on day 15. The initial biopsy and surgically removed tumor were evaluated to determine the proliferative index, percentage of cells positive for ER and PgR, and inhibin immunoreactivity. It was found that the proliferative index was reduced from 18% to 4% in r-hCG-treated patients ($p < 0.00006$). Expression of ER and PgR was decreased, and inhibin expression was significantly increased following the hormonal treatment. These changes were not observed in the placebo group. Hormonal profiles remained as those characteristic of postmenopausal women; r-hCG was well tolerated and no local or systemic side effects were seen at any time [67].

UNIFYING CONCEPTS

Breast cancer originates in undifferentiated terminal structures of the mammary gland. The terminal ducts of the Lob 1 of the human female breast that are the sites of origin of ductal carcinomas, are at their peak of cell replication during early adulthood, a period during which the breast is more susceptible to carcinogenesis. The susceptibility of Lob 1 to undergo neoplastic transformation has been confirmed by *in vitro* studies, which have shown that this structure has the highest proliferative activity and rate of carcinogen binding to the DNA. More importantly, when treated with carcinogens *in vitro* its epithelial cells express phenotypes indicative of cell transformation. These studies indicate that in the human breast the target cell of carcinogens is found in a specific compartment whose characteristics are the determinant factors in the initiation event (Figure 1). These target cells will become the stem cells of the neoplastic event, depending upon: [a] topographic location within the mammary gland tree, [b] age at exposure to a known or putative genotoxic agent, and [c] reproductive history of the host. The higher incidence of breast cancer observed in nulliparous women supports this concept, because it parallels the higher cancer incidence elicited by carcinogens in rodents when exposure occurs at a young age. In addition, it has been shown that early parity is associated with a pronounced decrease in the risk of breast cancer an additional live births confer greater risk reduction at an approximate rate of 10% per year. Thus, the protection afforded by early full-term pregnancy in women could be explained by the higher degree of differentiation of the mammary gland at the time in which an etiologic agent or agents act. Even though differentiation significantly reduces cell proliferation in the mammary gland, the mammary epithelium remains capable of responding with proliferation to given stimuli, such as a new pregnancy. Under these circumstances, however, the cells that are stimulated to proliferate are from structures that have already been primed, (or that have genomic changes that give these cells a specific signature), by the first cycle of differentiation, thus creating a second type of stem cells that are able to metabolize the carcinogen and repair the DNA damage induced more efficiently than the cells of the virginal gland, and are less susceptible to carcinogenesis, as it has been demonstrated in the rodent experimental system (Figure 1). However, a carcinogenic stimulus powerful enough may overburden the system, successfully initiating a neoplastic process. These conditions might explain the small fraction of women developing breast cancer after an early first full-term pregnancy, meaning completion of the first cycle of differentiation. The effect of pregnancy can be mimicked by gonadotropin hormones that we have found not only moved the stem cell to stage of stem cell 2 but also is able to act on the transformed cells and induced a differentiation effect indicating a therapeutic effect (Figure 1).

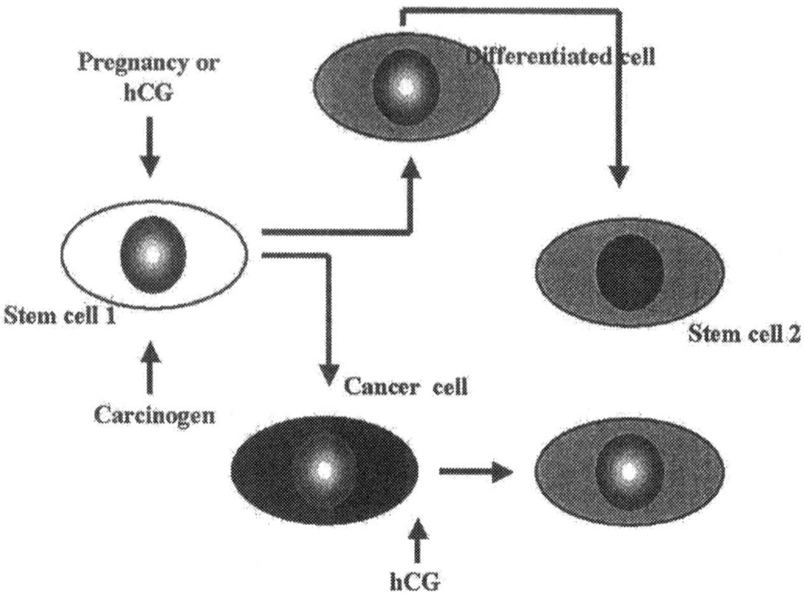

Figure 1. Evolution of the stem cell1 located in the lob.1 of the breast under the effect of the carcinogen evolving to a cancer cell or either stimulated by the differentiation effect of pregnancy or hCG inducing the stem cell 2. hCG also differentiates the cancer cell.

References

1. Greenle RT, Murray T, Boldin S, Wingo P. Cancer Statistics 2000. Ca Cancer J Clin 2000; 50:7-23.
2. Henderson BE, Ross RK, Pike MD. Hormonal chemoprevention of cancer in women. Science 1993;259:68-72.
3. MacMahon B, Cole P, Lin TM. et al. Age at first birth and breast cancer risk. Bull Natl Hlth Org 1970;43:209.
4. Vessey MD, McPherson K, Roberts MM, Neil A, Jones L. Fertility and the risk of breast cancer. Br J Cancer 1985;52:625-28.
5. Trapido EJ. Age at first birth, parity and breast cancer risk Cancer 1983;51:946-48.
6. Lambe M,. Hsieh CC, Chan HW, Ekbom A, Trichopoulos D, Adami HO. Parity, age at first and last birth, and risk of breast cancer: A population-based study in Sweden. Breast

Cancer Res Treat 1996;38: 305-11.
7. Wohlfahrt J, Melbye M. Age at any birth is associated with breast cancer risk. Epidemiology 2001;12:68-73.
8. Russo J, Tay LK, Russo IH. Differentiation of the mammary gland and susceptibility to carcinogenesis: A review. Breast Cancer Res Treat 1982;2:5-73.
9. Russo J, Russo IH. Development of the human mammary gland. In: Neville, MC, Daniel C, editors. The mammary gland. New York: Plenum Publishing, Inc., 1987: 67-93.
10. Russo J, Santen R, Russo IH. Hormonal control of the breast development. In: DeGroot LJ, Jameson LL, editors. Endocrinology (Fourth Edition). Philadelphia: W.B. Saunders Company, Vol.3, 2001:2181-88.
11. Russo J, Gusterson BA, Rogers AE, Russo IH, Welling SR, Van Zwieten MJ. Comparative study of human and rat mammary tumorigenesis. Lab Invest 1990;62:244-78.
12. Wellings SR, Jansen MM, Marcum RG. An atlas of sub-gross pathology of the human breast with special reference to possible pre-cancerous lesions. J Natl Cancer Inst 1975;55: 231-75.
13. Russo J, Russo IH. Influence of differentiation and cell kinetics on the susceptibility of the mammary gland to carcinogenesis. Cancer Res 1980;40:2677-87.
14. Tay LK, Russo J. 7, 12-dimethylbenz(a)anthracene (DMBA) induced DNA binding and repair synthesis in susceptible and non-susceptible mammary epithelial cells in culture. J Natl Cancer Inst 1981;67:155-61.
15. Tay LK, Russo J. Formation and removal of 7,12-dimethylbenz(a)anthracene-nucleic acid adducts in rat mammary epithelial cells with different susceptibility to carcinogenesis. Carcinogenesis 1981;2:1327-33.
16. Russo J, Reina D, Frederick J, Russo IH. Expression of phenotypical changes by human breast epithelial cells treated with carcinogens in vitro. Cancer Res 1988;48:2837-57.
17. Russo J, Calaf G, Russo IH. A critical approach to the malignant transformation of human breast epithelial cells. CRC Crit Rev Oncog 1993;4:403-17.
18. Russo J, Russo IH. Toward a physiological approach to breast cancer prevention. Cancer Epidemiol Biomarkers Prev 1994;3:353-64.
19. Russo J, Russo IH. Differentiation and Breast Cancer Development. In: Heppner G, editor. Advances in oncobiology. Vol. 2. Totowa, NJ: JAI. Press, Inc., 1998:1-10.
20. Russo J, Russo IH. Toward a unified concept of mammary tumorigenesis. Prog Clin Biol Res 1997;396:1-16.
21. Russo J, Ao X, Grill C, Russo IH. Pattern of distribution of cells positive for estrogen receptor α and progesterone receptor in relation to proliferating cells in the mammary gland. Breast Cancer Res Treat 1999;53:217-27.
22. Hu YF, Silva IDCG, Russo IH, Ao X, Russo J. A novel serpin gene cloned from differentiated human breast epithelial cells is a potential tumor suppressor. Proc Am Assoc Cancer Res 1998;39:114a.
23. Hu YF, Russo IH, Ao X, Russo J. Mammary-derived growth inhibitor (MDGI) cloned from human breast epithelial cells is expressed in fully differentiated lobular structure. Int J Oncol 1997;11:5-11.
24. Russo J, Rivera R, Russo J. Influence of age and parity on the development of the human

breast. Breast Cancer Res Treat 1992;23:211-18.

25. Russo J, Russo IH. Biological and molecular bases of mammary carcinogenesis. Lab Invest 1987;57:112-37.
26. Russo J, Russo IH. The cellular basis of breast cancer susceptibility. Oncol Res 1999;11: 169-78.
27. Russo J, Russo IH, Development pattern of human breast and susceptibility to carcinogenesis. Eur J Cancer Prev 1993;2:85-100.
28. Russo J, Romero AL, Russo IH. Architectural pattern of the normal and cancerous breast under the influence of parity. Cancer Epidemiol Biomarkers Prev 1994;3:219-24.
29. Russo IH, Russo J. Developmental stage of the rat mammary gland as determinant of its susceptibility to 7,12-dimethylbenz(a)anthracene. J Natl Cancer Inst 1978;61:1439-49.
30. Russo J, Hu YF, Yang X, Russo IH. Developmental, cellular and molecular basis of human breast cancer: J Natl Cancer Inst Monograph 27, 2000:17-38.
31. Russo J, Hu YF, Silva IDCG, Russo IH. Cancer risk related to mammary gland structure and development. Microsc Res Tech 2001;52:204-23.
32. Russo J, Russo IH. The pathway of neoplastic transformation. Radiat Res 2001;155:151-54.
33. Russo J, Russo IH. The cellular basis of breast cancer susceptibility. Oncol Res 1999;11: 169-78.
34. Russo J, Russo IH. DNA labeling index and structure of the rat mammary gland as determinants of its susceptibility to carcinogenesis. J Natl Cancer Inst 1978;61:1451-59.
35. Russo J, Wilgus G, Russo IH. Susceptibility of the mammary gland to carcinogenesis. Differentiation of the mammary gland as determinant of tumor incidence and type of lesion. Am J Pathol 1979;96:721-36.
36. Russo J. Basis of cellular autonomy in the susceptibility to carcinogenesis. Toxicol Pathol 1983;11:149-66.
37. Russo J, Saby J, Isenberg W, Russo IH. Pathogenesis of mammary carcinomas induced in rats by 7,12-dimethylbenz(a)anthracene. J Natl Cancer Inst 1977;59:435-45.
38. Russo J, Russo IH. Is differentiation the answer in breast cancer prevention? IRCS Med Sci 1982;10:935-41.
39. Russo IH, Russo J. Mammary gland neoplasia in long-term rodent studies. Environ Health Perspect 1996;104:938-67.
40. Russo IH, Koszalka M, Russo J. Human chorionic gonadotropin and rat mammary cancer prevention. J Natl Cancer Inst 1990;82:1286-89.
41. Russo IH, Koszalka M, Russo J. Comparative study of the influence of pregnancy and hormonal treatment on mammary carcinogenesis. Br J Cancer 1991;64:481-84.
42. Russo IH, Russo J. Role of hormones in cancer initiation and progression. J Mammary Gland Biol Neoplasia 1997;3:49-61.
43. Russo J, Russo IH. Human chorionic gonadotropin in breast cancer prevention In: Ethier SP, editor. Endocrine oncology. Totowa, NJ.: Humana Press Inc., 2000:121-36.
44. Russo IH, Russo J. Role of hCG and inhibin in breast cancer. Int J Oncol 1994;4:297-306.
45. Russo IH, Russo J. Hormonal approach to breast cancer prevention. J Cell Biochem 2000; 34(Suppl.):1-6.

46. Srivastava P, Russo J, Russo IH. Chorionic gonadotropin inhibits rat mammary carcinogenesis through activation of programmed cell death. Carcinogenesis 1997;18: 1799-1808.
47. Tay LK, Russo J. Effect of human chorionic gonadotropin on 7,12-dimethylbenz(a)anthracene-induced DNA binding and repair synthesis by rat mammary epithelial cells. Chem Biol Interact 1985;55:13-21.
48. De Waard F, Trichopoulos D. A unifying concept of the etiology of breast cancer. Int J Cancer 1988;41:666-69.
49. Hancock SL, Tucker MA, Hoppe RT. Breast cancer after treatment of Hodgkin's disease. J Natl Cancer Inst 1993;85:25-31.
50. Clemons M, Loijens L, Goss P. Breast cancer risk following irradiation for Hodgkin's disease. Cancer Treat Rev 2000;26:291-302.
51. Cutuli B, Borel C, Dhermain F, et al. Breast cancer occurred after treatment for Hodgkin's disease: Analysis of 133 cases. Radiother Oncol 2001;59:247-55.
52. Janov AJ, Tulecke M, O'Neill A, et al. Clinical and pathologic features of breast cancers in women treated for hodgkin's disease: A case-control study. Breast J 2001;7:46-52.
53. Morabia A, Bernstein M. A review of the relationship of active and passive smoking to breast cancer. J Women's Cancer 2000;2:1-9.
54. Gaffney DK, Hemmersmeier J, Holden J, et al. Breast cancer after mantle irradiation for Hodgkin's disease: Correlation of clinical, pathologic, and molecular features including loss of heterozygosity at BRCA1 and BRCA2. Int J Radiat Oncol Biol Phys 2001;49:539-46.
55. Jernstrom H, Lerman C, Ghadirian P, et al. Pregnancy and risk of early breast cancer in carriers of BRCA1 and BRCA2. Lancet 1999;354:1846-50.
56. Russo J, Lynch H, Russo IH. Mammary gland architecture as a determining factor in the susceptibility of the human breast to cancer. Breast J 2001;7:1-14.
57. Rebbeck TR. Inherited genetic predisposition in breast cancer. A population-based perspective. Cancer 1999;86:2493-501.
58. Russo J, Russo IH. Role of differentiation on transformation of human epithelial cells. In: D. Medina, et al., editors. Cellular and molecular biology of mammary cancer. New York: Plenum Press, 1987: 399- 417.
59. Calaf G, Alvarado ME, Bonney GE, Amfoh KK, Russo J. Influence of lobular development on breast epithelial cell proliferation and steroid hormone receptor content. Int J Oncology 1995;7:1285-88.
60. Russo J, Mills MJ, Moussalli MJ, Russo IH. Influence of human breast development on the growth properties of primary cultures. In Vitro Cell and Develop Biol 1989;25:643-49.
61. Nedermann P, Gallinari P, Lettieri T, et al. Cloning and expression of human G/T mistmatch-specific thymine DNA glycosylase. J Biol Chem1996;271:12767-74.
62. Wood RD, Mitchell M, Sgouros J, Lindahl T. Human DNA repair genes. Science 2001; 291:1284-89.
63. Phillips LS, Pao CI, Villafuerte BC. Molecular regulation of insulin-like growth factor-I and its principal binding protein, IGFBP-3. Prog Nucleic Acid Res Mol Biol 1998;60:195-265.

64. Oh Y. IGFBPs and neoplastic models. New concepts for roles of IGFBPs in regulation of cancer cell growth. Endocrine 1997;7:111-13.
65. Cubbage ML, Suwanichkul A, Powell DR. Insulin-like growth factor binding protein-3. Organization of the human chromosomal gene and demonstration of promoter activity. J Biol Chem 1990;265:12642-49.
66. Brotherick I, Robson CN, Bronell DA, et al. Cytokeratin expression in breast cancer: Phenotypic changes associated with disease progression. Cytometry 1998;32:301-8.
67. Russo J, Janssens J, Russo IH. Recombinant human chorionic gonadotropin(r-hCG) significantly reduces primary tumor cell proliferation in patients with breast cancer. Breast Cancer Res Treat 2000;64:161a.

Healthy Postmenopausal Women Receiving HRT Are Not at Risk for Early Coronary Events: Results from 2 Large Clinical Trials

Ginger D.Constantine, James H. Pickar, and Edward A. Trott

Introduction

Cardiovascular disease (CVD) is the most common and deadly disease among women, accounting for approximately 500,000 deaths annually, nearly twice the number of deaths from cancer [1]. The prevalence of CVD in women increases dramatically after menopause [1,2], when endogenous estradiol production by the ovaries significantly decreases. The concurrent increase in CVD risk and decrease in endogenous estrogens have led to the suggestion that exogenous estrogen can reduce the risk of CVD in postmenopausal women. Indeed, multiple studies have suggested that estrogen replacement therapy (ERT, unopposed estrogens) or hormone replacement therapy (HRT, estrogens in combination with a progestin) may reduce the risk of CVD in women [3-8]. Observational data from the large Nurses' Health Study of more than 70,000 healthy postmenopausal women indicate that HRT decreases the risk of cardiovascular events in women by as much as 40% [6]. In addition, a large randomized 3-year clinical trial with 875 healthy postmenopausal women showed significant improvement in cardiovascular parameters with HRT use [4].

In contrast, recent studies examining the efficacy of HRT for the secondary prevention of heart disease have not demonstrated a protective effect against recurrent coronary events [9,10] or atherosclerosis progression [11]. In the Heart and Estrogen/progestin Replacement Study (HERS), post-hoc analysis suggested that women with preexisting CVD who had received HRT were more likely to experience a cardiac event in the first year of therapy than patients who had received placebo [9]. A comparable examination of participants with coronary artery disease (CAD) in the Nurses' Health Study also indicated a higher rate of coronary events with short-term HRT use [12].

Methods

Because postmenopausal women aged 45 to 65 years are the primary users of HRT treatment, we sought to evaluate coronary events in this relevant population with special focus on the occurrence of cardiovascular adverse events within the first year of initiating ERT/HRT. The incidence of coronary events were evaluated in 2 large clinical studies of the effects of HRT in healthy postmenopausal women.

The effects of varying doses and regimens of HRT and placebo on coronary events were evaluated in 4,397 healthy postmenopausal women enrolled in 2 studies conducted between 1989 and 2001, the safety and efficacy of which have been reported [13-20]. The occurrence of nonfatal myocardial infarction (MI) and coronary heart disease (CHD) deaths during the first year of these 2 large primary-prevention clinical trials is the focus of this review. Secondary vascular outcomes of cerebrovascular events, deep vein thrombosis and thrombosis (DVT), and pulmonary embolism (PE) are also included.

STUDY DESIGNS

Women's HOPE Study. The 1-year core Women's HOPE study recruited healthy postmenopausal women for a randomized, double-blind, placebo-controlled trial to examine the safety and efficacy of 7 dose regimens of daily oral conjugated equine estrogens (CEE) with or without medroxyprogesterone acetate (MPA), or placebo, as shown in Table 1 [17].

The 1-year core study in Women's HOPE focused on menopausal symptoms and urogenital health [17], bleeding profiles [18], and endometrial effects [19]. Women were eligible for inclusion in the Women's HOPE study if they were between 40 and 65 years of age, had an intact uterus, had 12 months of amenorrhea, had no history of CVD, and were within 20% of normal body weight range. Initial screenings included a complete medical history and physical examination to ensure that inclusion/exclusion criteria were met [17].

A subset of 822 patients from the year 1 core Women's HOPE study participated in a 2-year osteoporosis and metabolic substudy to examine the safety and efficacy of the CE and MPA regimens in preventing postmenopausal osteoporosis and maintaining an acceptable metabolic profile.

Table 1. HOPE Study Dose Regimens[a,b,c]

		Dose (mg)	
Regimen	N	CEE[b]	CEE/MPA[b]
A	348	0.625	Placebo
B	331	Placebo	0.625/2.5
C	338	0.45	Placebo
D	340	Placebo	0.45/2.5
E	331	Placebo	0.45/1.5
F	326	0.3	Placebo
G	327	Placebo	0.3/1.5
H	332	Placebo	Placebo

a: All treatments were taken on cycle days 1 to 28; b: CEE = conjugated equine estrogens; MPA = medroxyprogesterone acetate; c: patient years of exposure = 2,082

Menopause Study Group Trial. Investigators began recruiting healthy postmenopausal women for the Menopause Study Group trial [13] in 1989 to evaluate the safety and efficacy of continuous and sequential regimens of 0.625 mg CEE plus 2.5, 5.0, or 10.0 mg MPA, as shown in Table 2.

Table 2. Menopause Study Group Trial Dose Regimens[a,b]

		Dose (mg)		
Regimen	n	CEE	MPA	Days of Use/Cycle
A	340	0.625	2.5	1-28
B	338	0.625	5.0	1-28
C	351	0.625	Placebo	1-14
		0.625	5.0	15-28
D	348	0.625	Placebo	1-14
		0.625	10.0	15-28
E	347	0.625	Placebo	1-28

a: CEE = conjugated equine estrogens; MPA = medroxyprogesterone acetate; b: patient years of exposure = 1,510

This randomized, double-blind study was conducted at 99 sites in the United States and Europe. The primary end point was the incidence of endometrial hyperplasia at 1 year [16]. Women were eligible for the study if they were between 45 and 65 years of age with an intact uterus, were within 20% of normal body weight range, and their last menstrual period had been at least 12 months before baseline screening. A complete medical history and physical examination were conducted to ensure that inclusion/exclusion criteria were met [13].

PROCEDURE

Patients were evaluated every 2-3 months and results of these evaluations were recorded in the individual's clinical case report form. If a patient had a cardiovascular event, it was reported to the sponsor and all adverse events were reported to the FDA in the United States and appropriate regulatory authorities in other countries. The principle investigator and medical monitor evaluated each reported vascular event and obtained supporting documents from these patients clinical report forms to confirm the identified vascular event.

Results

Baseline characteristics of the women in the 2 studies were similar, and consisted of healthy women averaging between 53.3 and 54.0 years of age and between 4.7 and 5.3 years postmenopause, as seen in Table 3.

Table 3. Baseline Characteristics of Postmenopausal Women in the Clinical Studies Reviewed

Study	Number	Age at Baseline	Years Since Menopause
Women's Health, Osteoporosis, Progestin, Estrogen (Women's HOPE) [17]	2673	53.3 ± 4.9	4.7 ± 4.2
Menopause Study Group (MSG) [13]	1724	54.0 ± 4.6	5.3 ± 1.3

The number of patients assigned to each treatment group was also similar across the studies (Tables 1 and 2).

NONFATAL MI AND CHD DEATHS

Among the 4,397 healthy patients who were enrolled in the 2 trials, there were no CHD fatalities. The only nonfatal MI occurred in 1 patient assigned to the placebo group in the Women's HOPE study. In 2,341 healthy postmenopausal women assigned to active treatment in the Women's HOPE study, there was no increase in the risk of primary CHD events compared with 332 patients assigned to placebo during the first year of HRT.

SECONDARY VASCULAR EVENTS

Individual data on patients who experienced secondary vascular events during the first year of the trials are presented in Table 4. There was no trend in event rate with HRT treatment regimen or duration of hormone use within the first year.

There was no difference in incidence rates among active treatment groups in the 2 clinical trials. The overall incidence of secondary vascular events was 195 per 100,000 patient-years of active treatment in the 2 studies.

Discussion

Cardiovascular disease has been shown to increase in women after menopause and is more prevalent among women who experience early menopause. Despite a large body of epidemiological evidence showing a decreased risk of heart disease for women taking either estrogen alone or estrogen combined with a progestin [5,6,21-24] data from large, randomized clinical trials of healthy postmenopausal women and HRT are limited and of relatively short duration.

Table 4. Secondary Vascular Events Observed

Study Event	Dose (mg)	Age (y)	Ht (in)	Wt (lb)
Women's HOPE Study (CEE/MPA)				
Stroke	0.625/2.5[a]	59	63	158
Stroke	0.625[a]	53	63	147
Transient ischemic attack	0.45/1.5[a]	56	66.5	177
Pulmonary embolism	0.45[a]	56	62.7	148
Deep vein thrombosis	0.45/1.5[a]	52	65.5	166
Menopause Study Group (CEE/MPA)				
Pulmonary embolism	0.625/5.0[b]	57	60.5	137.2
Cerebral aneurysm	0.625[a]	53	66.4	133.4

CEE = conjugated equine estrogens; MPA = medroxyprogesterone acetate. a: continuous (1-28); b: sequential (15-28).

The HERS study is the only large randomized trial that examined CHD and HRT, however, this was in older postmenopausal women (mean age = 66.7 years) with established coronary disease, i.e. secondary prevention [25]. Post-hoc analysis from HERS suggested an increased risk of cardiovascular events during the first year of HRT treatment for women with pre-existing CVD [9]. This may have been attributable to the unusual finding of a decreased risk of cardiovascular events in the HERS placebo patients who were ≥ 70 years old [26]. The CV event rate in these older women was actually less than that in participants who were 60 years of age or younger. This is unlike other cardiovascular trials that demonstrate increased CHD-related mortality and incidence of MIs in older women [27-30].

Despite the overall null results seen in HERS, the cardioprotective effect of HRT in postmenopausal women who are most likely to take these products has not been addressed, i.e. younger postmenopausal women without established CAD. The controversy surrounding the potential protective effects of HRT on cardiovascular disease is fueled by the favorable changes observed in lipids, lipoproteins, fibrinogen, plasminogen activator inhibitor-1 (PAI-1), antithrombin III, vascular reactivity, and antioxidant action after treatment with HRT [31, 32].

In this evaluation of 2 large randomized clinical trials, the cardiovascular effects of conjugated estrogens administered with and without a progestin are presented. The subjects enrolled in these trials were representative of the majority of HRT users, that is they were generally healthy postmenopausal women. In these studies, there were no first year coronary events, suggesting that HRT is safe in healthy postmenopausal women.

Of the secondary vascular events observed, none exceeded the incidence reported for a comparable population of non-HRT users. Because there were relatively few placebo patients in these trials, comparison was made to the expected incidence rate in the general population. The observed rate of 4.2 stroke-related events per 5,000 patient-years is not statistically different from the expected rate of 2.6 per 5,000 person-years within the general postmenopausal female population [29]. These data in healthy postmenopausal women agree with a report from the HERS trial that cerebrovascular events in postmenopausal women with established CVD are not related to HRT use [29].

There was an observed rate of 0.28 DVT per 1,000 patient-years in these trials that is less than the reported incidence of venous thrombosis (1.3 to 3.0 per 1,000 person-years) in postmenopausal women [33,34]. Previous studies have suggested a 2- to 3.5-fold increased risk of DVT among postmenopausal women using HRT [33-36]. In the 2 clinical trials, a 2-fold increase in the incidence of DVT was not observed in the healthy postmenopausal women studied.

Finally, the incidence rate of primary PE in a general population of women aged 50 to 59 years who never used HRT is 3 events per 5,000 person-years [37]. The observed rate of 2.8 PE per 5,000 patient-years in the 2 clinical trials indicated no increase in the rate of PE for these healthy postmenopausal women during 1 year of HRT treatment.

Healthy postmenopausal women who will benefit from HRT and their health care providers should be reassured that HRT did not increase the risk of CVD. These data demonstrate no increase in the rate of nonfatal MI or CHD-related death in healthy postmenopausal women 40 to 65 years of age during 1 year of treatment with commonly prescribed and lower doses of HRT. In addition, no increase in the rate of secondary vascular events was observed. These data support the cardiovascular safety of commonly prescribed and lower doses of HRT during the first year of therapy in healthy postmenopausal women.

References

1. American Heart Association. 2001 Heart and Stroke Statistical Update. Dallas, Texas: American Heart Association; 2001:1-32.
2. Kannel WB, Wilson PWF. Risk factors that attenuate the female coronary disease advantage. Arch Intern Med 1995;155:57-61.
3. Selzman CH, Whitehill TA, Shames BD, Pulido EJ, Cain BC, Harken AH. The biology of estrogen-mediated repair of cardiovascular injury. Ann Thorac Surg 1998;65:868-74.
4. Writing Group for the PEPI Trial. Effects of estrogen or estrogen/progestin regimens on heart disease risk factors in postmenopausal women: Postmenopausal Estrogen/Progestin Interventions (PEPI) Trial. JAMA 1995;273:199-208.
5. Barrett-Connor E, Grady D. Hormone replacement therapy, heart disease, and other considerations. Annu Rev Pub Health 1998;19:55-72.
6. Grodstein F, Stampfer MJ, Manson J, et al. Postmenopausal estrogen and progestin use and the risk of cardiovascular disease. N Engl J Med 1996;335:453-61.
7. Sullivan JM. Estrogen replacement therapy. Am J Med 1996;101:(4A)4A56S-4A59S.
8. Mendelsohn ME, Karas RH. The protective effects of estrogen on the cardiovascular system. N Engl J Med 1999;340:1801-11.
9. Hulley S, Grady D, Bush T, et al. Randomized trial of estrogen plus progestin for secondary prevention of coronary heart disease in postmenopausal women. JAMA 1998; 280:605-13.

10. Clarke S, Kelleher J, Lloyd-Jones H, Sharples L, Slack M, Schofield PM. Transdermal hormone replacement therapy for secondary prevention of coronary artery disease in postmenopausal women. Eur Heart J 2000;21:212.
11. Herrington DM, Reboussin DM, Brosnihan KB, et al. Effects of estrogen replacement on the progression of coronary-artery atherosclerosis. N Engl J Med 2000;343:522-29.
12. Grodstein F, Manson JE, Stampfer MJ. Postmenopausal hormones and recurrence of coronary events in the nurses' health study [abstract]. Circulation 1999;100(suppl):I-871.
13. Archer DF, Pickar JH, Bottiglioni F, for the Menopause Study Group. Bleeding patterns in postmenopausal women taking continuous combined or sequential regimens of conjugated estrogens with medroxyprogesterone acetate. Obstet Gynecol 1994;83:686-92.
14. Lobo RA, Pickar JH, Wild RA, Walsh B, Hirvonen E. Metabolic impact of adding medroxyprogesterone acetate to conjugated estrogen therapy in postmenopausal women. Obstet Gynecol 1994;84:987-95.
15. Archer DF, Pickar JH. Hormone replacement therapy: Effect of progestin dose and time since menopause on endometrial bleeding. Obstet Gynecol 2000;96:899-905.
16. Woodruff JD, Pickar JH. Incidence of endometrial hyperplasia in postmenopausal women taking conjugated estrogens (Premarin) with medroxyprogesterone acetate or conjugated estrogens alone. Am J Obstet Gynecol 1994;170:1213-23.
17. Utian WH, Shoupe D, Bachmann G, Pinkerton JV, Pickar JH. Relief of vasomotor symptoms and vaginal atrophy with lower doses of conjugated equine estrogens and medroxyprogesterone acetate. Fertil Steril 2001;75:1065-79.
18. Archer DF, Dorin M, Lewis V, Schneider DL, Pickar JH. Effects of lower doses of conjugated equine estrogens and medroxyprogesterone acetate on endometrial bleeding. Fertil Steril 2001;75:1080-87.
19. Pickar JH, Yeh I-T, Wheeler JE, Cunnane MF, Speroff L. Endometrial effects of lower doses of conjugated equine estrogens and medroxyprogesterone acetate. Fertil Steril 2001; 76:25-31.
20. Lobo RA, Bush T, Carr BR, Pickar JH. Effects of lower doses of conjugated equine estrogens and medroxyprogesterone acetate on plasma lipids and lipoproteins, coagulation factors, and carbohydrate metabolism. Fertil Steril 2001;76:13-24.
21. Grodstein F, Stampfer M. The epidemiology of coronary heart disease and estrogen replacement in postmenopausal women. Prog Cardiovasc Dis 1995;38:199-210.
22. Pedersen AT, Lidegaard O, Kreiner S, Ottesen B. Hormone replacement therapy and risk of non-fatal stroke. Lancet 1997;350:1277-83.
23. Petitti DB, Sidney S, Quesenberry CP, Bernstein A. Ischemic stroke and use of estrogen and estrogen/progestogen as hormone replacement therapy. Stroke 1998;29:23-28.
24. Falkeborn M, Persson I, Terént A, Adami H-O, Lithell H, Bergström R. Hormone replacement therapy and the risk of stroke. Follow-up of a population-based cohort in Sweden. Arch Intern Med 1993;153:1201-9.
25. Mosca L, Grundy SM, Judelson D, et al. AHA/ACC scientific statement: consensus panel statement. Guide to preventive cardiology in women. Circulation 1999;99:2480-84.
26. Simon JA, Hsia J, Cauley JA, et al. Postmenopausal hormone therapy and risk of stroke: The heart and estrogen-progestin replacement study (HERS). Circulation 2001;103:638-42.
27. Angerer P, Stork S, Kothny W, Schmitt P, von Schacky C. Effect of oral postmenopausal hormone replacement on progression of atherosclerosis: A randomized, controlled trial. Arterioscler Thromb Vasc Biol 2001;21:262-68.

28. Shepherd J, Cobbe SM, Ford I, et al. Prevention of coronary heart disease with pravastatin in men with hypercholesterolemia. N Engl J Med 1995;333:1301-7.
29. Grodstein F, Manson JE, Colditz GA, Willett WC, Speizer FE, Stampfer MJ. A prospective, observational study of postmenopausal hormone therapy and primary prevention of cardiovascular disease. Ann Intern Med 2000;133:933-41.
30. Pohjola S, Siltanen P, Romo M. Five-year survival of 728 patients after myocardial infarction: A community study. Br Heart J 1980;43:176-83.
31. Tikkanen MJ. Mechanisms of cardiovascular effects of estrogen and lipid-lowering therapies in postmenopausal women. Circulation 1996;93:1928-37.
32. Mathews KA, Kuller LH, Wing RR, Meilahn EN, Plantinga P. Prior to use of estrogen replacement therapy, are users healthier than non users? Am J Epidemiology 1996;143: 971-78.
33. Pérez Gutthann S, García Rodríguez LA, Castellsague J, Duque Oliart A. Hormone replacement therapy and risk of venous thromboembolism: Population based case-control study. BMJ 1997;314:796-800.
34. Kuller LH. Hormone replacement therapy and coronary heart disease. In: Robinson K, editor. Risk factor modification for cardiac disease. Philadelphia, Pennsylvania: WB Saunders Co; 2000:181-98.
35. Daly E, Vessey MP, Hawkins MM, Carson JL, Gough P, Marsh S. Risk of venous thromboembolism in users of hormone replacement therapy. Lancet 1996;348:977-80.
36. Jick H, Derby LE, Myers MW, Vasilakis C, Newton KM. Risk of hospital admission for idiopathic venous thromboembolism among users of postmenopausal oestrogens. Lancet 1996;348:981-83.
37. Grodstein F, Stampfer MJ, Goldhaber SZ, et al. Prospective study of exogenous hormones and risk of pulmonary embolism in women. Lancet 1996;348:983-87.

ORAL CONTRACEPTIVE USE AND RISK OF LOW BONE DENSITY IN WOMEN ATTENDING MENOPAUSE CLINICS IN ITALY

C. Donati Sarti, P. Monteleone, M. Gambacciani, F. Parazzini on behalf of the Progetto Menopausa Italia

Introduction

Osteoporosis is a major health care problem, which leads to a high incidence of spine, radial, and hip fractures. These are considered major causes of morbidity and mortality in the aging population. Bone mineral density (BMD) is an important determinant of fracture risk. It is now well recognized that a chronically hypoestrogenic state increases bone turnover that, in turn, causes a critical decrease in BMD [1-4]. This process is already present in perimenopausal oligomenorrheic women. Although hormone replacement therapy has been reported to prevent the reduction in bone density related to estrogen deficiency [5,6], these women cannot benefit from HRT and the sole supplementation of calcium at this phase is unable to arrest the loss in BMD. There are many studies in the literature reporting that the use of low-dose oral contraceptive (OC) administration may be an optimal preventive measure for perimenopausal decrease in radial [7] and vertebral [8] bone density. The observation of a protective effect of OC on the risk of hip fracture [9] is supported by the results of a longitudinal study, showing that, in perimenopausal oligomenorrheic women, the decrease in femoral bone density is reversed by the administration of a low-dose OC preparation [10]. In order to offer further data on this issue, we collected information in the framework of a large cross-sectional study on the characteristics of women around menopause attending a network of first level outpatient menopause clinics in Italy.

Methods

Between 1997 and March 2000, a large cross-sectional study was conducted on the characteristics of women around menopause attending menopause clinics all over Italy for general counseling about menopause or treatment of menopausal symptoms. Only those women who agreed to undergo strict follow-up during the study period were eligible for the study. The study protocol did not foresee any exclusion criteria. The study began in 1997 in 25 centers, which rose to 268 by March 1999. Of these, 63 were situated in northern Italy, 81, in central Italy and 124, in southern Italy. A total of 42,464 women (mean age 53) were studied during this period. All women were asked about their general characteristics, habits, reproductive and menstrual history. A problem-oriented medical history and a gynecological examination were also carried out. Laboratory and instrumental tests were requested on a clinical basis: BMD measurements were available in 25,016 cases, considered in this analysis. Low bone density (LBD) (osteopenia/osteoporosis) was defined according to WHO classification [11]. Postmenopausal women were defined as those subjects whose menstrual cycles had stopped more than one year before the interview.

BMD was measured in different centers and with different instruments (single photon absorptiometry, single and dual energy X-ray absorptiometry). However, most centers used dual energy X-ray absorptiometry, and anteroposterior measurement were performed in lumbar vertebral L2-L4 in about 60% of cases. In any case the inclusion in the analysis of terms for center or method of BMD evaluation did not change the OR estimates. Likewise, the analysis performed separately in strata of type of instruments and site of measurement (lumbar vertebral L2-L4, hip, forearm) consistently confirmed the results of the general analysis (data not shown).

The OR of low LBD were computed for various factors (age, age at menopause, body mass index, center, calendar year at interview, smoking, OC use), together with their 95% approximate confidence intervals (CI), using unconditional multiple logistic regression models. Two different models were performed, the first one controlling the effect of age only, the second one including all factors significantly associated with LBD in the age-adjusted analysis plus calendar year at interview and center. No marked differences emerged between the two models.

Results

Ever-OC use was reported in 2,886 cases (11.4%) women. The OR of osteopenia/osteoporosis was 0.89 (0.79-1.00) for ever-OC use in comparison with never-users. The OR of osteopenia/osteoporosis was 0.83 (95% CI 0.78-1.03) in women aged < 51 years, i.e. with more recent OC use.

Discussion

This large cross-sectional study, consistent with previous epidemiological studies in Italy, demonstrates that the use of OC in premenopausal Italian women may in part reverse the trend towards bone mineral loss, characteristic of this phase.

Potential limitations of the analysis may consist in the fact that BMD evaluation was requested by the gynecologist on a clinical basis, and according to the routine practice of each participating center. However, at the time of data collection the possible association between OC use and risk of osteoporosis was unknown to gynecologists as well as the women. Thus, it is unlikely that the request of BMD evaluation would have introduced a bias in the analysis of the association between OC use and risk of osteopenia/osteoporosis in women who underwent BMD evaluation.

The relation between ovarian function and bone turnover suggests that during the perimenopausal transition, subjects with low estrogen production may lose a substantial portion of bone before entering the menopause. In women with ovulatory disturbances, bone turnover is increased and BMD is lower than in normally cycling women [12]. A long cycle length may indicate anovulatory cycles, reflecting a hypoestrogenic condition. In these cases, administration of OC is capable of blocking increased bone loss and of restoring a normal BMD. In fact, all prospective studies in perimenopausal women [7,8,10,13] showed either maintenance of or increase in BMD among OC users, while a loss of BMD was observed in controls. Moreover, it seems that the longer women take OC, the greater the benefits in terms of BMD [14]. Michaelsson et al. [9] have recently suggested that OC use may reduce the risk of hip fractures, by reducing bone loss.

OC use is associated with a reduction in fracture risk if assumed after the age of forty but not in younger women. This is supported by the fact that BMD decreases when ovarian function becomes impaired [15-17], and therefore the use of OC may be effective in blocking the increase in bone turnover that follows the decline in ovarian estrogen production.

The estrogen in OC increases calcium absorption, decreases calcium loss, and has a direct inhibiting effect on bone resorption [18]. The potentially protective role of OC use on low bone density is biologically plausible, since OC represents a constant exposure to exogenous estrogens for the perimenopausal woman.

Acknowledgments

The Menopausa Italia Project is partially supported by Bracco Spa, Igea Srl, Menarini Srl, Novo Nordisk Farmaceutici Spa, Recordati Spa, Rottapharm Srl, Schering Spa, Schwarz Pharma Spa, Solvay Pharma Spa, Wyeth Lederle Spa, Theramex Spa.

References

1. Ott SM. Attainment of peak bone mass. J Clin Endocrinol Metab 1990;71:1082a-82c.
2. Geusens P, Dequeker J, Verstraeten A, Nijs J. Age-, sex-, and menopause-related changes of femur and peripheral bone: Population study using dual and single photon absorptiometry and radiogrammetry. J Nucl Med 1986;27:1504-9.
3. Riggs BL, Wahner HW, Dunn WL, Mazess RB, Offord KP, Melton LJ III. Differential changes in bone mineral density of the appendicular and axial skeleton with ageing. J Clin Invest 1981;67:328-35.
4. Gambacciani M, Spinetti A, De Simone L, et al. The relative contributions of menopause and aging to postmenopausal vertebral osteopenia. J Clin Endocrinol Metab 1993;77(11); 48-52.
5. Wallach S, Henneman P. Prolonged estrogen therapy in postmenopausal women. JAMA 1959;171:1637-41.
6. Lindsay R. Estrogen therapy in the prevention and management of osteoporosis. Am J Obstet Gynecol 1987;156:1347-56.
7. Gambacciani M, Spinetti A, Cappagli B, et al. Hormone replacement therapy in perimenopausal women with a low dose oral contraceptive preparation: Effects on bone

mineral density and metabolism Maturitas 1994;19:125-31
8. Gambacciani M, Spinetti A, Taponeco F, Cappagli B, Piaggesi L, Fioretti P. Longitudinal evaluation of perimenopausal vertebral bone loss: Effects of a low-dose oral contraceptive preparation on bone mineral density and metabolism. Obstet Gynecol 1994 Mar;83(3):392-6
9. Michaelsson K, Baron JA, Farahmand BY, Persson I., Ljunghall S. Oral-contraceptive use and risk of hip fractures: A case-control study. Lancet 1999;353:1481-84.
10. Gambacciani M, Ciaponi M, Cappagli B, Benussi C, Genazzani AR. Longitudinal evaluation of perimenopausal femoral bone loss: Effects of a low-dose oral contraceptive preparation on bone mineral density and metabolism. Osteoporosis International 2000;11: 544-48.
11. World Health Organization. Assessment of fracture risk and its application to screening for postmenopausal osteoporosis. WHO Technical Report Series 843. Geneva: WHO; 1994.
12. Perrone G, Galoppi P, Capri O, Anelli G, Borrello M, Zichella L. Lumbar and femoral bone density in perimenopausal women with irregular cycles. Int J Fertil Menopausal Stud 1995;May- June(3):120-25.
13. Haenggi W, Casez J-P, Birkhaeuser MH, et al. Bone mineral density in young women with long-standing amenorrhea: Limited effect of hormone replacement therapy with ethinylestradiol and desogestrel. Osteoporos Int. 1994;4:99-103.
14. Kritz-Silverstein D, Barrett-Connor E. Bone mineral density in postmenopausal women as determined by prior oral contraceptive use. Am J Public Health. 1993;83:100-102.
15. Rodin A, Murby B, Smith MA, et al. Perimenopausal bone loss in the lumbar spine and neck of femur: A study of 225 Caucasian women. Bone 1990;11:1-5.
16. Nilas L, Christiansen C. The pathophysiology of peri-and postmenopausal bone loss. Br J Obstet Gynaecol 1989;96:580-87.
17. Gambacciani M, Spinetti A, Taponeco F. Bone loss in perimenopausal women: A longitudinal study. Maturitas 1994;18:191-97.
18. Kleerekoper M, Brienza RS, Schultz LR, et al. Oral contraceptive use may protect against low bone mass. Arch Intern Med. 1991;151:1971-76.

LESS INVASIVE SURGERY IN STRESS INCONTINENCE

John Bidmead and Linda Cardozo

Introduction

Stress incontinence is a distressing symptom that has a major impact on a woman's quality of life. It has proved difficult to accurately establish the true incidence of genuine stress incontinence (GSI), but even the most conservative estimate is that one in ten women will suffer from GSI at some time. In the past many women have accepted urinary incontinence as an inevitable consequence of childbearing and aging but today more women are coming forward requesting treatment and anticipating prompt and effective management. A number of new surgical techniques have also been developed which aim to offer improved results with lower morbidity than conventional surgery.

Should these new procedures be adopted uncritically and who should be offering treatment to women with urinary incontinence?

Conventional Surgical Techniques for Treating GSI

Well over 150 operative procedures for stress incontinence have been described during the last hundred years. This reflects past uncertainty over the most effective treatment. The published results of various continence operations were examined in a meta-analysis by Jarvis in 1994 [1]. The results are shown in Table 1.

Table 1. Objective cure rates for first procedure and recurrent incontinence

Procedure	Mean (%) First Procedure	Mean (%) Recurrent Incontinence
Anterior vaginal repair	67.8	Not available
Burch Colposuspension	89.8	82.5
Needle suspension	86.7	86.4
Slings	93.9	86.1
Injectables	45.5	57.8

From Jarvis 1994[1]

Black and Downs in 1996 [2] and the American Urological Association in 1997 [3]

carried out further systematic reviews. As a result it became clear that suprapubic bladder neck suspensions and slings give the best results.

Recently Introduced Surgical Techniques

Attention has been directed at developing less invasive procedures, which will replicate the high cure rates but with reduced morbidity, hospital stay, and time taken to return to normal activities compared to conventional surgery.

LAPAROSCOPIC COLPOSUSPENSION

It is possible to perform colposuspension laparoscopically and in theory this should provide the same long-term success rates as an open colposuspension with reduced morbidity and quicker recovery. At present, however, the poorer long-term results and higher risk of urinary tract injury with the laparoscopic approach suggest that open colposuspension remains preferable. A large multi-centre randomized trial of laparoscopic and open colposuspension funded by the Medical Research Council (MRC) is underway. This will eventually provide definitive evidence of the role of laparoscopic surgery in this area.

BONE ANCHORS AND NEEDLE SUSPENSION TECHNIQUES

A number of techniques similar to conventional needle suspensions but using bone anchors to fix the upper ends of the sutures have been described. It was hoped that the bone anchors would improve the long-term results. The use of bone anchors, however, has been shown to cause osteomyelitis as a long-term complication without offering any clear advantages. Some longer-term reports are now being published showing medium-term failure rates similar to those of traditional needle suspensions [4]. Long-term follow-up does not demonstrate any advantage.

INJECTABLE PERIURIURETHRAL BULKING AGENTS

Injections of periurethral bulking agents are made under cystoscopic control. This can be performed under a short general anaesthetic or local anaesthetic so hospital stay and recovery time are short. Complications from periurethral injection are very uncommon.

A number of materials have been used for periurethral injection. One of the most common materials used is glutaraldehyde cross-linked bovine collagen (GAX Collagen) (Contigen, BARD, Crawley UK) [5]. Due the resorption of this material repeated injections may be necessary to sustain continence [6]. Another widely used injectable material consists of micronized silicone rubber particles (Macroplastique, Uroplasty, Reading, UK). Cure rates reported with Macroplastique are similar to those with Collagen.

Although injectable agents offer quick and easy treatment with low morbidity their longer-term results have been disappointing; most studies report cures in the region of 40-60% [7,8]. A recent longer-term study shows a cure rate of only 26% after five years [9].

Given the poor long-term results their use in fit, younger women is difficult to justify. While it might appear tempting to repeat injections every few years, this is not only extremely expensive but the long-term effects of repeated injection are unknown. Repeated injections might lead to fibrosis and denervation of the urethral sphincter, which would then be more difficult to treat with conventional surgery. They are, however, invaluable in the frail elderly, in the treatment of secondary incontinence in women who have undergone multiple failed procedures, or after radiotherapy where the urethra is fixed and scarred.

The Tension Free Vaginal Tape (TVT Procedure)

This is a technique developed in Sweden that has much in common with conventional sling techniques. The TVT is a knitted Prolene mesh tape placed at the mid-urethra [10]. The tape is inserted via a small vaginal incision and is self-retaining, needing no sutures. This is performed under local or regional anaesthesia allowing the position of the tape to be adjusted during a series of coughs. The most recent results demonstrate a promising 86% objective cure after three years [11]. Currently, large-scale randomized trials comparing the TVT and open colposuspension are underway.

A recent randomized multicentre study carried out in the U.K. compared the TVT with the current gold standard, the colposuspension [12]. The study involved 14 centers and recruited 344 women. The cure rate was similar in each treatment group, subjectively 66% (TVT) and 71%(colposuspension) and objectively 68% (TVT) and 66% (colposuspension). However, the mean duration of stay was significantly less in the TVT group: 2.2 days compared with 6.5 days in the colposuspension group. Seventy-six percent of the TVT group and 41% of the colposuspension group had returned to work by 6 weeks post-operatively. At six months all the patients in both groups considered themselves fit for normal activities.

Who Should Perform Surgery for Stress Incontinence?

Generalist gynecologists or urologists have traditionally performed surgery for stress incontinence. Throughout medicine there is now growing recognition that treatment in specialist units, with appropriate facilities and ancillary staff, gives the opportunity to improve outcomes in many areas. The treatment of stress incontinence, a benign condition, but one that has a major impact on the lives of many women, appears to be an area where treatment in specialist units can markedly improve the outcome.

A recent study undertaken by Black et al has highlighted this problem. This involved 38 gynaecologists and 11 urologists in the North Thames region from eighteen units [13,14]. Four hundred forty-two women having surgery for stress incontinence were recruited. Preoperative and postoperative data were obtained both from surgeons and from women. The results of this survey showed a marked discrepancy between previously published results and the women in the study, only 28% of whom reported subjective cure. It was also apparent that surgeon's perception of results differed from those of their patients, surgeons considered the outcome successful in 85% of cases. Results appear to be better after thorough preoperative assessment, by surgeons with special interest and training in this area and in a unit where appropriately trained, experienced, and motivated staff are available to provide support as part of a multidisciplinary team

Conclusions

Over the last one hundred years our understanding of the efficacy of the surgical methods available for treating female stress incontinence has improved. The relative cure rates along with the morbidity of these techniques have become more clearly defined. Colposuspension remains the most appropriate first-line treatment for the majority of women but the increasing range of surgical options allows tailoring of surgery to suit individual women.

It is also becoming clear that better results can be obtained when treatment of urinary incontinence is undertaken in units with a special interest in this area. Provision of specialist centers able to develop experience and expertise in the management of urinary incontinence would offer women the best chance of successful treatment.

Encouraging new techniques offering reduced morbidity continue to be developed but need careful evaluation before widespread use. Carefully conducted, large-scale, randomised trials with long-term follow-up should be undertaken before new techniques promising improved results replace tried and tested surgical treatments.

References

1. Jarvis GJ. Surgery for stress incontinence. Br J Obstet Gynaecol 1994:101;371-74.
2. Black NA, Downs SH. The effectiveness of surgery for stress incontinence in women: A systematic review. Br J Urol 1996;78:497-510.
3. Leach G, Dmochowski R, Appell R, et al. Female stress urinary incontinence guidelines. Panel summary report on surgical management of female stress urinary incontinence. J Urol 1997;158:875-80.
4. Schultheiss D, Hofner K, Oelke M, et al. Percutaneous bladder neck suspension with bone anchors: An improvement in the therapy of female stress urinary incontinence. Neurourol Urodyn 1998;17:457-58.
5. Kligman AM, Armstrong RC. Histological response to intra-dermal zyderm and zyplasy (gluteraldehyde cross-linked) collagen in humans. J Dermatol Surg Oncol 1986;12:351-57.
6. Monga AK, Robinson D, Stanton SL. Peri-urethral collagen injections for genuine stress incontinence: A two year follow-up. Br J Urol 1995;76:156-60.
7. Eckford SD, Abrams P. Para-urethral collagen implantation for female stress incontinence. Br JUrol 1991;68:586-89.
8. Khullar V, Cardozo LD, Abbott D, Anders K. GAX collagen in the treatment of urinary incontinence in elderly women: A two year follow-up. Br J Obstet & Gynaecol 1997;104: 96-99.
9. Gorton E, Stanton SL, Monga A, et al. Periurethral collagen injection: A long-term follow-up study. BJU Int 1999;84:966-71.
10. Petros P, Ulmsten U. Intravaginal slingplasty. An ambulatory surgical procedure for treatment of female urinary stress incontinence. Scand J Urol Nephrol 1995;29:75-82.

11. Ulmsten U, Johnson P, Rezapour M. A three year follow up of TVT for surgical treatment of female stress incontinence. Br J Obstet Gynecol 1999;106:345-50.
12. Ward K, Hilton P. A randomised trial of colposuspension and tension free vaginal tape (TVT) for primary genuine stress incontinence. Neurourol Urodyn 2000;19:386-87.
13. Black N, Griffiths J, Pope C, Bowling A, Abel P. Impact of surgery for stress incontinence on morbidity: cohort study. BMJ 1997;315:1493-98.
14. Hutchings A Griffiths J Black N. Surgery for stress incontinence: Factors associated with a successful outcome. Br J Urol 1998;82:634-41.

An Overview of Hormones and Brain Function

Barbara B. Sherwin

Introduction

During the past two decades, advances in basic neuroscience have provided a wealth of explanations for the manner in which steroid hormones may influence aspects of brain function. This has allowed researchers to begin to investigate changes in behavior that sometimes occur coincident with changes in hormone levels during various reproductive events. Ultimately, a better understanding of the mechanisms by which sex hormones influences brain function will allow us to prevent the occurrence of behavior disorders associated with changes in sex hormone production and/or to treat these disorders more effectively when they do occur.

Estrogen and Mood

The fact that the 2:1 female to male ratio in the incidence of major depressive disorders has been confirmed in numerous countries with diverse cultures decreases the likelihood that this excess of depressive disorders is primarily due to social factors. The possible role of biological factors in the etiology of depressive disorders in women is underlined by the fact that some women are at greater risk for the development of a depressive episode subsequent to changes in their sex hormone production during various reproductive events. For example, 35% of women report moderate affective and physical symptoms premenstrually while 3% experience severe symptoms at that time. Also, 50-70% of women experience postpartum "blues" and approximately 15% develop a major postpartum depression within the first 3 months following delivery [1]. Therefore, it seemed logical for investigators to attempt to determine how changing levels of sex hormones might increase a woman's risk for a major depressive episode.

The serotonin (5HT) hypothesis is still among the most prominent biological theories of depression. This theory holds that a deficiency in brain serotonergic activity increases vulnerability to depression. Such a deficit may be due to diminished availability of l-typtophan, the precursor of serotonin, impaired serotonin synthesis, release, reuptake or metabolism or serotonin postsynaptic receptor abnormalities [2]. Indeed, several lines of evidence suggest that estrogen may modulate the availability, the metabolism, and the transport of serotonin. First, it has been demonstrated in the rat that exogenous estrogen decreases monoamine oxidase (MAO), the enzyme that catabolizes serotonin in the amygdala and hypothalamus [3]. One of the end results of higher estrogen levels then, would be greater availability of brain serotonin and, consequently, more positive mood. Indeed, there is clinical evidence to support this theory [1].

A second mechanism that may explain the salutary effect of estrogen on mood is that tryptophan, the amino acid precursor of serotonin, is displaced from its binding sites to plasma albumin by estrogens *in vivo* and *in vitro* [4], thereby increasing the amount of free tryptophan that is able to enter the brain and be synthesized to serotonin. This, of course, would serve to increase the concentration of brain serotonin.

Finally, there is also evidence that estrogen can influence neurotransmitter receptors to affect mood. During long-term imipramine administration in rats, an estrogen-dependent decrease in 5HT2 receptor binding occurred in the frontal cortex [5]. Castration abolished this decline, which was reversed by estrogen or testosterone but not by dihydrotestosterone, which is nonaromatizable. A final mechanism by means of which estrogen could influence mood is concerned with its effect on tritiated imipramine binding sites which are endogenous binding sites on platelets and neurons that are thought to modulate the presynaptic uptake of serotonin in both tissues . A decrease in the density (Bmax) of these binding sites has been found in the brain and patelets of depressed patients [6]. In a prospective , randomized, controlled trial, we showed that women randomly treated with estrogen following their bilateral oophorectomy had significantly better mood scores and a higher Bmax of tritiated imipramine binding sites on platelets compared to those who received a placebo [7].

In summary, several mechanisms of action of estrogen have been described whose impact would be to upregulate the serotonergic system. To the extent that higher concentrations of serotonin in synaptic sites in areas of the brain that regulate affect act to enhance mood, then higher levels of estrogen should also induce more positive mood. Indeed, there is a considerable amount of evidence to show that estrogen enhances mood in women. It now seems clear that while physiological doses of estrogen given to postmenopausal women alleviate depressive symptoms, or dysphoria [8-11], these doses are without significant effect on the more profound mood disturbances that fulfill diagnostic criteria for a major depressive episode [12-13] Although large, physiological doses of estrogen are somewhat effective as a sole agent for the treatment of a major depressive disorder [14], the importance of this finding is theoretical rather than clinical since the side effects of these doses of estrogen far exceed the side effects that accrue to the newer, second-generation antidepressant drugs. Nonetheless, in a recent randomized, controlled trial, 85% of women with a minor depression and 79% of women with a major depression had full or partial remission of their depressed mood when they were treated with 0.05 mg/day transdermal estradiol [15]. However, other associated symptoms such as disturbed sleep, lack of energy, and emotional detachment were unaffected by this dose of estrogen suggesting that, while estrogen has antidepressant properties, physiological doses of estrogen alone are not sufficient to treat the entire range of symptoms in the major depressive syndrome.

Progesterone and Mood

Because postmenopausal women with an intact uterus are usually given a progestin along with estrogen in order to protect against endometrial hyperplasia, it is important to also consider the possible effects of progestins on the brain. Whereas estrogen increases the rate of degredation of MAO, the enzyme that catabolizes serotonin, progesterone increases the concentration of MAO thereby decreasing the amount of brain serotonin [3]. Indeed, in a randomized clinical trial, we showed that the addition of medroxyprogesterone acetate (MPA) to either of two doses of conjugated equine estrogen (CEE) attenuated the beneficial effect of estrogen on mood in a dose-dependent manner such that the higher the estrogen/MPA ratio, the more positive the mood [16]. These findings were confirmed in a meta-analysis of hormone replacement therapy and mood [17]and suggest that the negative influence of some progestins on mood should be considered in the treatment of postmenopausal women who have a history of depressive illness.

Estrogen and Cognition

It has by now been well demonstrated that estrogen has numerous effects on the neurochemistry and neuroanatomy of brain areas that underlie cognitive functions. For example, estrogen plays a role in protecting neurons from free-radical damage and in protecting dissociated hippocampal neurons against beta-amyloid toxicity [18]. In the hippocampus, estrogen also increases the concentration of choline acetyltransferase (ChAT), the synthetic enzyme for acetylcholine, which is the neurotransmitter that is most critical for memory [19]. In the CA 1 area of the hippocampus, estrogen has been shown to promote synaptogenesis [18] thereby enhancing neuronal communication in this area of the brain which is critically important for memory. These chemical and morphological influences of estrogen on critical brain areas provide biological plausibility for the notion that estrogen protects aspects of cognition in women.

Indeed, findings from numerous case-control, longitudinal and randomized controlled trials of ERT and cognitive functioning are now available. Although the findings are not absolutely consistent, perhaps due to the variety of populations studied and to the variety of instruments used to measure cognition across studies, there does seem to be a consensus that ERT protects short- and long-term memory and enhances the capacity for new learning in healthy aging women [see Ref. 20, for a review]. There is also evidence that ERT decreases the risk of Alzheimer's disease (AD) in older women by 29% to 34% [21] but is ineffective as a treatment for women with diagnosed AD when administered in physiological doses [22].

In summary, there is compelling evidence that sex hormones are neuroactive and can be powerful modulators of brain functions that subserve mood and cognition. Clinical trials of HRT in postmenopausal women demonstrate that these influences of sex hormones on brain mechanisms are manifest clinically as behavioral changes in some treated women. A greater understanding of the mechanisms of action of sex hormones on brain function that will eventually emanate from research studies currently underway will allow us to further enhance the quality of life for women during the latter one-third of their lifespan.

Acknowledgments

The preparation of this manuscript was supported by Grant No. MA-11623 from the Canadian Institute for Health Research.

References

1. Sherwin BB. Estrogen and refractory depression. In: Amsterdam J, editor. Advances in psychiatry and psychopharmacology, Volume 2. New York: Raven Press 1991: 209-18.
2. Maes M, Meltzer HY. The serotonin hypothesis of major depression. In: Bloom FE, Kupfer DJ, editors. Psychopharmacology: The fourth generation of progress. New York: Raven Press, 1995: 933-44.
3. Luine VN, Khylchevskaya RI, McEwen BS. Effects of gonadal steroids on activities of monoamine oxidase and choline acetylase in rat brain. Brain Res 1975;86:293-306.
4. Aylward M. Estrogens, plasma tryptophan levels in perimenopausal patients. In: Campbell S, editors. The management of the menopause and postmenopausal years. Baltimore: University Park Press, 1976; 135-47.
5. Kendall DA, Stancel GM, Enna SJ. The influence of sex hormones on antidepressant-induced alterations in neurotransmitter receptor binding. J Neurosci 1982;2:354-60.
6. Suranyi-Cadotte BE, Wood PL, Schwatz G, Nair PVN. Altered platelet ^{3}H-imipramine binding in schizoaffective and depressive disorders. Biol Psychiatry 1983;18:923-27.
7. Sherwin BB, Suranyi-Cadotte BE. Up-regulatory effect of estrogen on platelet 3H-imipramine bindings sites in surgically menopausal women. Biol Psychiatry 1990;28:339-48.
8. Sherwin BB. Affective changes with estrogen and androgen replacement therapy in surgically menopausal women. J Affect Disord 1988;14:177-87.
9. Ditkoff EC, Gary WG, Cristo M, Lobo RA. Estrogen improves psychological function in asymptomatic postmenopausal women. Obstet Gyneco 1991;78:991-95.
10. Sherwin BB, Gelfand MM. Sex steroids and affect in the surgical menopause: A double-blind, crossover study. Psychoneuroendocrinology 1985;10:325-35.
11. Palinkas LA, Barrett-Connor E. Estrogen use and depressive symptoms in postmenopausal women. Obstet Gynecol 1992;80:30-36.
12. Schneider MA, Brotherton PL, Hailes J. The effect of exogenous oestrogens on depression in menopausal women. Med J Aust 1977;2:162-63.
13. Shapira B, Oppenheim G, Zohar J, Segal M, Malach D, Belmaker RH. Lack of efficacy of estrogen supplementation to imipramine in resistant female depressives. Biol Psychiatry 1985;20:576-79.
14. Klaiber EL, Broverman DM, Vogel W, Kobayashi Y. Estrogen therapy for severe persistent depression in women. Arch Gen Psychiatry 1979;36:550-54.
15. Schmidt PJ, Nieman L, Danaceau MA, et al. Estrogen replacement in perimenopausal-related depression: A preliminary report. Am J Obstet Gynecol 2000;183:414-20.
16. Sherwin BB. The impact of different doses of estrogen and progestin on mood and sexual behavior in postmenopausal women. J Clin Endocrinol Metab 1991;72:336-43.
17. Zweifel JE, O'Brien WH. A meta-analysis of the effect of hormone replacement therapy

upon depressed mood. Psychoneuroendocrinol 1997;22:189-212.
18. Henderson VW. Estrogen replacement therapy for the prevention and treatment of Alzheimer's disease. CNS Drugs 1977;8:343-51.
19. Luine VN. Estradiol increases choline acetyltransferase activity in specific basal forebrain nuclei and projection areas of female rats. Exp Neurol 1985;80:484-90.
20. Sherwin BB. Estrogen effects on cognition in menopausal women. Neurology 1997;48 (Suppl.7):S21-S26.
21. LeBlanc ES, Janowsky J, Chan BK, Nelson HD. Hormone replacement therapy and cognition: A systematic review and meta-analysis. J Am Med Assoc 2001;285:1489-99.
22. Mulnard RA, Cotman CW, Kawas CW, et al. Estrogen replacement therapy for treatment of mild to moderate Alzheimer's disease. J Am Med Assoc 2000;283:1007-15.

Mechanisms of the Neuroprotective Effects of Estrogen

Silvia Belcredito, Elisabetta Vegeto, Clara Meda, and Adriana Maggi

Introduction

It is now well accepted that in mammals estrogen action extends far beyond the control of sexual functions. Apart from the regulation of reproductive functions and behavior, in fact, estrogen's direct involvement has been demonstrated in the differentiation of fetal brain [1], in the control of locomotion and the regulation of fine movements [2], in memory performance [3], and in temperature control [4]. Moreover, it is now well known that estrogen exerts beneficial effects throughout the entire organism, which quite abruptly cease in women at the beginning of menopause, leading to an increase in the onset of pathologies typical of the older years: osteoporosis, increased cardiovascular risk, chronic inflammatory disorders, and neurodegeneration, in which estrogen administration appears to actively provide benefit [5].

How estradiol can exert such a variety of effects is still unclear. One explanation can be found in the existence of two isoforms for estrogen receptors [6], which seem to mediate differential effects in the target cells [7]. On the other hand, estrogen receptors can evoke cellular responses also by working independently from ligand binding and interaction with DNA, as they are able to activate signal transduction pathways common to other molecules, the so called "cross-talk" modality [8]. Another less strongly evidence-based mechanism stands on the existence of membrane estrogen receptors, which however has not been sufficiently proven yet [9,10].

In the last few years our laboratory has been investigating the mechanisms of beneficial effects of estrogen on brain, demonstrated by both *in vitro* [11] and *in vivo* [12] experiments and in clinical trials [5]. In the brain, estrogen receptor expression is not restricted to neurons [13]. ERα was found in astrocytes and oligodendrocytes [14,15], both ERs were shown to be present in microglia, the resident macrophages of the central nervous system (CNS) [16], and neural stem cells (Pollio et al., unpublished results). Given the increasing importance of interactions among these different cell types in CNS, our attention was moved from neurons to glia, which appears to play an active role on neuronal functions, playing more than trophic and structural roles [17]. Here, we review our recent evidences on estrogen action in the brain, illustrating first our studies aimed at the identification of estrogen target genes, then our investigations of estrogen effects *in vivo*, which led to a novel hypothesis on the mechanism of estrogen neuroprotective action.

Estrogen: A Single Molecule for a Variety of Effects

The biological response to estradiol stimulation can be differentially modulated depending on a series of variables. Among these, estrogen receptor multiplicity was demonstrated in 1996, when ERβ was cloned [6], nine years later than ERα [18]. Both isoforms belong to the superfamily of steroid-thyroid hormone receptors [19], which behave as hormone-regulated transcription factors to modulate the expression of target genes. ERs reside in the nuclei of target cells and are transcriptionally inactive in the absence of ligand, because they are bound to inhibitory proteins (the heat shock proteins). Upon ligand binding, these proteins are released and the receptors are phosphorylated, dimerize (both homodimers and heterodimers have been recognized [20]), and bind conserved sequences named estrogen response elements (ERE) in the promoter of target genes. The newly formed complex recruits proteins of the preinitiation complex and induces transcription. After dimerization, estrogen receptors may influence transcription even without directly binding to DNA. ERs, in fact, can modulate other transcription factors activity, such as NF-κB and AP-1 [21,22]. To explain some rapid actions of estrogen, e.g. the modulation of intracellular levels of signaling molecules, the existence of estradiol-operated membrane receptors has been suggested [9,10], though no convincing evidence has been provided yet.

Besides this "classical" pathway, estrogen receptors can modulate gene expression also in a "nonclassical" way, which does not require the presence of receptor ligand. This mechanism takes advantage of a cross-talk between ERs and elements of other signaling pathways that originate when an extracellular signal activates its own membrane receptor. ERα can thus be activated in response to extracellular signals like dopamine, IGF-I, EGF, and cAMP [8]. This may happen by the phosphorylation of either the receptor molecule itself, or of coactivators/corepressors interacting with it. These differential activation pathways may play an important role in time- and tissue-dependent differential activation of ERs.

Identification of Estrogen Target Genes in Cells of Neural Origin

The influence that estrogen exerts on the brain originates very early in mammalian life. Estrogen in fact is involved in the differentiation of the CNS, both in females and in males, through mechanisms following both the classical and nonclassical pathways. In adult life, the effects of estrogen on the brain go far beyond the control of reproductive functions. It positively influences memory [3], affective behavior [23], and delays the onset of neurodegenerative disorders like Alzheimer's disease. At the molecular level, estrogen influences neural transmission by modulating the synthesis of various neurotransmitters and of molecules involved in their secretion [24-29]; it improves electrical conductivity in neurons, acting on oligodendrocyte metabolism [30]; it directs the secretion of endocrine peptides [31]; it increases the production of respiratory enzymes, thus modifying the energetic state of the cells [32]; it affects neural cytoarchitecture by facilitating the accumulation of cytoskeleton components [33,34]. As a result of all these subcellular events, or dependently on different phenomena, estrogen has been shown to increase neurons' viability in response to a series of toxic insults. While some groups attribute neuroprotective effects of estrogen to a classical genomic effect [35,36], others propose as important the antioxidant properties of 17β-estradiol, which would influence excitotoxic stressors like glutamate, free radicals, β-amyloid [37-39].

To gain an insight on the molecular details of the effect on neural cells of 17β-estradiol, we used a model system generated in our laboratory, the estrogen receptor-expressing neuroblastoma SK-ER3 cell line [40,41], to identify estrogen-regulated genes [42]. Among the numerous genes found to be transcriptionally regulated by 17β-estradiol, three were recognized as previously cloned genes: prothymosine-alpha (PTMA), involved in cell cycle progression and proliferation, and recently recognized to behave as an ER coactivator [43]; L7, another transcriptional coactivator [44]; and *bnip2* (formerly known as *nip2*). Initially we focused our attention on *bnip2*. Its transcript was down-modulated by 1 nM 17β-estradiol pretreatment in a time-dependent manner, with the maximal effect seen 6 hours after treatment. No difference was seen in *bnip2* mRNA levels when the parental cell line SK-N-BE was used, which does not express estrogen receptors [45].

bnip2 had been cloned a few years before as a member of a little family of three Bcl-2 interacting proteins (hence the name *b*cl-2 *n*ineteen kDa *i*nteracting *p*roteins) characterized by high homology with adenoviral protein E1B 19kDa [46]. Their homology with a proapoptotic gene product and their capability to interact with a well-known antiapoptotic molecule pointed to their involvement in cell death. Thus we studied *bnip2* influence on cell viability and proved a correlation between high levels of *bnip2* expression and cell death, by transient transfections and by investigating *bnip2* content in cells exposed to neurotoxic stimuli [46]. Interestingly, in co-transfection studies we showed that overexpression of *bcl-2* opposed *bnip2* proapoptotic activity [47].

To evaluate estrogen's role in this system, we challenged our experimental model with a well-known neurotoxic insult, that is glucose deprivation, described to induce apoptosis in cells of neural origin. Deficits in glucose metabolism have also been described in brains of individuals at risk for the onset of familial Alzheimer's disease [48]. We induced hypoglycemia in our cell system by replacement of normal culture medium with Locke's solution, a glucose-free medium. Together with a marked decrease in cell survival (50% versus control), we could observe a significant increase in endogenous *bnip2* mRNA levels (40% versus control), in both SK-ER3 and SK-N-BE cell lines. However, in SK-ER3 only did 17β-estradiol prevent *bnip2* up-regulation and maintain cell viability to control values (Figure 1) [45].

These results were then confirmed in primary cultures of neurons from both embryos (at E17) and adult rats. Again, 17β-estradiol prevented both the increase of *bnip2* mRNA levels and apoptosis. The effect is receptor-mediated, as the protective effect of the hormone could be abolished by pretreatment with ICI 182,780, a complete antagonist of ER, and is hormone specific, because no effect was seen when cells were treated with other steroidal hormones, such as glucocorticoids or progesterone [45].

Our study, born to identify estrogen-regulated genes, therefore led us to describe a potential mechanism through which 17β-estradiol is neuroprotective. Antiapoptotic properties of estrogen have often been ascribed to its antioxidant potential. These results add evidence to the genomic effect-based theory, by underlining that estrogen receptor is necessary in order to gain benefit, and that receptor binding to the ligand results in a transcriptional effect. They are therefore a good example of how the identification of genes regulated by a hormone can be the basis on which to build up a series of hypothesis that can shed a clearer light on hormone-mediated cellular events.

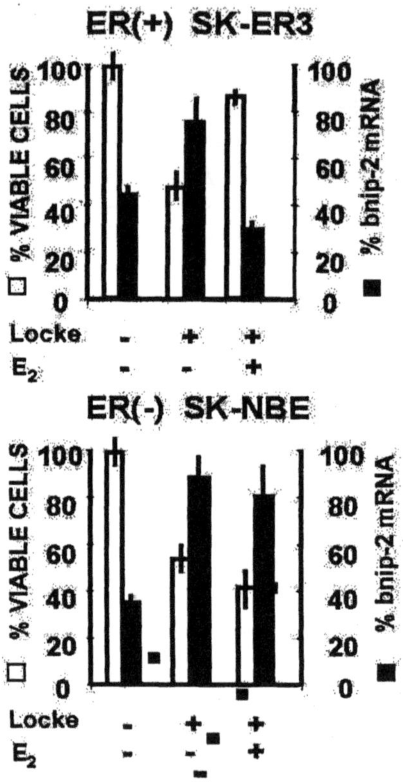

Figure 1. Glucose deprivation apoptotic effect is opposed by 17β-estradiol in ER (+) SK-ER3 cells (upper panel). No protective effect of estrogen can be seen in ER (-) SK-N-BE (lower panel). Comparably, *bnip2* is down-regulated by 17β-estradiol only in the presence of ERα (white columns: viable cells percentage; black columns: *bnip2* mRNA content, as assessed by Northern blot analysis).

Glia: Novel Targets for Estrogen Action

Though for many years glial cell were not considered to play an active role in steroid hormone effects on brain, recent results clearly show how physical and functional interactions between glia and neurons deeply influence brain physiology [17]. The hypothesis that glia could be directly influenced by steroid hormones, and by estrogen in particular, dates back to 1992, when estrogen binding properties were recognized on glial cells [14]. Two years later we identified ERα in both astrocytes and oligodendrocytes, thus providing the explanation to earlier studies showing a functional response of glial cells to estrogen [15]. Identifying estrogen receptor on glial cells meant that a new investigation field was opened; all the well-known effects of estrogen in brain could be reinterpreted taking into consideration the potential involvement of glia. Since then, several lines of evidence were provided to show how astrocytes are involved in brain sexual development, in synapse formation and synaptic plasticity, and in injury repair [17].

In addition to astroglia and oligodendroglia, however, a third glia subtype exists, which is actively involved in brain pathophysiology, that is microglia, and to which we turned our interest.

Microglia are the resident macrophages of the central nervous system. Like the other glial cells, they influence neural cells viability by producing growth factors and removing potentially toxic extracellular molecules, but their peculiarity stands in their macrophagic lineage. Upon appropriate stimuli, microglia becomes activated and starts secreting a series of inflammatory mediators, such as nitric oxide (NO), arachidonic acid derivatives, and cytokines, while they express different surface antigens and undergo morphological alterations that lead to their phenotypical activation. As macrophage-like cells, microglia have phagocytic properties, thus removes toxic debris from the extracellular space, and promotes tissue repair for the resolution of the inflammatory status. On the other hand, the prolonged microglia activation was proposed to convert its potential benefits into a noxious factor. Activated microglia has in fact been described as a hallmark of several neurodegenerative diseases (Parkinson's, Alzheimer's, Huntington's, prion diseases), in which inflammation seems to play an important role.

In our effort to recognize brain cells as targets of estrogen action, we asked whether microglia, similarly to the other glial cell types, express the estrogen receptors. If this was true, microglia could have represented a novel target for estrogen positive influence against neurodegeneration.

The hypothesis of estrogen receptor expression in microglia was also suggested by our previous observations of estrogen responsiveness in monocytes and macrophages [49].

Indeed we were able to show that ERα and ERβ are expressed in rat microglia in primary cultures [16]. The way was opened to the investigation of estrogen effects on microglia, both *in vitro* and *in vivo*.

17β-estradiol Blocks Morphological and Biochemical Microglia Activation Induced by Inflammatory Stimuli

To test microglial reactivity to pro-inflammatory stimuli, we chose LPS, a lipopolysaccharide present in the bacterial cell wall and known to induce strong microglia activation. This process induces a series of morphological modifications, leading from thin, mainly bipolar cells, to round, amoeboid-shaped cells, with a phenotype characteristic of phagocytic cells. Estradiol administration prevented any morphological modification induced by LPS. Indeed amoeboid cells were reduced by 70% and an intermediate phenotype was prevalent, characterized by short-branched cells, different from both the resting and the activated phenotype (Figure 2).

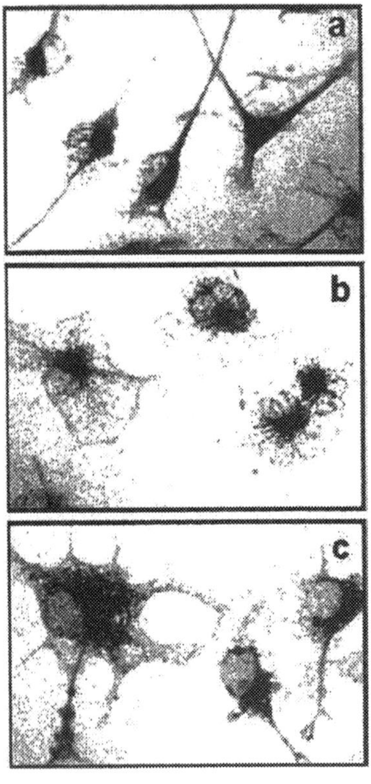

Figure 2. Photomicrographs of microglial cells treated for 16 hours with (a) vehicle, (b) LPS 0.5 μg/mL, (c) LPS 0.5 μg/mL with 1 nM 17β-estradiol given 4 hours before LPS. Staining is obtained with HRP-conjugated isolectin-B4 (which binds to specific glycoprotein residues expressed by macrophage-like cells) after exposure to HRP chromogen substrate DAB.

Morphological activation is the phenotypic counterpart of biochemical activation of microglia, which leads to production and secretion of the mediators of the inflammatory response. Among these, nitric oxide, prostaglandins, and matrix-metalloproteases (MMPs) seem to be the most active among the molecules of microglial origin which have been associated with microglia-induced neurotoxicity. Several studies, both *in vivo* and *in vitro*, show how the synthesis of the inducible form of nitric oxide synthase (iNOS) and the following NO release from microglia correlate with the progression of neurodegeneration [50]. Similarly, increased levels of prostaglandins and of their synthetic enzyme cyclooxygenase-2 (COX-2) have been associated to neurological disorders [51], in agreement with the result of clinical trials showing reduced incidence of Alzheimer's disease in patients treated with COX-2 inhibitors [52]. MMP-9, involved in both matrix and protein degradation, seems to be up-regulated by β-amyloid, which is among its molecular targets. This would give an explanation for MMP-9 up-regulation in Alzheimer's disease [53].

iNOS is expressed only in a small percentage of cells in the absence of inflammatory stimuli, as we verified by immunocytochemistry staining of microglia with an anti-iNOS antibody. However, after LPS exposure, number of iNOS positive cells increased up to 50%, consistently with the accumulation of NO_2^- in culture medium. Pretreatment with 17β-estradiol prevented both iNOS expression and NO_2^- accumulation in a dose-dependent manner, but only when it was given to cells 4 hours prior to LPS. Estradiol administration for shorter time intervals resulted in reduced protection. Protection completely waned when hormone was given to cells at the same time as LPS or later. This latter observation is in accordance with what seen in clinical trials, according to which the beneficial effects of estrogen on brain disappear if the inflammatory process has already settled. In fact positive effects of estrogen on memory or on cognitive performance, for example in women with AD, could not be demonstrated in women who had started taking hormone replacement therapy only after neurological problems had reached the clinical level [54]. Estrogen has otherwise been shown to be efficacious in delaying AD onset in women to whom hormones were given in early menopausal years [5].

A similar effect was demonstrated when we studied LPS effect on PGE_2 and MMP-9 production, both of which were significantly up-regulated. Again 17β-estradiol proved effective in reducing their levels, in a dose-dependent manner and when given 4 hours before LPS (Figure 3).

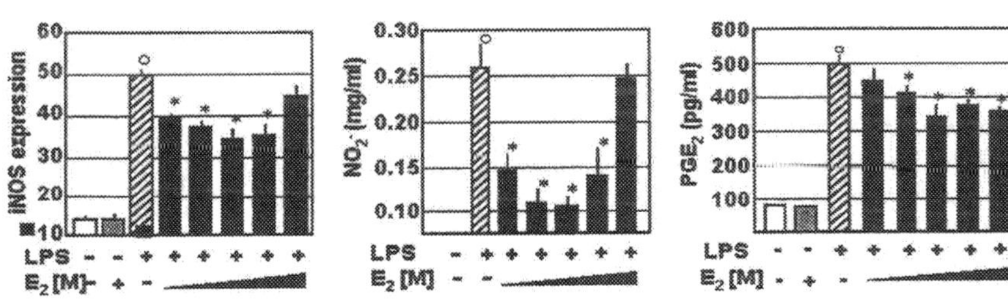

Figure 3. LPS-mediated induction of inflammatory mediators' synthesis is prevented by increasing concentrations of 17β-estradiol. From left to right: iNOS expression, assessed by immunocytochemistry against iNOS; NO_2^-, evaluated through Griess reaction on cell supernatants; PGE_2, quantitated in cell supernatants with plate-immobilized antibodies.

ICI 182,780 completely blocked estrogen action on each of the considered mediators, pointing to a receptor-mediated mechanism.

Estrogen: A New Class of Anti-inflammatory Drugs?

The hypothesis of a beneficial role of estrogen in inflammatory diseases goes against the traditional belief: the inflammatory-like action of estradiol in the ovarian follicle maturation has in fact led to think of this hormone as an inflammatory more than an anti-inflammatory agent. More recently, however, evidences have been provided consistent with the increased manifestation of inflammatory reaction in the absence of estrogen, which decreased again with estrogen replacement. This observation is also well reproduced in experimental models, such as carrageenan-induced pleurisy [55], endotoxin-induced uveitis [56], experimental encephalomyelitis and experimental adjuvant-induced arthritis [57], and cutaneous wound healing [58].

Apart from typical inflammation-based diseases, growing evidence supports the view of beneficial effects of estrogen on other pathologic conditions, for which no inflammatory etiology had been recognized, mediated through its anti-inflammatory characteristics.

Estrogen protection from cardiovascular diseases in women before menopause, for example, could be the result of its action on circulating monocytes. Estrogen inhibits the expression both of adhesion molecules, thus keeping monocytes from adhere and migrate through the endothelium of vessel walls, and of chemokines, which recruit leukocytes to the inflammation site.

Estrogen benefits on osteoporosis have been known for years now. Even if it is not immediately apparent, an inflammatory-like process is involved in the establishment of this pathology. Osteoblasts and osteoclasts, in fact, derive from the macrophage lineage and produce a series of pro-inflammatory cytokines (such as IL-1, IL-6, and TNFα), hematopoietic growth factors (M-CSF, macrophage colony stimulating factor) and differentiating agents (RANKL, receptor activator of NF-κB ligand), which guide bone remodeling in the presence of normal levels of estrogen [59]. The skeletal system undergoes a progressive deterioration in the elderly, in particular in women after menopause, because reduced estrogen levels cannot prevent excessive differentiation of osteoblasts into osteoclasts, and therefore bone resorption.

Microglia activation, and therefore an inflammatory state, has also been recognized in brains of patients affected by several neurodegenerative diseases, including Parkinson's disease, Alzheimer's disease, multiple sclerosis, AIDS dementia, Huntington's disease, Sandhoff disease, Lewy bodies dementia [60], thus substantiating the hypothesis that a chronic inflammatory reaction could be responsible for neural tissue degeneration.

Evidence of estrogen activity on brain inflammation *in vivo* in animal models are still scarce, though preliminary observations obtained from studies on experimental autoimmune encephalomyelitis (EAE) and on ischemic damage seem to support the anti-inflammatory hypothesis of estrogen action. Gender differences have in fact been reported in susceptibility to EAE, and ovariectomy is associated with a more severe form of the disease [57]. Similarly, estrogen has proven efficacy in reducing damage to brain tissue in several animal models of ischemia, due, at least in part, to its antioxidant properties, which limit the increase of free radicals that follows reperfusion, but also by reducing iNOS production [61].

Even with the evidence presented so far, however, it may be early to include estrogen among the anti-inflammatory drugs. It is however certain that its role on immune cells and on inflammatory mediators deserves consideration among the means with which estrogen exerts its protective effects on brain, together with its well-known antiapoptotic activity. Similarly to what happened in the investigation of antiapoptotic properties, also the study of estrogen anti-inflammatory activity will probably take advantage of looking for estrogen target genes, which will help comprehension of estradiol mechanism of action in order to design drugs that mimic positive estrogen action without inducing its negative side effects. A great help will come in future years from the use in research as well as in clinical practice of SERMs, the "selective estrogen receptor modulators," molecules endowed with estrogen receptor affinity, but whose estrogenic activity is made manifest only at selected levels, while they behave as antagonist at others. Their introduction into the clinical practice, in fact, would give women a new tool to face later years of their lives with the expectation of a healthier old age.

References

1. Arnold AP, Gorski RA. Gonadal steroid induction of structural sex differences in the central nervous system. Annu Rev Neurosci 1984;7:413-42.
2. Jarvik LF. Human intelligence: Sex differences. Acta Genet Med Gamellol 1975;24:189-211.
3. Luine VN. Steroid hormone influences on spatial memory. Ann N Y Acad Sci 1994;743: 201-11.
4. Charkoudian N, Stephens DP, Pirkle KC, Kosiba WA, Johnson JM. Influence of female reproductive hormones on local thermal control of skin blood flow. J Appl Physiol 1999; 87:1719-23.
5. Honjo H, Tanaka K, Kashiwagi T, et al. Senile dementia-Alzheimer's type and estrogens. Horm Metab Res 1995;27:204-7.
6. Kuiper GJ, Enmark E, Pelto-Huikko M, Nilsson G, Gustafsson J-Å. Cloning of a novel estrogen receptor expressed in rat prostate and ovary. Proc Natl Acad Sci USA 1996;93: 5925-30.
7. Patrone C, Vegeto E, Pollio G, Enmark E, De Curtis I, Gustafsson J-Å. Estradiol induces differential neuronal phenotypes by activating ERα or ERβ. Endocrinology 2000;141: 1839-45.
8. Picard D, Bunone G, Liu JW, Donzé O. Steroid-independent activation of steroid receptors in mammalian and yeast cells and in breast cancer. Biochem Soc Trans 1997;25:597-602.
9. Wong M, Moss RL. Electrophysiological evidence for a rapid membrane action of the gonadal steroid, 17β-estradiol, on CA-1 pyramidal neurons of the rat hippocampus. Brain Res 1991;543:148-52.
10. Pappas TC, Gametchu B, Watson CS. Membrane estrogen receptors identified by multiple antibody labeling and impeded-ligand binding. FASEB J 1995;9:404-10.
11. Behl C, Widmann M, Trapp T, Holsboer F. 17beta-estradiol protects neurons from oxidative stress-induced cell death in vitro. Biochem Biophys Res Commun 1995;216:473-82.

12. Toung TJK, Traystman RJ, Hurn D. Estrogen mediated neuroprotection after experimental stroke in male rats. Stroke 1998;29:1666-70.
13. Couse JF, Lindzey J, Grandien K, Gustafsson J-Å. Tissue distribution and quantitative analysis of estrogen receptor-alpha (ER-alpha) and estrogen receptor-beta (ER-beta) messenger ribonucleic acid in the wild-type and ER-alpha-knock out mouse. Endocrinology 1997;138:4613-21.
14. Jung-Testas I, Renoir M, Bugnard H, Greene GL, Beulieu EE. Demonstrations of steroid hormone receptors and steroid action in primary cultures of rat glial cells. J Steroid Biochem Mol Biol 1992;41:621-31.
15. Santagati S, Melcangi RC, Celotti F, Martini L, Maggi A. Estrogen receptor is expressed in different types of glial cells in culture. J Neurochem 1994;63:2058-64.
16. Vegeto E, Bonincontro C, Pollio G, et al. Estrogen prevents the lipopolysaccharide-induced inflammatory response in microglia. J Neurosci 2001;21:1908-18.
17. Garcia-Segura LM, Cardona-Gomez GP, Trejo JL, Fernandez-Galaz MC, Chowen JA. Glial cells are involved in organizational and activational effects of sex hormones in the brain. In: Matsumoto A, editor. Sexual differentiation of the brain. CRC Press, 2000:83-93.
18. Korke S, Sakai M, Muramatsu M. Molecular cloning and characterization of rat estrogen receptor cDNA. Nucleic Acids Res 1987;15:2499-2513.
19. Tsai MJ, O'Malley BW. Molecular mechanisms of action of steroid/thyroid receptor superfamily members. Annu Rev Biochem 1994;63:451-86.
20. Ogawa S, Inoue S, Watanabe T, et al. The complete structure of human estrogen receptor β (hERβ) and its heterodimerization with ERα in vivo and in vitro. Biochem Biophys Res Commun 1998;243:122-26.
21. Shyamala J, Guoit MC. Activation of κB specific proteins by estradiol. Proc Natl Acad Sci USA 1992;89:507-25.
22. Webb P, Nguyen P, Valentine C, et al. The estrogen receptor enhances AP-1 activity by two distinct mechanisms with different requirement for receptor transactivation functions. Mol Endocrinol 1999;13:1672-85.
23. Yaffe K, Sawaya G, Lieberburg I, Grady D. Estrogen therapy in postmenopausal women: Effects on cognitive function and dementia. JAMA 1998;279:688-95.
24. Rainbow TC, Degroff V, Luine VN, McEwen BS. Estradiol 17β increases the number of muscarinic receptors in hypothalamic nuclei. Brain Res 1980;198:239-43.
25. Hrusca RE, Pittman KT. Distribution and localization of estrogen-sensitive dopamine receptors in the rat brain. J Neurochem 1982;39:1418-23.
26. Wilkinson M, Herdon HJ. Diethylstilbestrol regulates the number of α- and β-adrenergic binding sites in incubated hypothalamus and amygdala. Brain Res 1982;248:79-85.
27. Ichida S, Tokunaga H, Oda Y, Fujita N, Hirata A, HataT. Increase of serotonin receptors in rat uterus induced by estradiol. J Biol Chem 1983;258:13438-43.
28. Maggi A, Perez J. Estrogen-induced up-regulation of gamma-aminobutyric acid receptors in the CNS of rodents. J Neurochem 1986;47:1793-97.
29. Gazzaley AH, Weiland NG, McEwen BS, Morrison JH. Differential regulation of NMDAR1 mRNA and protein by estradiol in the rat hippocampus. J Neurosci 1996;16: 6830-38.
30. Mor G, Nilsen J, Horvath T, et al. Estrogen and microglia: A regulatory system that affects the brain. J Neurobiol 1999;40:484-96.
31. Zyzek E, Dufy-Barbe L, Dufy B, Vincent JD. Short-term effect of estrogen on release of

prolactin by pituitary cells in culture. Biochem Biophys Res Commun 1981;102:1151-57.
32. Bettini E, Maggi A. Estrogen induction of cytochrome c oxidase subunit III in rat hippocampus. J Neurochem 1992;58:1923-29.
33. Sapino A, Pietribiasi F, Bussolati G, Marchisio PC. Estrogen- and tamoxifen-induced rearrangement of cytoskeletal and adhesion structures in breast cancer MCF-7 cells. Cancer Res 1986;46:2526-531.
34. Hsu LY, Frankel FR. Effect of estrogen on the expression of mRNAs of different action isoforms in immature rat uterus. J Biol Chem 1987;262:9594-9600.
35. Garcia-Segura LM, Cardona-Gomez P, Naftolin F, Chowen JA. Estradiol upregulates Bcl-2 expression in adult brain neurons. Neuroreport 1998;9:593-97.
36. Pike CJ. Estrogen modulates neuronal Bcl-Xl expression and β-amyloid-induced apoptosis: Relevance to Alzheimer's disease. J Neurochem 1999;72:1552-63.
37. Behl C, Widmann M, Trapp T, Holsboer F. 17-βestradiol protects neurons from oxidative stress-induced cell death in vitro. Biochem Biophys Res Commun 1995;216:473-82.
38. Goodman Y, Bruce AJ, Cheng B, Mattson, MP. Oestrogens attenuate and corticosterone exacerbates excitotoxicity, oxidative injury, and amyloid β-peptide toxicity in hippocampal neurons. J Neurochem 1996;66:1836-44.
39. Xu H, Gouras GK, Greenfield JP, et al. Estrogen reduces neuronal generation of Alzheimer beta-amyloid peptides. Nat Med 1998;4:447-51.
40. Ma ZQ, Spreafico E, Pollio G, et al. Activated estrogen receptor mediates growth arrest and differentiation of a neuroblastoma cell line. Proc Natl Acad Sci USA 1993;90:3740-44.
41. Agrati P, Garnier M, Patrone C, et al. SK-ER3 neuroblastoma cells as a model for the study of estrogen influence on neural cells. Brain Res Bull 1997;44:519-23.
42. Garnier M, Di Lorenzo D, Albertini A, Maggi A. Identification of estrogen-responsive genes in neuroblastoma SK-ER3 cells. J Neurosci 1997;17:4591-99.
43. Martini PGV, Delage-Mourroux R, Kraichely DM, Katzenellenbogen BS. Prothymosin alpha selectively enhances estrogen receptor transcriptional activity by interacting with a repressor of estrogen receptor activity. Mol Cell Biol 2000;20:6224-32.
44. Jackson TA, Richer JK, Bain DL, Takimoto GS, Tung L, Horwitz KB. The partial agonist activity of antagonist-occupied steroid receptors is controlled by a novel hinge domain-binding coactivator L7/SPA and the corepressors N-CoR or SMRT. Mol Endocrinol 1997; 11:693-705.
45. Meda C, Vegeto E, Pollio G, et al. Oestrogen prevention of neural cell death correlates with decreased expression of mRNA for the pro-apoptotic protein Nip-2. J Neuroendocrinol 2000;12:1051-59.
46. Boyd JM, Malstrom S, Subramanian T, et al. Adenovirus E1B-19kDa and Bcl-2 proteins interact with a common set of cellular proteins. Cell 1994;79:341-51.
47. Belcredito S, Brusadelli A, Maggi A. Estrogen, apoptosis and cells of neural origin. J Neurocytol 2000;29:359-65.
48. Kennedy AM, Frackowiak RSJ, Newman SK, et al. Deficits in cerebral glucose metabolism demonstrated by positron emission tomography in individual at risk of familial Alzheimer's disease. Neurosci Lett 1995;186:17-20.
49. Vegeto E, Pollio G, Pellicciari C, Maggi A. Estrogen and progesterone induction of survival of monoblastoid cells undergoing TNF-alpha-induced apoptosis. FASEB J 1999; 13:793-803.
50. Boje KM, Arora PK, Microglial-produced nitric oxide and reactive nitrogen oxides

mediate neuronal cell death. Brain Res 1992;587:250-56.
51. Shimizu T, Wolfe LS. Arachidonic acid cascade and signal transduction. J Neurochem 1990;55:1-15.
52. Mc Geer PL, Mc Geer EG. Anti-inflammatory drugs in the fight against Alzheimer's disease. Ann N Y Acad Sci 1996;777:213-20.
53. Gottshall PE. Beta-amyloid induction of gelatinase B secretion in cultured microglia: inhibition by dexamethasone and indomethacin. Neuroreport 1996;7:3077-80.
54. Mulnard RA, Cotman CW, Kawas C, et al. Estrogen replacement therapy for the treatment of mild to moderate Alzheimer disease: A randomized controlled trial. Alzheimer's Disease Cooperative Study. JAMA 2000;283:1007-15.
55. Cuzzocrea S, Santagati S, Sautebin L, et al. 17beta-estradiol antiinflammatory activity in carrageenan-induced pleurisy. Endocrinology 2000;141:1455-63.
56. Miyamoto M, Mandai M, Suzuma I, Suzuma K, Kabayashi K, Honda Y. Estrogen protects against cellular infiltration by reducing expression of E-selectin and IL-6 in endotoxin-induced uveitis. J Immunol 1999;163:374-79.
57. Jansson L, Olsson T, Holmdahl R. Estrogen induces a potent suppression of experimental autoimmune encephalomyelitis and collagen-induced arthritis in mice. J Neuroimmunol 1994;53:203-7.
58. Ashcroft GS, Greenwell-Wild T, Horan MA, Wahl SM, Ferguson MWJ. Topical estrogen accelerates cutaneous wound healing in aged humans associated with an altered inflammatory response. Am J Pathol 1999;155:1137-46.
59. Riggs BL. The mechanisms of estrogen regulation of bone resorption. J Clin Invest 2000; 106:1203-4.
60. Gonzales-Scarano F, Baltuch G. Microglia as mediators of inflammatory and degenerative diseases. Annu Rev Neurosci 1999;22:219-40.
61. Shi J, Bui JD, Yang S-H, et al. Estrogens decrease reperfusion-associated cortical ischemic damage. Stroke 2001;32:987-92.

NEUROSTEROIDS

Andrea Riccardo Genazzani, Francesca Bernardi, Martina Liut, M. Stomati, M. Pieri, and M. Luisi

Sources and Targets of Neurosteroids

Neurosteroids are steroids *de novo* synthesized in the brain or metabolized *in situ* by blood borne precursors. Neurosteroids influence brain function via both genomic and nongenomic mechanisms [1]; the first include the induction of progesterone receptors in cultured oligodendrocytes, the latter include the modulation of calcium channel and of chloride channel opening. Some neurosteroids act as GABA-A agonists, such as allopregnanolone and tetrahydrodesoxycorticosterone; others are GABA-A antagonists, such as DHEA and pregnanolone sulfate (Figure 1). Brain is the first known source of neurosteroids. Bixo et al. have evaluated women post-mortem concentrations of allopregnanolone in brain cortex, amygdala, hippocampus, caudate nucleus, putamen, thalamus, and the highest levels were observed in the substantia nigra and basal hypothalamus [2]. The regional differences in brain steroid levels imply different local mechanisms for steroid uptake and binding. Brain concentrations of allopregnanolone were significantly higher in fertile women at luteal phase than in postmenopausal controls; this may depend on ovarian steroid production, indicating that the secretion pattern during the menstrual cycle is reflected in the brain [2]. Δ5 androgens have also been measured in specific regions of cadaver brains and the central/plasmatic ratio of DHEA demonstrated a higher concentration of the steroid within the brain [1,3].

Allopregnanolone is also measurable in cerebrospinal fluid (CSF). Uzunova et al. have found that allopregnanolone concentration was about 60% lower in patients with major unipolar depression than in controls, while in the same patients, fluoxetine or fluvoxamine treatment normalized the CSF allopregnanolone content [4].

Other possible sources of allopregnanolone in women were investigated by evaluating the response of serum allopregnanolone to functional endocrine tests (gonadotropin-releasing hormone [GnRH] test; corticotropin-releasing hormone [CRH] test; adrenocorticotropin hormone [ACTH] test) [5] . Both GnRH test, and CRH or ACTH tests induce a significant rise in circulating allopregnanolone, suggesting that both ovary and adrenal are sources of this steroid [5]. Further origins of allopregnanolone cannot be excluded; in particular, testis, adipose tissue, and liver are under investigation.

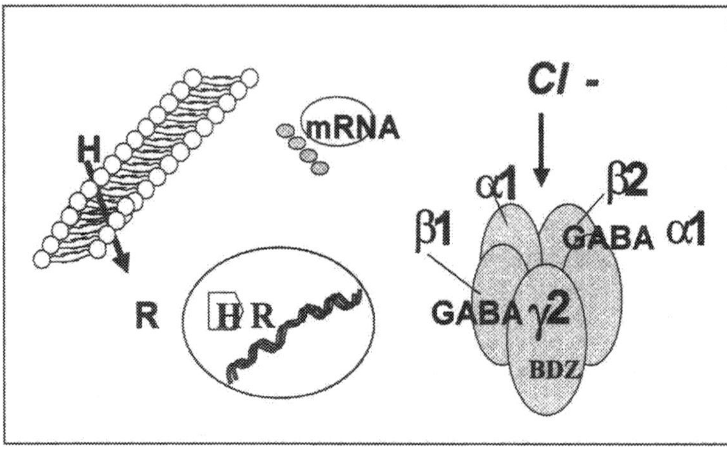

Figure 1. Mechanism of action of neurosteroids

Age-Related Changes

It has been reported that allopregnanolone levels do not vary during the two first years of life while they increase during puberal development both in boys and in girls, in a Tunner stage-related manner, indicating an involvement of allopregnanolone in the neuroendocrine modifications in the puberal period [6]. In addition a progressive increase in progesterone and DHEA levels during puberty has been described in both sexes [6]. Increased levels of adrenal androgens seem to have a role in the sexual development during early stages of puberty constituting the so called adrenarche [7]. In this period, serum DHEA and DHEAS levels induce pubic and axillary hair growth. The increase of DHEA levels begins before than that of testosterone and is not regulated by ACTH or cortisol. The mechanism for the enhanced androgen secretion during the early phase of puberty remains obscure but it is clear that this event is also correlated with behavioral changes [8].

It is well known that pubertal transition affects psychological distress of adolescents: the onset of puberty itself is a novel event that calls for psychological adaptation, physical maturation, and fertility [9]. Neurosteroids may be involved in the complex neuroendocrine modifications occurring during this period.

Serum allopregnanolone levels shows an age-related decrease in men, with lowest levels after 60 years of age. Preliminary data show that in postmenopausal women allopregnanolone levels are similar to those observed during fertile women during follicular phase and are significantly lower than those of women during luteal phase, because the lack of ovarian activity [5]. However, in women, allopregnanolone concentrations do not vary with increasing age [5]. Clinical experiments, performed on a great number of patients, are ongoing to confirm these evidences and to clarify the effects of hormonal replacement therapy in early and late postmenopause and in the elderly.

It is well known that DHEA levels decrease with age both in men and in women

[10,11]. In humans DHEA and DHEAS are the major adrenal cortex products, and the circulating levels of both Δ5 steroids show selective changes during lifetime, reaching their highest values around 25 years of age. After the third decade of life, a progressive decline of the synthesis of the Δ5-androgens is described in both sexes; after 70 years of age DHEA(S) levels are maintained at 20% or less of the maximum plasma concentrations, while cortisol levels remain unchanged [11]. The decline in Δ5-androgens and the parallel increase in cortisol/DHEA(S) ratio has been proven to be in part responsible of the physiological and/or pathological age-associated changes. Epidemiological studies have shown a relationship between the progressive decrease of circulating DHEA(S) levels and the increase of cardiovascular morbidity in men [12], the risk of breast cancer in women [13] and the impairment of the immune competence in both sexes [14]. Clinical studies have investigated the effects of DHEA(S) administration in men and women of different age. The first trials reported metabolic effects, which are different and not comparable both in young and old men and women treated with high doses of DHEA (1,600 mg/daily) [15]. In other studies the use of a lower dose of DHEA (50-100 mg/daily) lead to a restoration in circulating DHEA and DHEAS levels to physiological values [16], associated with a 2-fold increase in circulating levels of androgens (androstenedione, testosterone, and dihydrotestosterone) and estrogens (estradiol and estrone), and no changes in sex hormone-binding globulin levels (SHBG) in women [17]. A single oral dose (500 mg) of DHEA, 60 minutes before sleeping, induced a significant increase in rapid eye movement (REM) sleep, that appears to be implicated in memory processes [18,19].

Neurosteroids and Reproductive Function

Fertile Life

The changes of brain allopregnanolone concentration in female rats during the estrous cycle and the effect of intracerebroventricular injection of allopregnanolone or of its antiserum on ovulatory rat function suggest a correlation between brain allopregnanolone and reproductive function. In fact, the intracerebroventricular injection of allopregnanolone is able to reduce ovulation rate while the injection of an antiserum directed against allopregnanolone increase ovulation rate in rats [20]. In humans, modifications of circulating allopregnanolone levels throughout menstrual cycle and pregnancy have been reported. Allopregnanolone levels are higher in luteal than in follicular phase and these modifications have been related to the changes in mood and activity observed during menstrual cycle [21].

Dehydroepiandrosterone is not influenced by gonadotropin levels, since only random fluctuations of plasma DHEA levels have been observed during the cycle [22]. An involvement of allopregnanolone in the pathogenesis of premenstrual syndrome [23] has been hypothesized. Initial studies showed no variations of serum allopregnanolone levels in the luteal phase of PMS patients with respect to controls, although higher luteal phase allopregnanolone levels were associated with improved symptom ratings in PMS patients [24]. Our data [23] sustain the low levels of allopregnanolone in the luteal phase of women with PMS when compared to controls, while progesterone levels seem to be significantly lower in both phases of the menstrual cycle in PMS patients. These data are indicative of an impaired synthesis of this hormone on behalf of the corpus luteum or other steroidogenic organs (adrenals, liver, and adipose tissue). A GnRH injection during the luteal phase prompted a low allopregnanolone and progesterone response in women with PMS with respect to controls [25], reinforcing the concept that some sort of deficiency in corpus luteum function and synthesis of allopregnanolone and progesterone may underlie PMS. In addition, recent reports sustain that the biological key to the initiation of premenstrual syndrome may also be found in the altered "genomic" effects on behalf of this neurosteroid at the central level [26]. Another hypothesis is that progesterone metabolism may be altered in the brain, being transformed preferentially into an anxiogenic neurosteroid rather than into the anxiolytic allopregnanolone in women with PMS [27].

It is possible to hypothesize an involvement of androgens in the pathophysiology of premenstrual syndrome. DHEA levels were found to be significantly higher in PMS subjects than in controls, around ovulation [28] and, thus, may be in part responsible for premenstrual irritability and dysphoria. In conclusion, the onset of premenstrual anxiety symptoms may result from the interplay of neurosteroids with opposite GABAA-receptor activity within the central nervous system.

Hypothalamic amenorrhea (HA) is a functional disorder characterized by an altered GnRH pulsatility [29], improper pulsatile gonadotropin secretion (FSH and LH) and, in turn, altered ovarian steroidogenesis. Women with HA, despite the high ACTH and cortisol levels and, therefore, hypothalamus-pituitary-adrenal axis hyperactivity, are characterized by low allopregnanolone basal levels, most probably due to an impairment of both adrenal and ovarian synthesis. The blunted response of ACTH, allopregnanolone and cortisol to CRH indicate that women with hypothalamic amenorrhea have a reduced sensitivity and/or expression of CRH receptor [30] (Figure 2).

Anorexia nervosa is one of the leading causes of hypothalamic amenorrhea, being accompanied by disorders in GnRH pulsatile secretion [31]. Furthermore, when administered to rats, allopregnanolone determines hyperphagia [32]. Our data show that serum allopregnanolone levels are significantly higher in patients with anorexia nervosa than in normal fertile women [31]. Allopregnanolone may be involved in appetite control; the elevation of allopregnanolone levels in women with anorexia nervosa may represent a specific stimulus for hunger and therefore food intake. On the other hand, high circulating allopregnanolone may be the effect of an intense stress response which is typical of anorexia nervosa.

Pregnancy

Concerning pregnancy, maternal serum allopregnanolone and progesterone levels rise significantly throughout gestation in healthy pregnant women [33]. No marked changes are found at delivery, except for a significant decrease of maternal and cord serum allopregnanolone levels during emergency cesarean section. Furthermore, serum allopregnanolone levels are significantly higher in patients with chronic hypertension, with or without preeclampsia, than in healthy pregnant women. The changes in these two hormones in maternal and umbilical cord serum are correlated with gestation, but not with parturition, neither in healthy women nor in hypertensive patients. The role of allopregnanolone in pregnancy remains uncertain. Allopregnanolone may play a role in uterine kinetics [34,35]. Maternal anxiety may be related to serum allopregnanolone levels, given the potent anxiolytic effect of this neuroactive steroid [36]. The evidence of increased level of serum allopregnanolone in hypertensive pregnant women is of great interest in view of the possible role of progesterone in vascular tension during pregnancy.

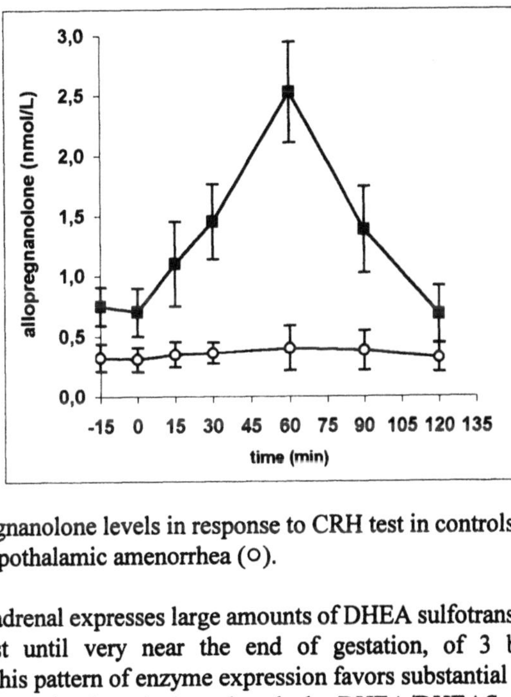

Figure 2. Allopregnanolone levels in response to CRH test in controls (■) and in patients suffering from hypothalamic amenorrhea (○).

The fetal adrenal expresses large amounts of DHEA sulfotransferase and minimal amounts, at least until very near the end of gestation, of 3 beta-hydroxysteroid dehydrogenase. This pattern of enzyme expression favors substantial secretion of DHEA and DHEAS with minimal cortisol produced; the DHEA/DHEAS serves as the major precursor for placental estrogen formation in human pregnancy [10]. The mean plasma concentration of DHEAS in 10 normal pregnant women decreased in early gestation to minimum levels at week 38. At delivery there was a 2-fold increase in plasma DHEAS. The peak levels of DHEAS at admission to the delivery room reflect increased maternal and fetal stress with the onset of labor [37]. Distressed infants have lower serum levels of DHEA and higher levels of corisol than control infants [38]. It also seems that higher levels of DHEA are associated with a better mood during pregnancy [39].

MENOPAUSE

Concerning menopause, several studies suggest that the reduction of 17,20 desmolase activity, the enzyme that governs the biosynthesis of the Δ5-adrenal pathway, may provoke modifications in DHEA(S) synthesis [11]. At present it is unknown whether changes of plasma DHEA(S) levels can directly affect CNS functions. In experimental animals, DHEA treatment induced a memory-enhancing effect [18]. *In vitro* studies suggest a neurotrophic effect on neurons and glial cells [18]. In postmenopausal women, the daily administration of DHEA (50 mg/day) for three months induced an improvement in psychological and physical well-being [16]. Recently, it has been shown that the oral administration of DHEA (50 mg/daily) for three months determined an increase in well-being and mood only in women but not in men [19].

In order to clarify the effects on the neuroendocrine functions, our group has recently investigated the effects of DHEA and DHEAS supplementation on the opiatergic tonus in postmenopausal women. In particular, the attention was focused on β-endorphin (β-EP), an important and biologically active endogenous opioid peptide, having behavioral, analgesic, thermoregulatory, and neuroendocrine properties. In postmenopausal women a decrease in plasma β-EP levels has been demonstrated. In fertile subjects, naloxone, an opioid receptor antagonist, and clonidine, an α_2-presynaptic receptor agonist, bolus injection increases β-EP levels. In postmenopause, a lack of response of β-EP to clonidine and to naloxone occurs and these findings suggest a postmenopausal impairment of adrenergic and opiatergic receptors in modulating β-EP release. HRT restores basal plasma β-EP levels to those present in fertile women as well as the β-EP response to clonidine and naloxone [40].

DHEA oral administration (50 or 100 mg/day) increases basal plasma levels of androgens and estrogens, indicating that the Δ5-androgen and its sulphate conjugated ester may be converted into active steroids [15,18]. The increase of basal plasma β-EP levels after the first month of DHEAS therapy support an estrogen-like effect of the molecule on CNS. The treatment with DHEA(S) induces a restoration of the β-EP response to clonidine, naloxone or fluoxetine tests, respectively, suggesting a restored neuroendocrine control of α2-adrenergic, opioidergic, and serotonine receptors on the anterioro-pituitary β-EP secretion. The modulation of the neuroendocrine pathways after DHEAS supplementation may be mediated by a specific estrogenic action of DHEAS metabolites or, alternatively by a similar receptorial specificity of DHEAS and estro-progestin compounds on opiatergic and adrenergic neurons. In conclusion, the present findings suggest that both the Δ-5 androgens, and or their metabolites, may be considered one of neuroendocrine correlates of the DHEA(S)-induced psychological and physical improvements. In postmenopausal women, the levels of allopregnanolone are similar to follicular phase levels present in fertile women. The age-related decrease in progesterone levels is not paralleled by a similar decrease in allopregnanolone levels, suggesting that ovarian progesterone is not the major determinant of circulating allopregnanolone in this phase of a woman's life [5]. Our preliminary unpublished results indicate that HRT is able to increase allopregnanolone levels in postmenopausal subjects but further data obtained in a larger population are necessary to give sure information concerning this interesting issue.

Mood, Behavior, and Cognitive Performances

Purdy et al. [41] first found an increase in the brain and plasma levels of allopregnanolone in rats after exposure to swim stress, and they hypothesized that allopregnanolone may be involved in adaptive response to stress. Moreover, it has been shown that pretreatment with high doses of allopregnanolone significantly decreased corticotropin-releasing factor release evoked by pharmacologic challenges in hypothalamic explants [42]. Swim stress determines a significant increase of allopregnanolone and pregnanolone in rat frontal cortex [43]. In addition it has been demonstrated that the acute footshock stress is able to induce greater percentage increase in the cortical concentration of allopregnanolone in isolated rats than in group-housed rats, indicating that these animals, having lower allopregnanolone basal levels, show a exasperated response to stressful stimuli [44].On the other hand, it has been hypothesized that the involvement of allopregnanolone in seizures may enter in stress-related responses of organism against cerebral damage. In fact it has been demonstrated that there are changes in serum allopregnanolone levels after epileptic seizure. In a recent study several blood samples were drawn immediately, 15 minutes, and 6 hours after a seizure in seven fertile females with partial epilepsy [45]. Allopregnanolone increases in serum during the first 15 minutes after partial seizures and decreases after 6 hours. These data suggest that allopregnanolone might play a role in inhibiting the spread of epileptic discharge. If data of elevation of allopregnanolone after epileptic seizures were confirmed as specific, this steroid could be considered a marker of epileptic seizures. However, it cannot be ruled out that the increase in allopregnanolone represents a nonspecific reaction of the organism to stress.

An involvement of $GABA_A$ receptors in anxiety and depression has been demonstrated; in fact, such conditions are characterized by a GABAergic hypotone and by an hyperactivity of hypothalamic-pituitary-adrenal axis [46]. In fact, low levels of allopregnanolone have been reported in cerebrospinal fluid of depressed patients and that fluoxetine or fluvoxamine administration in these patients is able to increase allopregnanolone levels, while progesterone and pregnanolone do not undergo modifications [4]. On the contrary, Strohle et al. have reported high levels of pregnanolone and pregnanolone sulphate in depressive-anxiety disorders [47]. DHEA and DHEAS levels also vary in depression and in patients who show aggressive behavior [47,48].

Neurosteroids may be also implicated in the memory mechanisms that modulate the acquisition and loss of memory, suggesting that the reduced memory performance occurring in humans with aging could be related to a modification of steroidogenesis. It is known that DHEA and DHEAS improve long-term memory and diminish amnesia in mice and enhance neuronal and glial survival and differentiation in cultures of embryonic mouse brain cells [49]. The administration of DHEA improves physical and psychological well-being and cognitive performances in aged subjects [11]. The mechanism(s) of DHEA-mediated neuroprotection are unclear: probably, DHEA antagonizes some deleterious effects of cortisol which cause progressive hippocampal damage and cognitive impairment in dementia [50-52].

The hypothesis that allopregnanolone might be involved in modulating cognitive function is supported by the evidence that conditions characterized by modifications in behavior, mood, and cognitive performances, such as menstrual cycle, pregnancy, and aging, are associated with changes in allopregnanolone levels [5,24,53]. Allopregnanolone and DHEA levels are reduced both in Alzheimer's and in vascular dementia; on the other hand, CRH administration determines an increase in allopregnanolone levels lower than this observed in control subjects [54] (Figure 3). It is possible to hypothesize that in dementia the low allopregnanolone levels are a consequence of the low CRH levels that may explain also the low DHEA levels observed. On the other hand, both the AUC of DHEA and allopregnanolone response to CRH have been described to be reduced in dementia indicating that these patients had an impairment in the total neuroendocrine balance capacity involving DHEA and allopregnanolone secretion. In conclusion, these evidences support the concept that dementia per se, independently of the nature, may be the result of an altered stress response, and the modifications in the circulating levels of allopregnanolone, a stress-related steroid hormone, might enter in this view. Therefore, it will be of interest to study the role of allopregnanolone in the complex way leading from stress to cognition, possibly via the interplay between brain CRH and CRH-related peptides.

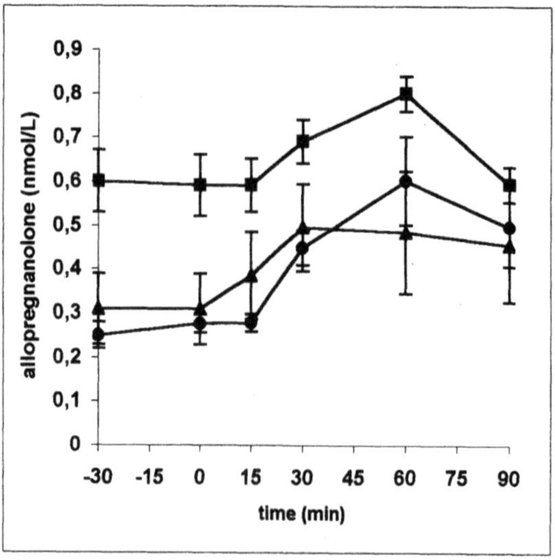

Figure 3. Allopregnanolone levels in response to CRH in controls (■) and in patients suffering from Alzheimer's disease (●) and vascular dementia (▲).

References

1. Mellon SH. Neurosteroids: Biochemistry, modes of action, and clinical relevance. J Clin Endocrinol Metab 1994:78:1003-8.
2. Bixo M, Andersson A, Winblad B, Purdy RH, Backstrom T. Progesterone, 5alpha-pregnane-3,20-dione and 3alpha-hydroxy-5alpha-pregnane-20-one in specific regions of the human female brain in different endocrine states. Brain Res 1997 Aug 1;764(1-2):173-78.
3. Majewska MD, Demirgoren S, Spivak CE, London ED. The neurosteroid DHEA is an allosteric antagonist of the GABAA receptor. Brain Res 1990;526:143-46.
4. Uzunova V, Sheline Y, Davis JM, et al. Increase in the cerebrospinal fluid content of neurosteroids in patients with unipolar major depression who are receiving fluoxetine or fluvoxamine. Proc Natl Acad Sci USA 1998 Mar 17;95(6):3239-44.
5. Genazzani AR, Petraglia F, Bernardi F, et al. Circulating levels of allopregnanolone in humans: Gender, age and endocrine influences. J Clin Endocrinol Metab 1998;83:2099-210.
6. Holst J., Backstrom T., Hammerbsck S., von Schoultz B. Progestogen addition during estrogen replacement therapy-effects opn vasomotor symptoms and mood. Maturitas 1989; 11:13-19.
7. Hopper BR, Yen SC. Circulating concentrations of dehydroepiandrosterone and dehydroepiandrosterone sulfate during puberty. J Clin Endocrinol Metab 1975;40:458-61.
8. Reiter EO, Fuldauer VG, Root AW. Secretion of the adrenal androgen, dehydroepiandrosterone sulfate, during normal infancy, childhood, and adolescence, in sick infants, and in children with endocrinologic abnormalities. J Pediatr 1977;90:766-70.
9. Xiaojia G, Conger RD, Elder GH. Coming of age too early: Pubertal influences on girls' vulnerability to psychological distress. Child Develop 1996;67:3386-3400.
10. Parker CR Jr. Dehydroepiandrosterone and dehydroepiandrosterone sulfate production in the human adrenal during development and aging. Steroids. 1999 Sep;64(9):640-47.
11. Liu CH, Laughlin GA, Fischer UG, Yen SSC. Marked attenuation of ultradian and circadian rhythms of dehydroepiandrosterone in postmenopausal women: Evidence for a reduced 17,20-Desmolase enzymatic activity.J Clin Endocrinol Metab 1990;71(4):900-906.
12. Barret-Connor E, Khaw K, Yen SSC. A prospective study of DS mortality and cardiovascular disease. N Engl J Med 1986;315:1519-24.
13. Helzlsouer KJ, Gordon GB, Alberg A, Bush TL, Comstock GW. Relationship of prediagnostic serum levels of DHEA and DS to the risk of developing premenopausal breast cancer. Cancer Res 1992;52:1-4.
14. Thoman ML, Weigle WO. The cellular and subcellular bases of immunosenescence. Adv Immunol 1989;46:221-61.
15. Mortola JF, Yen SSC. The effects of oral dehydroepiandrosterone on endocrine-metabolic parameters in postmenopausal women. J Clin Endocrinol Metab 1990;71:696-704.
16. Morales AJ, Nolan JJ, Nelson JC, Yen SSC. Effects of replacement dose of dehydroepiandrosterone in men and women of advancing age. J Clin Endocrinol Metab 1994;78:1360-770.
17. Stomati M, Rubino S, Spinetti A, et al. Endocrine, neuroendocrine and behavioural effects of oral dehydroepiandrosterone sulphate supplementation in postmenopausal women. Gynecol Endocrinol 1999;13:15-25.

18. Thijssen JHH, Nieuwenhuyse H. DHEA: A comprehensive review. New York: The Parthenon Publishing Group, 1999.
19. Wolf OT, Neumenn O, Helhammer DH, et al. Effects of a two-week physiological dehydroepiandrosterone substitution on cognitive performance and well-being in healthy elderly women and men. J Clin Endocrinol Metab 1997;82:2363-67.
20. Genazzani AR, Palombo MA, de Micheroux AA, et al. Evidence for a role for the neurosteroid allopregnanolone in the modulation of reproductive function in female rats. Eur J Endocrinol 1995;133:375-80.
21. Genazzani AR, Petraglia F, Bernardi F, et al. Circulating levels of allopregnanolone in humans: Gender, age, and endocrine influences. J Clin Endocrinol Metab 1998;83:2099-2103.
22. Vermeulen A, Verdonck L. Plasma androgen levels during the menstrual cycle. Am J Obstet Gynecol 1976;125:491-94.
23. Monteleone P, Luisi S, Tonetti A, et al. Allopregnanolone concentrations and premenstrual syndrome. Eur J Endocrinol 2000;142;269-73.
24. Schmidt PJ, Purdy RH, Moore PH, et al. Circulating levels of anxiolytic steroids in the luteal phase in women with premenstrual syndrome and in control subjects. J Clin Endocrinol Metab 1994;79:1256-60.
25. Monteleone P, Luisi S, Tonetti A, et al. Allopregnanolone concentrations and premenstrual syndrome. Eur J Endocrinol. 2000 Mar;142(3):269-73.
26. Smith SS, Gong QH, Hsu F-C, et al. $GABA_A$ receptor α4 subunit suppression prevents withdrawal properties of an endogenous steroid. Nature 1998;392:926-30.
27. Berga SL. Understanding premenstrual syndrome. Lancet 1998;351:465-66.
28. Eriksson E, Sundblad C, Lisjo P, Modigh K, Andersch B. Serum levels of androgens are higher in women with premenstrual irritability and dysphoria than in controls. Psychoneuroendocrinology.1992 May-Jul;17(2-3):195-204.
29. Meczekalski B, Tonetti A, Monteleone P, et al. Hypothalamic amenorrhea with normal body weight: ACTH, allopregnanolone and cortisol responses to corticotropin-releasing hormone test. Eur J Endocrinol. 2000 Mar;142(3):280-85.
30. Petraglia F, Sutton S, Vale W, Plotsky P. Corticotropin releasing factor decreases plasma luteinizing hormone levels in female rats by inhibiting GnRH release into hypophyseal-portal circulation. Endocrinology 1987;120:1083-88.
31. Monteleone P, Luisi M, Colurcio B, et al. Plasma levels of neuroactive steroids are increased in untreated women with anorexia nervosa or bulimia nervosa. Psycosomatic Medicine 2001;63:62-68.
32. Chen SW, Rodriguez L, Davies MF, Loew GH. The hyperphagic effect of 3 alpha-hydroxylated pregnane steroids in male rats. Pharmacol Biochem Behav 1996 Apr;53(4): 777-82.
33. Luisi S, Petraglia F, Benedetto C, et al. Serum allopregnanolone levels in pregnant women: Changes during pregnancy, at delivery and in hypertensive patients. J Clin Endorinol Metab 2000;83:2733-49.
34. Putnam CD, Brann DW, Kolbeck RC, Mahesh VB. Inhibition of uterine contractility by progesterone and progesterone metabolites: Mediation by progesterone and gamma amino butyric acidA recpetor systems. Biol Reprod 1991;45:266-72.
35. Majewska MD, Vaupel DB. Steroid control of uterine motility via gamma-aminobutyric acidA receptors in the rabbit: A novel mechanism? J Endocrinol 1991;13:427-34.
36. Bitran D, Shiekh M, MacLeod M. Anxiolytic effect of progesterone is mediated by the

neurosteroid allopregnanoloneregnanolone at brain GABAa receptors. J Neuroendo 1995; 7:171-77.

37. Buckwalter JG, Stanczyk FZ, McCleary CA, et al. Pregnancy, the postpartum, and steroid hormones: effects on cognition and mood. Psychoneuroendocrinology. 1999 Jan;24(1):69-84.

38. Peter M, Dorr HG, Sippell WG. Changes in the concentrations of dehydroepiandrosterone sulfate and estriol in maternal plasma during pregnancy: A longitudinal study in healthy women throughout gestation and at term. Horm Res 1994;42(6):278-81.

39. Parker CR Jr, Favor JK, Carden LG, Brown CH. Effects of intrapartum stress on fetal adrenal function. Am J Obstet Gynecol 1993 Dec;169(6):1407-11.

40. Stomati M, Bersi C, Rubino S, et al. Neuroendocrine effectsof different estradiol-progestin regimens in postmenopausal women. Maturitas 1997;28:127-35.

41. Purdy RH, Morrow AL, Moore PH, et al. Stress-induced elevations of γ-aminobutyric acid type A receptor-active steroids in the rat brain. Proc Natl Acad Sci USA 1991;8:4553-57.

42. Patchev VK, Shoaib M, Holsboer F, et al. The neurosteroid tetrahydroprogesterone counteracts corticotropin-releasing hormone induced anxiety and alters the release and gene expression of corticotropin-releasing hormone in the rat hypothalamus. Neuroscience 1994;62:265-71.

43. Vallee M, Rivera JD, Koob GF, Purdy RH, Fitzgerald RL. Quantification of neurosteroids in rat plasma and brain following swim stress and allopregnanolone administration using negative chemical ionization gas chromatography/ mass spectrometry. Anal Biochem 2000 Dec 1;287(1):153-66.

44. Serra M, Pisu MG, Lettera M, et al. Social isolation-induced decreases in both the abundance of neuroactive steroids and GABA(A) receptor function in rat brain. J Neurochem 2000 Aug;75(2):732-40.

45. Galli R, Luisi M, Pizzanelli C, et al. Circulating levels of allopregnanolone, an anticonvulsant metabolite of progesterone, in women with partial epilepsy in the postcritical phase. Epilepsia 2001;42(2):216-219.

46. Berretini WH, Post RM. Gaba in affective illness. In: Post RM, Ballanger JC, editors. Ineurobilogy of mood disorders. Williams and Wilkins, Baltimore; 1984, 673-685.

47. Strohle A, Romeo E, Hermann B, et al. Concentrations of 3α-reduced neuroactive steroids and their precursors in plasma of patients with major depression and after clinical recovery. Biol Psychiatry 1999;45:274-77.

48. van Goozen SHM, Matthys W, Cohen-Kettenis PT, Thijssen JHH, van Engeland II. Adrenal androgens and aggression in conduct disorder prepubertal boys and normal controls. Biol Psychiatry 1998;43:145-53.

49. Roberts E. Dehydroepiandrosterone (DHEA) and its sulphate (DHEAS) as neural facilitators: effects on brain tissue in culture and on memory in young and old mice: A cyclic GMP hypothesis of action of DHEA and DHEAS in nervous system and other tissues. In: Kalimi M, Regelson W, editors. The biologic role of dehydroepiandrosterone. Berlin, Walter de Gruyter;1990, 13-42.

50. Sapolsky RM, Krey LC, McEwen BS. The neuroendocrinology of stress and aging: the glucocorticoid cascade hypothesis. Endocr Rev 1986;7:284-301.

51. Wolkowitz OM, Reus VI, Manfredi F, Roberts E. Antiglucocorticoid effects in Alzheimer's disease (reply). Am J Psychiatry 1992;149:1126.

52. Svec F, Lopez A. Antiglucocorticoid actions of DHEA and low concentrations in Alzheimer's disease (letter). Lancet 1989;2:1335-36.

53. Majewska MD. Neurosteroids: Endogenous bimodal modulators of the GABA-A receptor. Mechanism of action and physiological significance. Progress in Neurobiology 1992,38: 379-95.

54. Bernardi F, Lanzone A, et al. Allopregnanolone and dehydroepiandrosterone response to corticotropin-releasing factor in patients suffering from Alzheimer's disease and vascular dementia. Eur J Endocrinol 2000;142:466-71.

RANDOMIZED TRIALS OF ESTROGEN FOR MEMORY AND DEMENTIA

Victor W. Henderson

Introduction: Memory and Dementia

It is well-documented that memory and other cognitive skills decline with age, beginning in midlife and progressing thereafter [1]. Among the different kinds of memory affected by aging, long-term memory [2] is the most important. Long-term memory is often evaluated by delayed recall tasks, in which new information is presented for learning, followed some minutes later by the conscious recall of this information. In contrast, short-term memory is assessed by recall several seconds after new information is presented. Separate distinction is sometimes made between memory for verbal information and memory for information not easily described by words (for example, a visual pattern).

Dementia is an age-associated disorder in which impairments in memory and other cognitive skills have dropped to a level where social or occupational functioning is substantially affected. After about age 65 years, the prevalence of dementia increases with advancing age, at least until about the tenth decade of life [3]. Although there are many specific causes of dementia, in most countries the most common etiology is Alzheimer's disease [4]. This disorder is characterized by the insidious onset of memory loss and other cognitive symptoms that relentlessly worsen over a period of years. Alzheimer's disease is 1.5 to 3 times more common among women than men [5], largely because of sex differences in longevity, but also in part because women may be more affected by recognized Alzheimer risk factors [6,7].

Memory and Dementia: Possible Relation to Estrogen

Menopause is associated with sharp declines in concentrations of circulating estrogen, and this change has the potential to affect the central nervous system [8]. In the brain as in other target organs, estrogen interacts with specific intranuclear receptors [9], as well as putative receptors located within cell membranes [10].

In some rodent models, estrogen replacement after ovariectomy appears to enhance learning and memory [11,12]. Several estrogen actions may account for these effects. Estrogen promotes the formation of new neurons in a portion of the hippocampus [13], a brain region essential to long-term memory [2]. In the hippocampus, estrogen also enhances synaptic plasticity and long-term potentiation [14], physiological processes believed to underlie long-term memory. Further, in experimental brain-lesion models, estrogen helps protect against the loss of acetylcholine [11,15], a neurotransmitter important in learning and memory.

There is additional laboratory evidence that estrogen has the potential to impact favorably on Alzheimer's disease. Estrogen reduces the formation of β-amyloid, an abnormal protein deposited in Alzheimer brain [16]. Further, as recently reviewed [8], estrogen is neuroprotective and neurotrophic, reduces oxidative damage, influences neurotransmitter systems impaired in Alzheimer's disease, modulates the immune system, and enhances cerebral blood flow.

Clinical Trials of Estrogen and Memory

Serum estrogen concentrations in menopausal women do not appear to be closely related to memory [17,18], although one study reported a positive association between estrogen concentrations and verbal memory but an inverse association with nonverbal memory [19]. Several cross-sectional and longitudinal analyses of community-dwelling older women have suggested that the use of menopausal estrogen therapy, with or without a progestin, enhances or maintains memory test performance [20-22], but the absence of an estrogen effect is also reported [23-26].

Whether there is a causal link between estrogen and memory is better answered by data from randomized controlled trials than from observational studies. For postmenopausal women, it would be useful to distinguish between trials of estrogen designed to prevent or retard the gradual loss of memory skills associated with aging and trials designed to boost current memory abilities. Unfortunately, no clinical trails have yet examined the former possibility.

Several short-term, randomized, placebo-controlled, double-blind trials have considered the effects of estrogen on long-term memory after abrupt menopause induced by oophorectomy or, somewhat analogously, temporarily induced by the pharmacological suppression of ovarian function. Other short-term clinical trials have examined whether estrogen might augment memory scores in women months or years after their menopause. Results of these trials are summarized in Table 1. Information on other trials is provided in recent reviews [27-29].

Eight randomized controlled trials studies have examined estrogen effects on long-term memory [30-37] (Table 1). Six of these included tests of verbal memory, and an equal number included nonverbal memory tests. Strictly speaking, memory is not measured in isolation from other cognitive processes. Depending on the particular memory test, language, visuoperceptual, and visuoconstructive (drawing) abilities might have an impact on test scores. In addition, performance on long-term memory tasks can be influenced by attention, motivation, and executive function (i.e. the ability to categorize and organize stimuli, and rehearsal strategies).

Long-term memory is sometimes assessed immediately after information is presented, where "immediate" is taken to mean assessments that begin within about half a minute of stimulus presentation. However, immediate recall scores reflect contributions of long-term memory only when the amount of information exceeds what can be maintained in short-term memory. Further, immediate recall is especially vulnerable to disturbances in attentional and executive processes [38]. Delayed recall is thus a more valid measure of long-term memory. This important distinction between immediate and delayed recall is often overlooked when estrogen effects on long-term memory are considered. The following discussion separates findings from verbal and nonverbal tasks, as well as findings from immediate recall and delayed recall tasks.

Estrogen and Verbal Memory

Two kinds of verbal memory tasks are reported in randomized controlled trials of estrogen (Table 1): paragraph learning and paired associate learning. The first task involves the oral or written presentation of a short paragraph-length story; subjects are later asked to recall contents of the story. For verbal paired associate learning, the examiner first reads aloud a list of word pairs. Memory is assessed when the examiner provides one word from a pair and asks the subject to recall the second word.

Delayed recall of verbal material was assessed in five randomized controlled trials [32,33,35-37] (Table 1). Three trials involved paired associate learning in older women who had experienced menopause months or years before [35-37]. Estrogen had no effect on memory in these studies. Two other studies involved women who had undergone acute surgical menopause (hysterectomy and oophorectomy) [32] or reversible ovarian suppression by a pharmacological agent [33]. In the first of these special populations, estrogen prevented a decline in paired associate learning but had no effect on paragraph learning [32], and in the second estrogen improved paragraph delayed recall but not paired associate delayed recall [33].

Immediate recall, an indirect measure of verbal long-term memory, has been assessed in five studies [31-33,35,37] (Table 1). For paired associate learning, no estrogen effect was reported in a two-week study [35] and a nine-month study [37] of older postmenopausal women. In contrast, studies of acutely menopausal women indicated a benefit of estrogen when subjects were assessed with the immediate recall of written [31] and oral [32,33] paragraph information and with the immediate recall of verbal paired associates [32,33].

Estrogen and Nonverbal Memory

Nonverbal memory is often assessed with visual reproductions. For this type of psychometric task, a figural design is presented for visual inspection and then removed from sight. The subject is then required to draw the figure from memory, either immediately or after a delay. Commonly used tasks are the Visual Reproduction Test from the Wechsler Memory Scale (or one of its revised versions) and the Benton Visual Retention Test. In randomized controlled trials using a visual reproduction task, immediate [32-34] and delayed [32,33] figural recall was unaffected by estrogen administration. Similarly, no effect is reported in studies using different nonverbal memory tests. These other tasks have involved the immediate recall of spatial location in a manual maze [30],

Table 1. Randomized Double-blind, Placebo-controlled Trials of Estrogen for Long-term Memory in Women Without Dementia

			Verbal memory		Nonverbal memory	
Study and Study design	Subjects; Subject number; Mean age	Treatment Duration	Delayed recall / Results	Immediate recall / Results	Delayed recall / Results	Immediate recall / Results
Vanhull & Demol, 1976 [30] Parallel groups	Postmenopausal nuns; 29 randomized, 26 completed; 58 years	3 months				(1) Visual reproduction / No between-group differences (2) Manual labyrinth / No between-group differences
*Sherwin, 1988 [31] Crossover	Acute surgical menopause, hysterectomy and oophorectomy for benign conditions; 20 completed; 45 years	3 months		Paragraph recall / Between-group difference favored estrogen		
Phillips & Sherwin, 1992 [32] Parallel groups	Acute surgical menopause, hysterectomy and oophorectomy for benign disease; 31 recruited, 19 completed; 48 years	2 months	(1) Paragraph recall / No within-group difference (2) Paired associates / Decline within placebo group	(1) Paragraph recall / Increase within estrogen group (2) Paired associates / Decline within placebo group	Visual reproduction / No within-group change	Visual reproduction / No within-group change
Sherwin & Tulandi, 1996 [33] Parallel groups	Infertility due to leiomyomata; acute pharmacological ovarian suppression with leuprolide acetate; 20 randomized, 19 completed; 34 years	8 weeks	(1) Paragraph recall / Increase within estrogen group (2) Paired associates / No within-group change	(1) Paragraph recall / Increases within estrogen group (2) Paired associates / Increases within estrogen group	Visual reproduction / No within-group change	Visual reproduction / No within-group change
Polo-Kantola et al., 1998 [34] Crossover	Healthy, with prior hysterectomy; 68 randomized, 62 completed; 56 years	3 months				Visual reproduction / No between-group difference
Wolf et al., 1999 [35] Parallel groups	Healthy postmenopausal, natural or surgical; 40 randomized, 38 completed; 69 years	2 weeks	Paired associates / No between-group difference	Paired associates / No between-group difference	Spatial (map) memory / No between-group difference	Spatial (map) memory / No between-group difference

Table 1, continued. Randomized Double-blind, Placebo-controlled Trials of Estrogen for Long-term Memory in Women Without Dementia

			Verbal memory		Nonverbal memory	
Study and Study design	Subjects; Subject number; Mean age	Treatment Duration	Delayed recall / Results	Immediate recall / Results	Delayed recall / Results	Immediate recall / Results
Duka et al., 2000 [36] Parallel-groups	Healthy postmenopausal, natural or surgical; 40 randomized, 37 completed; 69 years	3 weeks	Paired associates with pictured objects / No between-group difference on primary analysis			Pattern location paired associates / No between-group differences on 2 primary analyses
Binder et al., 2001 [37] Parallel groups	Healthy postmenopausal, natural or surgical; 67 randomized, 52 completed; 81 years	9 months	Paired associates / No between-group difference	Paired associates / No between-group difference		

*There were a total of five treatment groups, with results from the estrogen and placebo groups shown here. Treatment allocation was randomized, but it is not stated whether the study was conducted in a blinded manner. Analyses were based on study completers [32].

the immediate and delayed recall of map routes [35], and immediate recall on a paired associate task involving a visual pattern and a spatial location [36] (Table 1).

ESTROGEN AND MEMORY: CONCLUDING COMMENTS

It is difficult to draw strong conclusions from clinical trial data on estrogen and memory. Most studies have not adhered to a more rigorous intention-to-treat analysis. Treatment durations have varied from as short as two weeks to as long as nine months, and estrogen dosages and preparations have varied. In older postmenopausal women, studies of verbal delayed recall (all of which were negative) have used transdermal estradiol [35,36] or oral conjugated estrogens [37]. Trials in women after acute menopause have used intramuscular estradiol [31,32] or oral conjugated estrogens [33]. In most studies, small sample sizes have limited the statistical power to detect modest estrogen effects that might be present. For example, in one negative study, a *post hoc* analysis that combined a verbal memory measure with two measures from a nonverbal memory task indicated a beneficial estrogen effect, even though no significant effect had been discerned in primary analyses [36]. Within studies, results are sometimes inconsistent (positive on one delayed recall measure but not on a second measure) [32,33], a discrepancy that might reflect low statistical power, psychometric properties of the test instruments, or chance.

The most promising findings are from clinical trials of women who have suffered an abrupt loss of ovarian function [31-33], and it is possible that estrogen effects on memory are clinically evident only in the acute setting. Alternatively, and of greater public health concern, it is possible that estrogen effects are evident only when treatment has not been preceded by prolonged estrogen deprivation. These same studies in acutely menopausal women also imply an interaction with the modality of material to be learned (verbal versus visuoperceptual), with apparent estrogen effects confined to verbal memory. Conclusions on modality specificity must be drawn cautiously, however, as psychometric properties of verbal and nonverbal memory tasks are not comparable.

Clinical Trials of Menopausal Estrogen Therapy and Dementia

Very few studies have considered potential effects of estrogen on dementing disorders other than Alzheimer's disease. There is, however, great interest in estrogen and Alzheimer's disease. Case-control and cohort studies generally suggest an overall protective effect of menopausal estrogen therapy on Alzheimer risk [39-44], but there are exceptions [45,46]. Randomized controlled trials of estrogen for Alzheimer's disease prevention are in progress [47,48].

In contrast to the dearth of clinical trial data on primary prevention, six randomized, double-blind, placebo-controlled clinical trials have examined estrogen effects in women diagnosed with Alzheimer's disease [49-54] (Table 2).These studies were organized after observational studies [55] and several pilot trials [56] implied a role for estrogen in Alzheimer therapy. Most clinical trials have not used long-term memory as a primary outcome when assessing estrogen in this illness.

Table 2. Randomized Double-blind, Placebo-controlled Trials of Estrogen for the Treatment of Alzheimer's Disease

Study and Study design	Alzheimer subjects; Subject number; Mean Age	Treatment duration	Primary outcome measures / Results	Other tests of long-term memory / Results	Selected results of other tests
Honjo et al., 1993 [49] Parallel groups	Nursing home residents with dementia; 14 randomized, 14 completed; 83 years	3 weeks	(1) Revised Hasegawa Dementia Scale / Improvement within estrogen group; between-group difference favored estrogen (2) New Screening Test for Dementia / Improvement within estrogen group; no between-group differences (3) Mini-Mental State examination / Improvement within estrogen group; no between-group differences		
Asthana et al., 1999 [50] Parallel groups	Mild to moderate dementia; 14 randomized, 12 completed; 79 years	8 weeks	Comprehensive neuropsychological battery with 7 tasks and 16 measures, each assessed at 1, 3, 5, and 8 weeks / Between-group differences favored estrogen on the number of self-corrections in interference condition of the Stroop Color-Word Test, and delayed cued recall of the Selective Reminding Test; no between-group differences on 14 other cognitive measures		No between-group differences on 2 psychometric measures of dementia severity
Henderson et al., 2000 [51] Parallel groups	Mild to moderate dementia; 42 randomized, 36 completed; 78 years	16 weeks	Cognitive subscale of the Alzheimer's Disease Assessment Scale / No between-group difference	(1) Paragraph delayed recall / No between-group differences (2) Paragraph immediate recall / No between-group differences (3) Visual reproduction delayed recall / No between-group differences (4) Visual reproduction immediate recall / No between-group differences	No between-group differences on global staging and functional skills; Between-group differences favored placebo for 1 of 13 other cognitive measures

Table 2. continued. Randomized Double-blind, Placebo-controlled Trials of Estrogen for the Treatment of Alzheimer's Disease

Study and Study design	Alzheimer subjects; Subject number; Mean Age	Treatment duration	Primary outcome measures / Results	Other tests of long-term memory / Results	Selected results of other tests
Mulnard et al., 2000 [52] Parallel groups, Intention-to-treat analyses	Mild to moderate dementia with prior hysterectomy; 120 randomized, 97 completed; 75 years	12 months	Global staging / No between-group difference	(1) Face recognition / No between-group differences (2) Visual delayed non-match to sample recognition /) No between-group differences	No between-group differences on 2 psychometric measures of dementia severity; Between-group differences favored placebo on a secondary global staging score; No between-group differences on 3 measures of daily activities; Between-group differences favored placebo on 2 of 9 other cognitive measures
Wang et al., 2000 [53]	Mild to moderate dementia; 50 randomized, 47 completed; 72 years	12 weeks	(1) Cognitive Abilities Screening Instrument / No between-group differences (2,3) Two global staging tests / No between-group differences		
Asthana et al., 2001 [54] Parallel groups	Mild to moderate dementia; 20 randomized, 20 completed; 80 years	8 weeks	Outcome measures at 3,5, and 8 weeks: (1) Time to complete interference condition of Stroop Color-Word Test / Between-group differences favored estrogen (2) Total (immediate + delayed) recall on Selective Reminding Test / Between-group differences favored estrogen	(1) Paragraph recall (immediate + delayed) / No between-group differences (2) Visual paired associates (immediate recall) /) No between-group differences (3) Spatial location recall / No between-group differences	No between-group differences on 2 psychometric measures of dementia severity, on a global staging score, or 2 measures of functional skills; Between-group differences favored estrogen for 2 of 9 other cognitive measures, including a visual reproduction task that combined recall and copy conditions

Three clinical trials were interpreted by their authors as supporting a clinically-important effect of estrogen in Alzheimer's disease [49,50,54] and three others were not [51-53] (Table 2). Positive trials were of shorter duration (3 to 8 weeks versus 12 weeks to 12 months), involved fewer subjects (12 to 20 women versus 42 to 120 women), and have relied on outcome measures that are less often used in Alzheimer clinical trials. Two of the positive trials, conducted by the same investigators, used transdermal estradiol [50,54], whereas one positive trial [49] and the three negative trials [51-53] used oral conjugated estrogens. In addition to these peer-review reports, findings from two other randomized trials have been partially described in the literature: a negative trial of 8 women using low-dose transdermal estradiol [57] and a positive trial of 20 women using oral conjugated estrogens [58]. Long-term memory does not appear particularly affected by estrogen (Table 2), but long-term memory is severely reduced early in the disease course, and floor-effects might mask any estrogen benefit.

ESTROGEN AND ALZHEIMER'S DISEASE: CONCLUDING COMMENTS

Clinical trial data address only the issue of Alzheimer treatment; there are not yet clinical trial data for primary prevention. The number of treatment trials is small, sample sizes are small to moderate, and not all studies used intention-to-treat analyses. Treatment durations have ranged from only 3 weeks to as long as 12 months. Based on clinical trial results summarized in Table 2, it might be inferred that efficacy might differ among different estrogen formulations or routes of administration. However, the weight of the evidence, and this evidence is not yet conclusive, indicates that estrogen does not have a clinically important effect on dementia symptoms. The possibility that estrogen may enhance cognitive effects of cholinergic therapy in Alzheimer's disease [59] remains to evaluated in randomized clinical trials. Observational reports that implied estrogen might have a large effect on Alzheimer symptoms [55] well may have reflected unrecognized biases, which are avoided in randomized trials. However, for some women in these observational studies, long-term estrogen use antedated clinical manifestations of Alzheimer's disease, and the possibility that the disease course in these women was indeed milder is cannot be directly answered by clinical trials initiated only after the onset of dementia symptoms.

References

1. Storandt M. Longitudinal studies of aging and age-associated dementias. In: Boller F, Grafman J, editors. Handbook of Neuropsychology, vol. 4. New York: Elsevier, 1991.
2. Squire LT, Zola-Morgan S. The medial temporal lobe memory system. Science 1991;253: 1380-86.
3. Ritchie K, Kildea D. Is senile dementia "age-related" or "ageing-related"? Evidence from meta-analysis of dementia prevalence in the oldest old. Lancet 1997;346:931-34.
4. van Duijn CM. Epidemiology of the dementias: Recent developments and new approaches. J Neurol Neurosurg Psychiatry 1996;60:478-88.
5. Jorm AF, Korten AE, Henderson AS. The prevalence of dementia: A quantitative integration of the literature. Acta Psychiatr Scand 1987;76:465-79.

6. Bretsky PM, Buckwalter JG, Seeman TE, et al. Evidence for an interaction between apolipoprotein E genotype, gender, and Alzheimer disease. Alzheimer Dis Assoc Disord 1999;13:216-21.
7. Farrer LA, Cupples LA, Haines JL, et al. Effects of age, sex, and ethnicity on the association between apolipoprotein E genotype and Alzheimer disease. JAMA 1997;278: 1349-56.
8. Henderson VW. Hormone therapy and the brain: A clinical perspective on the role of estrogen. New York: Parthenon Publishing, 2000.
9. Shughrue PJ, Lane MV, Merchenthaler I. Comparative distribution of estrogen receptor-α and -β mRNA in the rat central nervous system. J Comp Neurol 1997;388:507-25.
10. Wong M, Thompson TL, Moss RL. Nongenomic actions of estrogen in the brain: physiological significance and cellular mechanisms. Crit Rev Neurobiol 1996;10:189-203.
11. Singh M, Meyer EM, Millard WJ, Simpkins JW. Ovarian steroid deprivation results in a reversible learning impairment and compromised cholinergic function in female Sprague Dawley rats. Brain Res 1994;644:305-12.
12. Fader AJ, Hendricson AW, Dohanich GP. Estrogen improves performance of reinforced T-maze alternation and prevents the amnestic effects of scopolamine administered systemically or intrahippocampally. Neurobiol Learn Memory 1998;69:225-40.
13. Tanapat P, Hastings NB, Reeves AJ, Gould E. Estrogen stimulates a transient increase in the number of new neurons in the dentate gyrus of the adult female rat. J Neurosci 1999; 19:5792-5801.
14. Foy MR, Henderson VW, Berger TW, Thompson RF. Estrogen and neural plasticity. Curr Dir Psychol Sci 2000;9:148-52.
15. Luine V. Estradiol increases choline acetyltransferase activity in specific basal forebrain nuclei and projection areas of female rats. Exp Neurol 1985;89:484-90.
16. Petanceska SS, Nagy G, Frail D, Gandy S. Ovariectomy and 17β-estradiol modulate the levels of Alzheimer's amyloid β peptides in brain. Neurology 2000;54:2212-17.
17. Portin R, Polo-Kantola P, Polo O, et al. Serum estrogen level, attention, memory and other cognitive functions in middle-aged women. Climacteric 1999;2:115-23.
18. Barrett-Connor E, Goodman-Gruen D. Cognitive function and endogenous sex hormones in older women. J Am Geriatr Soc 1999;47:1289-93.
19. Drake EB, Henderson VW, Stanczyk FZ, et al. Associations between circulating sex steroid hormones and cognition in normal elderly women. Neurology 2000;54:599-603.
20. Kampen DL, Sherwin BB. Estrogen use and verbal memory in healthy postmenopausal women. Obstet Gynecol 1994;83:979-83.
21. Jacobs DM, Tang MX, Stern Y, et al. Cognitive function in nondemented older women who took estrogen after menopause. Neurology 1998;50:368-73.
22. Maki PM, Zonderman AB, Resnick SM. Enhanced verbal memory in nondemented elderly women receiving hormone-replacement therapy. Am J Psychiatry 2001;158:227-33.
23. Barrett-Connor E, Kritz-Silverstein D. Estrogen replacement therapy and cognitive function in older women. JAMA 1993;269:2637-41.
24. Schmidt R, Fazekas F, Reinhart B, et al. Estrogen replacement therapy in older women: a neuropsychological and brain MRI study. J Am Geriatr Soc 1996;44:1307-13.
25. Szklo M, Cerhan J, Diez-Roux AV, et al. Estrogen replacement therapy and cognitive functioning in the Atherosclerosis Risk in Communities (ARIC) study. Am J Epidemiol 1996;144:1048-57.

26. Hogervorst E, Boshuisen M, Riedel W, et al. The effect of hormone replacement therapy on cognitive function in elderly women. Psychoneuroendocrinology 1999;24:43-68.
27. Haskell SG, Richardson ED, Horwitz RI. The effect of estrogen replacement therapy on cognitive function in women: A critical review of the literature. J Clin Epidemiol 1997;50: 1249-64.
28. Yaffe K, Sawaya G, Lieberburg I, Grady D. Estrogen therapy in postmenopausal women. JAMA 1998;279:688-95.
29. Hogervorst E, Williams J, Budge M, et al. The nature of the effect of female gonadal hormone replacement therapy on cognitive function in post-menopausal women: A meta-analysis. Neuroscience 2000;101:485-512.
30. Vanhulle G, Demol R. A double-blind study into the influence of estriol on a number of psychological tests in post-menopausal women. Consensus on menopause research: A summary of international opinion. Baltimore: University Park Press, 1976:94-99.
31. Sherwin BB. Estrogen and/or androgen replacement therapy and cognitive functioning in surgically menopausal women. Psychoneuroendocrinology 1988;13:345-57.
32. Phillips SM, Sherwin BB. Effects of estrogen on memory function in surgically menopausal women. Psychoneuroendocrinology 1992;17:485-95.
33. Sherwin BB, Tulandi T. "Add back" estrogen reverses cognitive deficits induced by a gonadotropin releasing hormone agonist in women with leiomyomata uteri. J Clin Endocrinol Metab 1996;81:2545-49.
34. Polo-Kantola P, Portin R, Polo O, et al. The effect of short-term estrogen replacement therapy on cognition: a randomized, double-blind, cross-over trial in postmenopausal women. Obstet Gynecol 1998;91:459-66.
35. Wolf OT, Kudielka MB, Hellhammer DH, et al. Two weeks of transdermal estradiol treatment in postmenopausal elderly women and its effect on memory and mood: Verbal memory changes are associated with the treatment induced estradiol levels. Psychoneuroendocrinology 1999;24:727-41.
36. Duka T, Tasker R, McGowan JF. The effects of 3-week estrogen hormone replacement on cognition in elderly healthy females. Psychopharmacology 2000;149:129-39.
37. Binder EF, Schechtman KB, Birge SJ, et al. Effects of hormone replacement therapy on cognitive performance in elderly women. Maturitas 2001;38:137-46.
38. Cherry BJ, Buckwalter JG, Henderson VW. Better preservation of memory span relative to supraspan immediate recall in Alzheimer's disease. Neuropsychologia; in press.
39. Henderson VW, Paganini-Hill A, Emanuel CK, et al. Estrogen replacement therapy in older women: Comparisons between Alzheimer's disease cases and nondemented control subjects. Arch Neurol 1994;51:896-900.
40. Paganini-Hill A, Henderson VW. Estrogen replacement therapy and risk of Alzheimer's disease. Arch Intern Med 1996;156:2213-17.
41. Tang M-X, Jacobs D, Stern Y, et al. Effect of oestrogen during menopause on risk and age at onset of Alzheimer's disease. Lancet 1996;348:429-32.
42. Kawas C, Resnick S, Morrison A, et al. A prospective study of estrogen replacement therapy and the risk of developing Alzheimer's disease: The Baltimore Longitudinal Study of Aging. Neurology 1997;48:1517-21.
43. Baldereschi M, Di Carlo A, Lepore V, et al. Estrogen replacement therapy and Alzheimer's disease in the Italian Longitudinal Study on Aging. Neurology 1998;50:996-1002.
44. Slooter AJ, Bronzova J, Witteman JC, et al. Estrogen use and early onset Alzheimer's disease: A population-based study. J Neurol Neurosurg Psychiatry 1999;67:779-81.

45. Brenner DE, Kukull WA, Stergachis A, et al. Postmenopausal estrogen replacement therapy and the risk of Alzheimer s disease: A population-based case-control study. Am J Epidemiol 1994;140:262-67.
46. Seshadri S, Zomberg GL, Derby LE, et al. Postmenopausal estrogen replacement therapy and the risk of Alzheimer's disease. Arch Neurol 2001;58:435-40.
47. Vickers MR. The MRC long-term randomised control trial of hormone replacement therapy: background, design and objectives. J Br Menopause Soc 1996;2(3):9-13.
48. Shumaker SA, Reboussin BA, Espeland MA, et al. The Women's Health Initiative Memory Study (WHIMS): A trial of the effect of estrogen therapy in preventing and slowing the progression of dementia. Controlled Clin Trials 1998;19:604-21.
49. Honjo H, Ogino Y, Tanaka K, et al. An effect of conjugated estrogen to cognitive impairment in women with senile dementia Alzheimer's type: A placebo controlled double blind study. J Jpn Menopause Soc 1993;1:167-71.
50. Asthana S, Craft S, Baker LD, et al. Cognitive and neuroendocrine response to transdermal estrogen in postmenopausal women with Alzheimer's disease: Results of a placebo-controlled, double-blind, pilot study. Psychoneuroendocrinology 1999;24:657-77.
51. Henderson VW, Paganini-Hill A, Miller BL, et al. Estrogen for Alzheimer's disease in women: randomized, double-blind, placebo-controlled trial. Neurology 2000;54:295-301.
52. Mulnard RA, Cotman CW, Kawas C, et al. Estrogen replacement therapy for treatment of mild to moderate Alzheimer disease: A randomized controlled trial. JAMA 2000;283:1007-15.
53. Wang PN, Liao SQ, Liu RS, et al. Effects of estrogen on cognition, mood, and cerebral blood flow in AD: A controlled study. Neurology 2000;54:2061-66.
54. Asthana S, Baker LD, Craft S, et al. High-dose estradiol improves cognition for women with AD: Results of a randomized study. Neurology 2001;57:605-12.
55. Henderson VW, Watt L, Buckwalter JG. Cognitive skills associated with estrogen replacement in women with Alzheimer's disease. Psychoneuroendocrinology 1996;21:421-30.
56. Henderson VW. Estrogen replacement therapy for the prevention and treatment of Alzheimer's disease. CNS Drugs 1997;8:343-51.
57. Fillit H. Estrogens in the pathogenesis and treatment of Alzheimer's disease in postmenopausal women. Ann NY Acad Sci 1994;743:233-38.
58. Birge SJ. The role of estrogen in the treatment of Alzheimer's disease. Neurology 1997;48 (Suppl.7):S36-S41.
59. Schneider LS, Farlow MR, Henderson VW, Pogoda JM. Effects of estrogen replacement therapy on response to tacrine in patients with Alzheimer's disease. Neurology 1996;46: 1580-84.

ESTROGEN AND ANDROGEN: MOOD, SEXUAL FUNCTION, AND QUALITY OF LIFE IN THE MENOPAUSAL WOMAN

Jeanne Leventhal Alexander, Krista Kotz, and Susan Davis

Introduction

Biological changes at menopause play a significant role in quality of life. Changes in hormone levels and other physiologic changes need to be addressed. However, biological problems rarely exist in the absence of psychological, sociocultural and interpersonal issues. Generally, a dynamic interaction exists between physiologic and nonphysiologic changes during this stage of life.

Gonadal Hormones – Sources, Actions and Changes at Menopause

SOURCES OF GONADAL HORMONES

Estradiol, progesterone, and testosterone are often considered the "classic" gonadal steroids. These hormones are derived from cholesterol and are structurally very similar. The main sources for circulating steroids are gonads and adrenal glands, but they can be synthesized in other tissues [1].

ACTIONS OF GONADAL HORMONES ON THE BRAIN

Gonadal steroids have two types of action on the brain: 1) activational effects, which are acute, temporary actions of hormones, and 2) organizational effects, which refers to the ability of the gonadal steroids, when acting on the brain during brief developmental windows, to permanently alter the structure or functional potential of the brain [2,3].

Gonadal steroids influence cell activity by genomic or nongenomic activity. Nongenomic activity is mediated by direct action of the hormone at the cell membrane. Genomic activity refers to influences through protein synthesis. Steroid hormones bind to the hormone-binding domain of the receptor. This complex binds to DNA, which activates the genome, producing an mRNA transcript, which encodes a variety of enzymatic, structural, and receptor proteins [2]. The vast array of proteins regulated through the gonadal hormone genomic activity permit these hormones to influence virtually all aspects of neurotransmitter formation and activity [4].

Two classes of intracellular estrogen receptors have been identified: alpha and beta (ERα and ERβ); different estrogens have different binding affinities for ERα and ERβ. Since the distribution of these receptors differs in different tissues, estrogen has selective actions in various target tissues. The brain also has receptors for androgens. In addition to different receptors, there are numerous ways in which cell-specific estrogen effects are realized [3].

The relationship between gonadal steroids and mood and behavior is very complex, and depends on many variables, including: stage of development, age, exposure to other steroids, stress, individual differences in metabolism, past experience, environment, and social context [1,2].

CHANGES IN GONADAL HORMONES AT MENOPAUSE

Hormonal changes are marked during menopause. Circulating levels of testosterone tend to decline prior to the menopause with little change across the menopause transition [5,6].

In women not taking exogenous estrogen, sex hormone binding globulin (SHBG) tends to decline. About one third of this decline may be explained by serum estradiol and body mass index (BMI). This may result in a small rise in free testosterone [6]. The months preceding the last menstrual period can be a time of of fluctuating estradiol levels such that many women experience symptoms of estrogen excess, namely mastalgia and menorrhagia mixed in with vasomotor symptoms of estrogen deficiency. Overall serum levels of estradiol begin to decline and FSH begins to increase about two years before the last menstrual period. Estradiol and estrone both decrease in parallel fashion during the postmenopausal period. Some women experience relative estradiol deficiency at mid-cycle and during the late luteal phase due to a low estrogen to progesterone ratio. Serum levels of progesterone are low in the postmenopausal years. ($\leq$ 2 nmol/l) [7].

Menopause and Mood

ACTIONS OF GONADAL HORMONES ON MOOD SYSTEMS IN THE BRAIN

Gonadal steroids affect serotonin activity in the brain. Estradiol is capable of modulating serotonergic activity through a variety of mechanisms [4]. Estrogen has been shown to effect tryptophan metabolism in women [8, 9]. In rat brains, estrogen decreases serotonin receptors acutely, followed by (48-72 hours later) a selective increase in serotonin receptors in those brain regions known to contain estrogen receptors (hypothalamus, preoptic area, and amygdala) [10]. Some studies suggest that estrogen increases monoamine oxidase activity [11]. Others suggest that estrogen decreases monoamine oxidase activity [3] . Estrogen has been shown to have activity in all brain areas.

Rodent studies show effects of testosterone on the following systems: serotonin, dopamine, acetylcholine, norepinephrine, γ-amino butyric acid (GABA), vasopressin, oxytocin, neurokinin, and cholecystokinin. These effects have been shown to take place in several areas of the brain, including the cortex, amygdala, hippocampus, and hypothalamus

[2]. Testosterone decreases metabolism of epinephrine by monoamine oxidase [12].

Progesterone has been shown to decrease extracellular serotonin in ovariectomized rats *in vivo* [13].

Effects of Gonadal Hormones on Mood

Evidence suggests that estrogen enhances mood and may have an impact on verbal memory. During the climacteric, estrogen replacement is reported to diminish anxiety, and improve mood and mental well-being [3,14,15].

Progesterone has also been shown to affect mood. Progesterone is primarily metabolized to allopregnanolone or pregnenolone within the brain. Allpregnanolone and allotetrahydro DOC bind $GABA_A$ receptors sterioselectively and with high affinity resulting in benzodiazepine and barbiturate-like effects. Pregnenolone, pregnenolone sulphate, and DHEAS antagonize $GABA_A$ receptors and are proconvulsant in laboratory animals [16]. Increased levels of progesterone have been shown to modulate the serotonergic system and have been associated with dysphoric moods, irritability, perhaps due to pregnenolone excess and dizziness, drowsiness, and deep sleep possibly due to preferential metabolism to allopregnanolone [17,18].

Testosterone may also influence mood. However the mood effects that are directly due to androgen action, and those that are a consequence of aromatization of testosterone to estradiol need to be elucidated. Clinically, a negative correlation between circulating testosterone levels and severity of depression has been observed in several studies [2]. Well-being and depressed mood scores were shown to improve with the addition of testosteone to oral estrogen progestin therapy in surgically postmenopausal women [19].

β-endorphin has well-known behavioral and neuroendocrine properties [20]. This hormone produces euphoria and tranquility, through mechanisms that have been incompletely elucidated but probably involve complex interactions with other central nervous system neurotransmitters [21]. Levels of β-endorphin change throughout an individual's life span, increasing progressively from childhood through a woman's reproductive years, after which they decline through to old age [22]. Experiments suggest that this reduction may be due to the decline in sex steroids with age. Treatment of gonadectomized rats with either estradiol benzoate or testosterone propionate restores β-endorphin levels to those in intact animals [23]. The effects of conjugated equine estrogens (CEE) on β-endorphin and β-lipotrophin (LPH) have been compared with placebo in symptomatic postmenopausal women. After 4 months, CEE increased plasma levels of β-endorphin and β-LPH versus placebo, and enhanced mood [24].

Sexual Functioning at Menopause

In addition to changes in mood, many women experience changes in sexual function at menopause. Several variables affect sexual functioning during this time of life, including: the process of aging, hormonal changes, hormone therapy, partner availability, relationship issues, the presence or absence of psychiatric disorders, psychological barriers, cultural issues, general medical well-being, and previous sexual functioning [25].

The incidence of sexual problems in the population is high, and increases with aging [26,27]. Sexual complaints are relatively common among menopausal women. In a study of 178 women attending a menopause clinic in London, 86% reported some sort of sexual problem [28]. A clinic population is different than the general population in that they tend to have more menopausal complaints, which is what brings them to the clinic in the first place. However, this study shows that of a group of women who have menopausal complaints, sexual problems affect the vast majority. Of the 178 women in this study, over 30% reported vaginal dryness, and just as common was touch impairment. Twenty-three percent were nonorgasmic secondary to other problems, 18.5% experienced vaginismus, and 17.4% had a loss of clitoral sensation.

Sexual functioning involves the peripheral nervous system, the central nervous system, and the cardiovascular system. Changes in gonadal hormones affect sexual functioning in several ways. They have an impact on sensory function, sexual drive or libido, central and peripheral nerve transmission, and discharge, peripheral blood flow, and the capacity to develop muscle tension [29].

Reduced Estrogen and Sexual Function

Classic estrogen deficiency symptoms, namely hot flashes and night sweats compromise well-being and libido. In addition, decreasing estrogen in menopause impacts the integrity of the tissues of the female reproductive tract. Dyspareunia occurs as a result of decreased vaginal lubrication and atrophic vaginitis. Decreased blood flow to the reproductive organs results in diminished vasocongestion [30]. With the loss of ovarian hormones, many other changes occur in the genital structures, including: progressive ischemia, thinning of the barrier layers of skin and mucous membrane tissues, loss of subcutaneous fat, flattening of the labia majora, and shrinkage of the introitus, labia minora, clitoris, uterus, and vagina [31]. Extragenital changes also occur, including a loss of pelvic muscle tone, decrease in intraurethral pressure, thinning of the mucous membrane lining the urethra and bladder, and decrease in the size of the bladder. These changes can directly cause problems in sexual function, and they can indirectly lead to a fear of sexual relations.

More generally, decreased estrogen levels can reduce the capacity to develop muscle tension [29]. Vasocongestion also decreases with age and reductions in estrogen [30].

Sexual response is generated by sensory stimulation. Nerve function is also altered in hypoestrogenic states. Postmenopausal women have been reported to have signs and symptoms of peripheral neuropathy, including numbness, itching, clothing intolerance, and increased two-point discrimination thresholds There is no strong evidence that these symptoms are specific to the menopause transition. Touch receptor zones along the pudendal nerve distribution path of the rat have been shown to become smaller after oophorectomy and expand with the administration of estradiol [32]. Estrogen enhances vibration sense, taste and smell [33-35]. The change in peripheral nervous function can lead to touch avoidance.

In summary, postmenopausal estrogen therapy is likely to alleviate dyspareunia, restore sexual interest and capacity for sexual pleasure in a significant proportion of women, obviating the need for further pharmacological intervention.

Reduced Androgens and Sexual Function

Declines in androgen levels can result in declines in sexual desire [36,37]. The adrenal glands produce dehydroepiandrosterone (DHEA), androstenedione, and to a limited extent, testosterone, and are the only source of DHEA sulfate (DHEAS). DHEA and DHEAS production by the adrenals declines with age, unrelated to menopause. Adrenal androgens are the primary precursors for estrone and estradiol biosynthesis in postmenopausal women [38-40]. The extent to which the postmenopausal ovary is a major source of androgen production is highly controversial [41]. Testosterone also appears to influence pelvic blood flow and vaginal arousal response [42].

Changes in Sex Hormone Binding Globulin and Sexual Function

Under normal physiological conditions only 1- 2% of total circulating testosterone is free or biologically available. The rest is bound by sex hormone binding globulin (SHBG) and albumin, with SHBG binding 66% of total circulating testosterone [7]. The binding affinity for steroids bound by SHBG is DHT > testosterone > androstenediol > estradiol > estrone [43]. SHBG also weekly binds DHEA, but not DHEA-S [43]. Therefore variations in the plasma levels of SHBG impact significantly on the amount of free, or bioavailable testosterone [43]. Different formulation and modes of administration of exogenous estrogens affect sex hormone binding globulin (SHBG) differently. Oral estrogens appear to have the greatest impact, but the impact is not clinically significant in all women. SHBG varies according to medical conditions, weight, as well as other factors [44]. SHBG is lower with obesity, androgen excess (for example polycystic ovarian syndrome) and hypothyroidism. On the other hand, SHBG is higher in fasting, anorexia nervosa, thyrotoxicosis, and cirrhosis.

Slater and others have demonstrated that oral micronized estradiol as well as CEE significantly increase SHBG whereas transdermal estradiol in doses as high as 100 mcg/day has minimal effect [45]. Some progestins affect SHBG as well. While derivatives of norprogesterone do not influence SHBG, derivatives of nortestosterone, such as norethisterone and norgestrel, decrease SHBG levels [46].

Relationship Issues and Sexual Function

Aside from biological changes, relationship issues affect sexual functioning. The availability of a partner becomes a challenge as women get older. In a study of 745 older women, only 53% of women age 60-74 years had a sexual partner [47]. For those with a partner, marital problems is one of the most common causes of a decline in sexual activity. It is important, however, to distinguish between acute and chronic marital problems. Acute changes in sexual activity can cause marital difficulties, but these difficulties will resolve with a return to normal sexual activity. A chronic lack of sexual activity is rarely a function of physiologic changes due to age or menopause.

The changes in sexual functioning with age and menopause are often insidious. A woman often does not realize she has lost the appetite for sexual activity; slowly, subtle changes develop in the sexual relationship. Marriage is often affected, if not destabilized. Also, a loss of self-esteem can change the marital dynamic and lead to a decrease in physical touching by the couple.

Attitudes about sexual activity vary between women with and without partners. A study of older women found that over half of women with partners (and about 40% without partners) say that sexuality is a critical part of a good relationship [47]. Interestingly, while only 10% of women without partners say that sexual activity is important to quality of life, half of women with partners say that it is. Over 20% of women without partners say that they do not particularly enjoy sex, while a little over 10% of women with partners say so.

PSYCHOLOGICAL ISSUES AND SEXUAL FUNCTION

Psychological issues also have an impact on sexual function. Depression and anxiety disorders are under-treated illnesses in general and are more prevalent in women. Many women will present in the menopausal and postmenopausal years with an untreated dysthymia, a new episode of depression, or untreated anxiety disorder. These disorders can have an impact on sexual functioning alone or in concert with the effects of declining gonadal hormones [48].

With decreased gonadal hormones in the later years, atrophic changes occur in the breasts and genital structures. These changes, along with the loss of menses can alter a woman's body image and result in a decreased sexual response. A slowed and often incomplete response to sexual stimulation of the postmenopausal woman can lead to anxious watching of oneself and one's partner during sexual activity. This is called "spectatoring."

Other psychological issues arise which can affect sexual functioning at menopause. Some women were raised to believe that sexual relationships end to a certain age or with menopause. Women who did not find sex pleasurable earlier in life may look forward to ceasing sexual activity after the menopause. Women with problems in their marital relationship may have built up resentment towards their spouse, and menopause may give them permission to decline sex [49].

Previous sexual functioning has been shown to be a predictor for menopausal sexual functioning. Koster and Garde examined sexual wellness of Danish women ages 40, 45, and 51. They used interviews and questionnaires to show that current frequency of sexual desire was highly correlated with former sexual activity. In addition, they found that anticipated decline in sexual desire predicted a decline in sexual desire [50].

SOCIOLOGIC AND CULTURAL ISSUES AND SEXUALITY

Societal attitudes towards sex in the midlife affects sexual behavior. A woman's postmenopausal value as a sexual person increases or decreases depending on the society in which she lives. In a Nigerian study, most of the women became sexually abstinent at menopause. In contrast, another study shows that older women in almost 25% of primitive societies were less inhibited, became more sexually active, and were more attractive to young men [29].

MEDICAL PROBLEMS AND SEXUAL FUNCTION

Physical health can affect a woman's ability to participate in sexual relations. Co-existing medical illnesses may have an impact. The geriatric patient is more likely to have chronic diseases, and is more likely to be prescribed drugs that interfere with sexual functioning. The postmenopausal patient is more likely to undergo surgical procedures that result in bodily disfiguration. Limitations of cardiovascular and pulmonary function can also affect sexuality [51].

Algorithms for the Health Care Provider

MANAGING MOOD PROBLEMS

Stepwise treatments of estrogen, androgen, and antidepressants, if needed, along with behavioral interventions will help achieve the highest level of wellness with the least invasive intervention. Androgen, as well as estrogen, can lead to increased quality of life in many women; however, all women do not necessarily need systemic use of these gonadal hormones. Individualized care is vital as each woman has different needs and will require different treatments.

The availability of a team approach using psychiatry, internal medicine, and OB/Gyn will help in those cases whose etiology is more complex.

ANDROGEN THERAPY AND SEXUAL FUNCTION

Androgen therapy in menopausal women may provide several benefits. It may improve sexuality through increased sexual desire, arousal, and sexual fantasies [52, 53]. Depression may be lessened, and mood enhanced. It has been suggested that cognition may be improved with androgen therapy in menopausal women; however, there is no data to support this.

MANAGING CHANGES IN SHBG

Some solutions are available to these changes in SHBG levels due to hormone replacement therapy. All women should have SHBG levels measured if they have had a libido and mood problem which existed prior to oral estrogen treatment. If SHBG is significantly elevated then the first intervention should be to change therapy to nonoral estrogen. The patient should be reviewed after several weeks as it will take at least 8 or more weeks for the

SHBG to fall. If despite this change free testosterone remains low and symptoms persist, the use of micronized estradiol with methyl testosterone should be considered.

MANAGING SEXUAL FUNCTION

Always consider and treat biologic causes for the change in sexual function using estrogen and testosterone where indicated. Assume hypoestrogenemia first and treat with estrogen +/- progestin therapy. If libido is not improved, consider the addition of testosterone, beginning at low doses, with early and frequent follow up for side effects.

Consider and address nonbiologic causes. If psychiatric illness is found, refer the patient to psychotherapy or psychiatry where appropriate. Discuss with the couple the interplay of how physiologic changes affect relationship issues. Guide the patient towards addressing interpersonal issues concurrent with using hormone replacement therapy for physiologic issues. Biologic treatment in the absence of behavioral change is often not effective. Address the impact of physiologic problems on the sexual relationship, help the couple demystify their sexuality and be more flexible with their sexual scripts. Help the couple to have broader definitions of sexual goals, such as, increased affiliative behavior, increased well-being, and increased sexuality.

Conclusions

SEXUAL FUNCTION

Sexual problems in the postmenopause are widespread. Sexual behavior is complex and is often affected by a number of factors. Estrogen has its major impact on the anatomic and physiologic aspects of sexual behavior as well as mood and well-being.

Testosterone has its major impact on the motivational or libidinal aspects of sexual behavior, such as desire and fantasies, as well as on peripheral responses. SHBG, which is affected by many medications and changes in hormone levels, may affect treatment when it significantly increases. Depression, anxiety disorders, and marital discord are relatively common during this time of life and may affect sexual function as well.

MOOD

Gonadal steroids effect several mood-related systems in the brain. Circulating levels of these hormones change with age and the menopausal transition. During perimenopause and the postmenopausal period, women may benefit from receiving estrogen and/or androgen replacement therapy. If this does not result in an adequate response, antidepressant therapy can also be used where appropriate. Along with these treatments, behavioral interventions can be highly beneficial. In complicated cases, a team approach is ideal, which would include psychiatry, internal medicine, and Ob/Gyn.

References

1. Schmidt PJ, Rubinow DR, Neuroregulatory role of gonadal steroids in humans. Psychopharmacol Bull 1997;33(2):219-20.
2. Rubinow DR, Schmidt PJ. Androgens, brain, and behavior. Am J Psychiatry 1996;153(8): 974-84.
3. Henderson VW. Hormone therapy and the brain. New York: The Parthenon Publishing Group, 2000: 12-14,20-21,27-30..
4. Rubinow DR, Schmidt PJ, Roca CA. Estrogen-serotonin interactions: Implications for affective regulation. Biol Psychiatry 1998;44(9):839-50.
5. Zumoff B, et al. Twenty-four-hour mean plasma testosterone concentration declines with age in normal premenopausal women. J Clin Endocrinol Metab 1995;80(4):1429-30.
6. Burger HG, et al. A prospective longitudinal study of serum testosterone, dehydroepiandrosterone sulfate, and sex hormone-binding globulin levels through the menopause transition. J Clin Endocrinol Metab 2000;85(8):2832-38.
7. Rannevik G, et al. A longitudinal study of the perimenopausal transition: Altered profiles of steroid and pituitary hormones, SHBG and bone mineral density. Maturitas 1995;21(2): 103-13.
8. Price J, Thornton M, Mueller L. Tryptophan metabolism in women using steroid hormones for ovulation control. Am J Clin Nutr 1967;20(5):452-56.
9. Adams PW, et al. Effect of pyridoxine hydrochloride (vitamin B 6) upon depression associated with oral contraception. Lancet 1973;1(7809):899-904.
10. Biegon A, McEwen BS. Modulation by estradiol of serotonin receptors in brain. J Neurosci 1982;2(2):199-205.
11. Chakravorty SG, Halbreich U. The influence of estrogen on monoamine oxidase activity. Psychopharmacol Bull 1997;33(2):229-33.
12. Bukhari AR, Guessab A, Nicol ML. Hormone mediated changes in monoamine stores and regulation of enzymes of biosynthesis and metabolism in the rat adrenal gland. Influence of progesterone, estradiol, ACTH and testosterone administration. Steroids 1981;38(1):1-10.
13. Farmer CJ, et al. In vivo evidence for progesterone dependent decreases in serotonin release in the hypothalamus and midbrain central grey: relation to the induction of lordosis. Brain Res 1996;711(1-2):84-92.
14. Ditkoff EC, et al. Estrogen improves psychological function in asymptomatic postmenopausal women. Obstet Gynecol 1991;78(6):991-95.
15. Sherwin BB. Hormones, mood, and cognitive functioning in postmenopausal women. Obstet Gynecol 1996;87(2 Suppl.):20S-26S.
16. Smith SS, et al. GABA(A) receptor alpha4 subunit suppression prevents withdrawal properties of an endogenous steroid. Nature 1998;392(6679):926-30.
17. Dennerstein L, et al. Hormone therapy and affect. Maturitas 1979;1(4):247-59.
18. Holzbauer M. Physiological aspects of steroids with anaesthetic properties. Med Biol 1976;54(4):227-42.
19. Shifren JL, et al. Transdermal testosterone treatment in women with impaired sexual function after oophorectomy [see comments]. N Engl J Med 2000;343(10):682-88.
20. Adler MW, Opioid peptides. Life Sci 1980;26(7):497-510.
21. Mani SK, Mitchell A, O'Malley BW. Progesterone receptor and dopamine receptors are required in Delta 9- tetrahydrocannabinol modulation of sexual receptivity in female rats.

Proc Natl Acad Sci USA 2001;98(3):1249-54.
22. Facchinetti F, et al. Different patterns of central and peripheral beta EP, beta LPH and ACTH throughout life. Peptides 1983;4(4):469-74.
23. Petraglia F, et al. Effect of gonadectomy and gonadal steroid replacement on pituitary and plasma beta-endorphin levels in the rat. Endocrinology 1982;111(4):1224-29.
24. Genazzani AR, et al. Steroid replacement treatment increases beta-endorphin and beta-lipotropin plasma levels in postmenopausal women. Gynecol Obstet Invest 1988;26(2): 153-59.
25. Pariser SF, JA Niedermier. Sex and the mature woman. J Womens Health 1998;7(7):849-59.
26. Bachmann GA, Leiblum SR, Grill J. Brief sexual inquiry in gynecologic practice. Obstet Gynecol 1989;73(3 Pt 1):425-27.
27. Frank E, Anderson C, Rubinstein D. Frequency of sexual dysfunction in "normal" couples. N Engl J Med 1978;299(3):111-15.
28. Sarrel PM, Whitehead MI. Sex and menopause: Defining the issues. Maturitas 1985;7(3): 217-24.
29. Sarrel PM. Sexuality in the middle years. Obstet Gynecol Clin North Am 1987;14(1):49-62.
30. Sarrel PM. Sexuality and menopause. Obstet Gynecol 1990;75(4Suppl):26S-30S; discussion 31S-35S.
31. Lang WR, Aponte GE. Gross and microscopic anatomy of the aged female reproductive organs. Clin Obstet Gynecol 1967;10(3):454-65.
32. Kow L, Pfaff D. Effects of oestrogen treatment on the size of receptive field and response threshold of pudendal nerve in the female rat. Neuroendocrinology 1973;13:299-313.
33. Gescheider GA, et al. Effects of the menstrual cycle on vibrotactile sensitivity. Percept Psychophys 1984;36(6):586-92.
34. Parlee MB. Menstrual rhythms in sensory processes: A review of fluctuations in vision, olfaction, audition, taste, and touch. Psychol Bull 1983;93(3):539-48.
35. Sarrel P, Marks L, Schwartz-Giblin S. Sex hormones and senses. In: Zichella L, Whitehead M, van Keep P, editors. The climacteric and beyond. Park Ridge, New Jersey: Parthenon Publishing, 1988:137-44.
36. Sherwin BB, Gelfand MM. The role of androgen in the maintenance of sexual functioning in oophorectomized women. Psychosom Med 1987;49(4):397-409.
37. Sarrel D, Dobay B, Wiita B. Estrogen and estrogen-androgen replacement in postmenopausal women dissatisfied with estrogen-only therapy. Sexual behavior and neuroendocrine responses. J Reprod Med 1998;43(10):847-56.
38. Longcope C, Hunter R, Franz C. Steroid secretion by the postmenopausal ovary. Am J Obstet Gynecol 1980;138(5):564-68.
39. Botella-Llusia J, Orio-Bosch A, Sanchez-Garrido F, Tresguerres JA. Testosterone and 17 beta oestradiol secretion of the human ovary. II Normal postmenopausal women, postmenopausal women with endometrial hyperplasia and postmenopausal women with adenocarcinoma of the endometrium. Maturitas 1980;2(1):7-12.
40. Lucisano A, et al. Ovarian and peripheral plasma levels of progestogens, androgens and oestrogens in post-menopausal women. Maturitas 1984;6(1):45-53.
41. Couzinet B, et al. The postmenopausal ovary is not a major androgen-producing gland. J Clin Endocrinol Metab 2001;86(10):5060-66.
42. Tuiten A, et al. Time course of effects of testosterone administration on sexual arousal in

women. Arch Gen Psychiatry 2000;57(2):149-53;discussion 155-56.
43. Dunn JF, Nisula BC, Rodbard D. Transport of steroid hormones: Binding of 21 endogenous steroids to both testosterone-binding globulin and corticosteroid-binding globulin in human plasma. J Clin Endocrinol Metab 1981;53(1):58-68.
44. Pugeat M, et al. Clinical utility of sex hormone-binding globulin measurement. Horm Res 1996;45(3-5):148-55.
45. Slater C.C, et al. Markedly elevated levels of estrone sulfate after long-term oral, but not transdermal, administration of estradiol in postmenopausal women. Menopause 2001;8(3): 200-3.
46. Simon J, et al. Differential effects of estrogen-androgen and estrogen-only therapy on vasomotor symptoms, gonadotropin secretion, and endogenous androgen bioavailability in postmenopausal women. Menopause 1999;6(2):138-46.
47. NFO Research, Inc. AARP/Modern maturity sexuality study. Sept/Oct 1999.
48. Jensvold M. Psychopharmacology and women: Sex, gender, and hormones. Washington, D.C.: American Psychiatry Press, Inc, 1996: 85,233,241,261.
49. Barbach L. Sexuality through the menopause and beyond. Menopause Management 1996; 5(5):18-21.
50. Koster A, Garde K. Sexual desire and menopausal development. A prospective study of Danish women born in 1936. Maturitas 1993;16(1):49-60.
51. Mooradian AD. Geriatric sexuality and chronic diseases. Clin Geriatr Med 1991;7(1):113-31.
52. Davis SR, McCloud PI, Strauss BJG, Burger H. Testosterone enhances estradiol's effects on postmenopausal bone density and sexuality. Mauritas 1995;21:227-36.
53. SherwinBB. Affective changes with estrogenand androgen replacement therapy in surgically menopausal women. J Affect Disord 1988;14:177-87.

WOMEN'S HEALTH AND MENOPAUSE: A COMPREHENSIVE APPROACH

Nanette K. Wenger

Introduction

During the past century the percentage of women older than 50 years of age has tripled. In the same time period, the mean life expectancy of women has increased from 50 to 81.7 years. Menopause offers the primary care health provider an opportunity to assess a woman's health, her concerns, and her needs for health promotion and disease prevention measures.

This session summarizes the components of an international position paper that provides evidence-based recommendations to guide clinical practice designed to enhance menopausal health. It is a cooperative venture of the National Heart, Lung, and Blood Institute (NHLBI) and the Office of Research on Women's Health (ORWH) at the U.S. National Institutes of Health (NIH), Bethesda, Maryland, USA and the Giovanni Lorenzini Medical Science Foundation of Milan, Italy.

The Process 1998-2001

Given the escalating population of menopausal women and the improved options for healthy menopausal years, an international panel of experts on menopausal health was selected and assigned the task of preparing evidence-based background chapters, the topics of which are outlined subsequently. The format of the chapters and scope of content were delineated at initial Panel meetings. The individual chapters, prepared by Panel members and invited authors, evaluated published research studies to determine relevant background information and compiled strategies for management. These were reviewed by internationally acknowledged leaders in their fields. The chapter authors subsequently incorporated the comments, queries, and additions based on their assessments. The composite monograph, consisting of the revised chapters, was then submitted to an international panel of experts. As previously, the subsequent comments, queries, and additions were incorporated in the appropriate chapters. Finally, a full Panel meeting reviewed the revised chapters and assessed the comments received from all the experts who had been invited to review initial drafts of either the individual chapters or the document in its entirety. Concomitantly and subsequently, a science writer interacted with each group of chapter authors. The authors of each chapter highlighted the key points that required incorporation into an Executive Summary. Levels of evidence (see subsequently) were delineated for the major recommendations. As well, the chapter authors prioritized future research needs in their specific domains.

Chapter Topics

Chapter topics addressed menopause and aging; symptoms in the menopause; sociocultural issues in menopause; the physiologic role of estrogen and estrogen receptors; the pharmacologic modulation of estrogen receptor activity; sexuality; cardiovascular and pulmonary disease; osteoporosis and oral bone loss in aging women: risks and therapy; gynecologic and urologic aspects of menopause; menopausal hormone therapy; related therapies and cancer epidemiology; menopause and disorders of neurological function, mental health and the eye; and a final chapter presenting a comprehensive approach to best clinical practice.

Executive Committee and Panel

Nanette K. Wenger, M.D., USA served as the Chair of the Panel and Editor of the monograph. The Co-Chairs and Co-Editors were Rodolfo Paoletti, M.D., Italy; Claude J.M. Lenfant, M.D., USA; and Vivian W. Pinn, M.D., USA.

The Panel Members included:

Elizabeth Barrett-Connor, MD, USA
Martin H. Birkhäuser, MD, Switzerland
Louise A. Brinton, PhD, USA
Aila Collins, PhD, Sweden
Peter Collins, MD, UK
Pier Giorgio Crosignani, MD, Italy
Lorraine Dennerstein, MBBS, PhD, DPM, Australia
Bruce Ettinger, MD, USA
Jan-Åke Gustafsson, MD, PhD, Sweden
Victor W. Henderson, MD, MS, USA
Susan Hendrix, DO, USA
Carlo LaVecchia, MD, Italy
Robert Lindsay, MD, PhD, USA
Adriana Maggi, PhD, Italy
Joan A. McGowan, PhD, USA
Anne McTiernan, MD, PhD, USA
Maryann Redford, DDS, MPH, USA
Susan M. Resnick, PhD, USA
Jacques E. Rossouw, MD, USA
Sherry Sherman, PhD, USA

Non-Panel Co-Authors

Additional authors who were invited to contribute to the chapters were:

Janet R. Gutherie, PhD, Australia
Barbara E.K. Klein, MD, PhD, USA
Stefan Nilsson Dr Med Sci, Sweden
Nanette Santoro, MD, USA

Special Acknowledgments

The Panel and the clinical community owe a debt of gratitude to those who gave of their time and expertise for their thoughtful comments and additions to the initial version of the chapters and for their dedication to the enhancement of menopausal health.

The experts who reviewed the individual chapters included:

Beth Alder, PhD, UK
Gloria A. Bachmann, MD, USA
Linda Cardozo, MD, UK
Sir Richard Doll, UK
Timothy M.M. Farley, PhD, Switzerland
Marcha Flint, PhD, USA
Silvia Franceschi, MD, France
Ulysses J. Gaspard, MD, PhD, Belgium
Anna Glasier, MD, PhD, UK
Elina Hemminki, MD, PhD, Finland
Myra S. Hunter, PhD, UK
Won-Whe Kim, MD, Korea
Britt-Marie Landgren, MD, PhD, Sweden
Lenore Manderson, PhD, Australia
Olav Meirik, MD, PhD, Chile
Daniel R. Mishell Jr., MD, USA
Bert O'Malley, MD, USA
Bent Ottesen, MD, Denmark
David Purdie, MD, UK
Lawrence G. Raisz, MD, USA
B. Lawrence Riggs, MD, PhD, USA
Henri Rochefort, MD, PhD, France
Giuseppe Rosano, MD, PhD, Italy
Raymond Rosen, PhD, USA
Karin Schenk-Gustafsson, MD, PhD, Sweden
Peter Schmidt, MD, USA
Ethel Siris, MD, USA
Sven O. Skouby, MD, Denmark
Leon Speroff, MD, USA
John C. Stevenson, MBBS, UK
David W. Sturdee, MD, UK
Cornelia Van Duijn, MD, The Netherlands
Nancy Woods, PhD, RN, USA

Those who reviewed the composite document were:

Takeshi Aso, MD, PhD, Japan
Giuseppe Benagiano, MD, Italy
Henry Burger, MD, PhD, Australia
Desmond Julian, MD, UK
Peter Kenemans, MD, PhD, The Netherlands
Luella Klein, MD, USA
Rogerio Lobo, MD, USA
Michael Mendelsohn, MD, USA
Henri Rozenbaum, MD, France
Goran Samsioe, MD, Sweden
Isaac Schiff, MD, USA
Piero Sismondi, MD, PhD, Italy
Wulf H. Utian, MD, USA
Nelson Watts, MD, USA

Special acknowledgment is warranted to Suzanne S. Hurd, MD, USA for her initial chairing of the project and for her scientific organizational skills; and to Ruth Johnsson Hegyeli, MD, USA for serving as the liaison between the Panel and the US National Institutes of Health, providing invaluable expert counsel. Also acknowledged with gratitude are the contributions of Silvia Belcredito, Italy; Cristina Bolsi, Italy; Andrea Cignarella, Italy; Anna Cozzi, Italy; Emanuela Folco, Italy; Ann S. Jackson, USA; Anna Miniotti, Italy; and Nancy Morris, USA.

Grading of Evidence

The grading of evidence used throughout the monograph for the recommendations promulgated by Expert Panel were based on the following categorization:

Evidence Category	Sources of Evidence	Definition
A	Randomized, controlled trials (rich body of data)	Evidence is from endpoints of well-defined randomized, controlled trials (or trials that depart only minimally from randomization) that provide a consistent pattern of findings in the population for which the recommendation is made. Category A therefore requires substantial numbers of studies involving substantial numbers of participants.
B	Randomized, controlled trials (limited body of data)	Evidence is from endpoints of intervention studies that include only a limited number of randomized, controlled trials, post hoc or subgroup analysis of randomized, controlled trials, or meta-analysis of randomized, controlled trials. In general, category B pertains when few randomized trials exist, they are small in size, and the trial results are somewhat inconsistent, or the trials were undertaken in a population that differs from the target population of the recommendation.
C	Nonrandomized trials and/or observational studies	Evidence is from outcomes of uncontrolled or nonrandomized trials or from observational studies.
D	Expert judgment	Expert judgment is based on the authors' synthesis of evidence from research described in the literature that does not meet the above-listed criteria, taking into consideration critical advice by other members of the international panel of experts, external referees, and external reviewers. The category is used only in cases in which the provision of some guidance was deemed valuable but an adequately compelling clinical literature addressing the subject of the recommendation was deemed insufficient to justify placement in one of the other categories (A through C)

Source: [Modified from] National Institutes of Health. Clinical Guidelines on the Identification, Evaluation, and Treatment of Overweight and Obesity in Adults. The Evidence Report. NIH pub. No. 98-4083. Bethesda, MD: National Institutes of Health, 1998.

Dissemination of Information

The monograph is scheduled for publication in early 2002. It reviews the spectrum of evidence to provide a multidisciplinary global approach to the enhancement of menopausal health, with consideration of sociocultural concerns and economic issues. The volume describes and references relevant clinical information, and provides evidence-based recommendations for best clinical practice. Importantly, this monograph is not copyrighted because the goal is that the materials be reproduced in individual countries for appropriate global dissemination. Further, it is hoped that expansion of specific topics will occur worldwide in appropriate professional journals.

The dissemination of information will be furthered by presentations at topic-related scientific meetings. A public/patient education companion document is planned.

As life expectancy continues to increase, the challenge will be to improve the quality of women's aging years. Better management of the symptoms and health risks associated with menopause is an important component of enhancing that quality of life.

GYNECOLOGIC AND UROGYNECOLOGIC ASPECTS OF MENOPAUSE

Susan L. Hendrix, PierGiorgio Crosignani, and Vivian W. Pinn

Introduction

Together with vasomotor symptoms, menstrual cycle irregularities are often one of the first signs of the menopausal transition. These cycle changes can occur ten years before the last menstrual period [1]. Distinguishing between hormonally induced bleeding versus uterine bleeding representing a premalignant, malignant, or a structural lesion can be difficult. Changes in frequency, duration, and volume of bleeding become clinically manifest as hypomenorrhea, oligomenorrhea, spotting, metrorrhagia, menorrhagia, menometrorrhagia, and polymenorrhea [2].

Menstrual and Endometrial Changes

Dysfunctional uterine bleeding is abnormal uterine bleeding with no organic cause and is a diagnosis of exclusion. Fifty percent of episodes occur between the ages of 40 and 50 [3]. It is caused by estrogen secretion sufficient to stimulate endometrial growth but insufficient to induce a midcycle surge of luteinizing hormone. In older women, follicular capacity is diminished leading to decreased estradiol and progesterone secretion. Luteal phase length is shortened with resultant menstrual irregularities. The relative lack of progesterone causes abnormal endometrial development resulting in uterine bleeding abnormalities.

Although endometrial atrophy is the most common histologic finding in women after the menopause, proliferative and secretory changes are common [4]. Endometrial hyperplasia is commonly found in perimenopausal women (6-13%) [5] and in women presenting with abnormal bleeding (4-30%) [6]. Endometrial hyperplasia can be simple or complex and when atypia is present, it represents a precursor for endometrial cancer. Most hyperplasia without atypia regresses and hyperplasia with atypia can regress [7].

Menstrual cycle irregularities and endometrial hyperplasia without atypia can be treated with the administration of progestins. Options include medroxyprogesterone acetate 10 mg, micronized progesterone 300 mg daily for 10 days per month, or combination oral contraceptives administered for 6 months. Mild atypia can be treated with the same regimens, while moderate to severe atypia requires more potent progestin treatment such as megestrol acetate 40-160 mg per day [8]. Repeat sampling 3 to 6 months after initiation of therapy is necessary to ensure resolution of the hyperplasia.

Risk factors for endometrial cancer include diabetes, hypertension, unopposed estrogen use, chronic anovulation, obesity, and estrogen-producing ovarian tumors. The association between unopposed estrogen use and endometrial cancer risk is well described [9,10]. Cancer of the endometrium is found in < 10 percent of those who are bleeding before the menopause, but in about 25% of those who are menopausal [11]. Because bleeding is a sign of possible endometrial abnormality, perimenopausal bleeding should be considered secondary to malignancy until proved otherwise.

Long-term continuous combined hormonal replacement therapy has been associated with endometrial cancer [12,13], however it is more frequent with cyclic use of progestins than with continuous combinations [10]. Tamoxifen has been associated with the development of endometrial carcinoma [14]. This was described as a 3-fold risk in women over fifty participating in the Breast Cancer Prevention Trial [15]. The effects of raloxifene appear to be different from tamoxifen. In a one-year randomized trial, no increase in endometrial thickness, hyperplasia, or malignancy was found in the women on raloxifene [16].

Bleeding During Hormone Replacement Therapy

Uterine bleeding due to HRT is a cause of patient concern [17], inconvenience [18,19], and discontinuation of use [20,21]. Bleeding during HRT may be related to the specific regimen. Other causes of bleeding during hormone replacement are failure of compliance (missed tablets, failure to change patch), absorption problems (intestinal problems, change in diet, use of antibiotics, defective patch compliance, skin problems), endometrial pathology (atrophy, polyps, submucosal leiomyoma, hyperplasia, adenocarcinoma), myometrial pathology, and drug use (anticoagulants, steroids, barbiturates, chemotherapy).

About 95% of women receiving sequential combined HRT will experience withdrawal bleeding after the progestin phase. About 6% will not bleed at all; the likelihood of no bleeding is higher in older age[22]. Bleeding during the estrogen-only phase is more likely associated with endometrial pathology [2]. Bleeding before day 11 of progestin treatment is correctable by a higher progestin dose [2]. Breakthrough bleeding may be caused by benign hyperplasia or atrophic endometrium but if no endometrial pathology is present may indicate an insufficient estrogen dosage [2].

Continuous administration of a progestin in combination with estrogen has been used to prevent the cyclic withdrawal bleeding associated with HRT [23]. Nevertheless, 50% of women have irregular bleeding, particularly during the first months [24]. Bleeding is usually slight, and the incidence of episodes decreases rapidly with time. Bleeding usually disappears within 1 year [20].

Diagnosis and Management of Abnormal Uterine Bleeding

Endometrial sampling remains the gold standard for diagnosing endometrial pathology. Measurement of endometrial thickness is a noninvasive clinical indicator of endometrial normality. Studies comparing ultrasonographic measurement of endometrial thickness with histopathologic findings on biopsy in women experiencing uterine bleeding showed endometrial thickness < 4 mm to correlate with atrophic endometrium and thickness > 4-7 mm to correlate with increased incidence of endometrial pathology in both groups [25]. Most importantly, measuring endometrial thickness in asymptomatic women is not predictive of endometrial pathology[26]. More recently, sonohysterography, which is less invasive and less expensive than hysteroscopy, has been proposed as a better method for the morphologic evaluation of the endometrium [27].

Clinical management of abnormal uterine bleeding in perimenopausal patients depends on the clinical and pathologic diagnosis. Options include observation, specific changes in the treatment regimen, or surgery.

Genital Atrophy And Vulvovaginal Complaints

Vulvovaginal complaints are very common in menopausal women [28]. The most common complaint is vaginal dryness. The loss of lubrication causes symptoms of vaginismus and dyspareunia. Estrogen is efficacious in treatment, and local estrogens are as effective as systemic in the therapy of genital atrophy [29].

Urinary Tract and Pelvic Floor

Estrogen deficiency causes atrophic changes of the urethral epithelium and the submucosa. In addition, urethral atrophy theoretically predisposes to ascending infection, which constitute a major problem in elderly women [30]. It is important to identify patients with recurrent infections because of the significant morbidity, which includes risk for renal impairment. Urinary tract infections are usually secondary to stepwise colonization of the vaginal introitus and urethral mucosa by organisms from the rectal flora. In theory, estrogen replacement therapy reduces urinary tract infections in postmenopausal years probably by its support of normal vaginal flora [31]. However, a recent randomized controlled trial of continuous combined hormone therapy did not reduce the frequency of urinary tract infections in postmenopausal women [32].

Pelvic organ prolapse has been reported with several selective estrogen receptor modulators (SERMs) removed from development [33]. In a large cross-sectional study of postmenopausal women, past or current use of estrogen did not increase the risk for uterine prolapse, cystocele, or rectocele [34]. In three clinical trials of raloxifene, safety data showed no increase in risk for pelvic floor surgery [35].

Urinary Incontinence

Urinary incontinence (UI) is a common but poorly understood problem. The International Continence Society defines incontinence as involuntary loss of urine that is objectively demonstrable and is a social or hygienic problem [36]. The relationship between menopause and urinary incontinence is unknown and not well studied. Although many experts quote menopause as a major risk factor for both stress and urge incontinence, there has been limited data to support this. It is theorized that the lack of estrogen in menopause can result in thinning of the lining of the urethra, which causes improper closure [37]. Estrogen deficiency also makes the bladder muscles weaken. The combination of a thin, injury-prone urinary tract and weak bladder muscles can cause the urethra to open unexpectedly during physical activity, leading to stress incontinence.

Established urinary incontinence can usually be divided into one of four major types: stress incontinence, urge incontinence (detrusor overactivity or instability), mixed incontinence, and overflow incontinence. These disorders often have classic histories, or typical physical findings. Neurogenic incontinence may be related to defects in the nervous system, which conducts urination signals between the bladder and the brain.

Stress incontinence is diagnosed when the pressure inside the bladder exceeds the pressure in the urethra in the absence of a detrusor contraction. Patients typically describe losses of small volumes of urine with activities resulting in transiently increased intra-abdominal pressure (coughing, sneezing, running, laughing, etc.). Physical examination may reveal evidence of pelvic relaxation, such as cystocele with urethral hypermobility, rectocele, and/or uterine prolapse. Urine loss can usually be demonstrated with coughing while the patient is in the supine position.

Urge incontinence is diagnosed when the detrusor muscle contracts, spontaneously or on provocation, during the filling phase of the bladder, while the woman is attempting to inhibit micturition. Urge incontinence is more common in older adults. Patients with detrusor overactivity have early, forceful detrusor muscle contractions, well before the bladder is full. This creates a sensation of urinary urgency and frequency. Patients with detrusor overactivity tend to lose moderate to occasionally large volumes of urine. If the detrusor contraction is strong enough to overcome the urethral resistance, incontinence occurs. The diagnosis of detrusor overactivity is made primarily by history and confirmed with urodynamic testing. There are no pathognomonic findings on physical examination although a careful pelvic and rectal examination and neurologic screening can occasionally reveal anatomic abnormalities (e.g. uterine prolapse, fecal impaction) or evidence of neurologic disease.

Mixed incontinence is a combination of both stress and urge incontinence, and is most common in older women.

Evaluation and treatment for incontinence is dependent on the type of incontinence and the person's age, medical history, and desires for therapy. The assessment for incontinence should include a history, physical examination, and mental, functional, and environmental assessments.

Urodynamic assessment includes a group of tests that measure bladder function. Multi-channel urodynamic studies include uroflow, cystometrogram, urethral pressure profiles, and electromyogram. These studies document bladder pressure and capacity; muscle contractibility; urethral length, and sphincter control, and are performed under the auspice of a gynecologist specializing in the disorders of the pelvic floor or an urologist. These studies should be done if surgery on the pelvic floor is being considered for urinary incontinence.

Treatment for incontinence depends on the type of incontinence, its causes, and the capabilities of the patient. Urge incontinence may be treated with a muscarinic receptor antagonist or anticholinergenic medications. Estrogen, either oral or vaginal, until recently has been thought to improve incontinent episodes either alone or in conjunction with other treatments for postmenopausal women with incontinence. Two short-term clinical trials found no significant difference between treatment and control groups in the number on incontinent episodes at 3 and 6 months of follow-up [38,39]. A randomized long-term clinical trial found HRT to be associated with worsening of urinary incontinence [40].

Future Needs

The determinants of endometrial function need to be better defined. There is a need for additional noninvasive methods for the diagnosis of endometrial pathology. More sensitive methods to determine estrogen effects at the tissue level need to be developed. Future clinical trials need to assess the relationship between estrogens, progestins, SERMs and pelvic organ prolapse. Future preclinical studies need to investigate if estrogens, progestins, or SERMs modify or otherwise affect collagen increasing the elasticity of the pelvic floor tissues and increasing the risk for pelvic organ prolapse. The actual effect of estrogen on incontinence needs to be better characterized.

References

1. Treolar AR, Bounton RE, Behn BG, Brown BW. Variation of the human menstrual cycle through reproductive life. International Journal of Infertility 1967;12:77-79.
2. Kenemans P, Barentsen R, van de Weijer P. Practical HRT. Bussum, The Netherlands: Medicom Europe BV, 1995;169:30.
3. March CM. Bleeding problems and treatment. Clin Obstet Gynecol 1998;41:928-39.
4. Trevoux R, de Brux J, Bergeron C. Biology of normal aging endometrium. In: Lorrain J, Plouffe L Jr, Ravnikar V, Speroff L, Watts N, editors. Comprehensive management of menopause. Clinical perspectives in obstetrics and gynecology. New York: Springer-Verlag, 1994;246-53.
5. Archer DF, McIntyre-Seltman K, Wilborn WW Jr, et al. Endometrial morphology in asymptomatic postmenopausal women. Am J Obstet Gynecol 1991;165:317-20.
6. Silverberg SG. Hyperplasia and carcinoma of the endometrium. Semin Diagn Pathol 1988; 5:135-53.
7. Mishell DR Jr, et al. In: Comprehensive gynecology. 3rd ed. St. Louis, Mo: Mosby-Year Book, Inc., 1997:867-73.
8. MacKay HT. Gynecology. In: Tierney LM Jr, McPhee SJ, Papadakis MA, editors. Current medical diagnosis and treatment 1998. 37th ed. Stamford, Conn: Appleton and Lange, 1998:691-732.
9. The Writing Group for the PEPI Trial. Effects of hormone replacement therapy on endometrial histology in postmenopausal women. The Postmenopausal Estrogen/Progestin Interventions (PEPI) Trial. JAMA 1996 Feb 7;275(5):370-75.
10. Weiderpass E, Adami HO, Baron JA, et al. Risk of endometrial cancer following estrogen replacement with and without progestins. J Natl Cancer Instit 1999:91;1131-37.
11. March CM. Bleeding problems and treatment. Clin Obstet Gynecol 1998;41:928-39.

12. Beresford SA, Weiss NS, Voigt LF, McKnight B. Risk of endometrial cancer in relation to use of oestrogen combined with cyclic progestagen therapy in postmenopausal women. Lancet 1997;349:458-61.
13. Jain MG, Rohan TE, Howe GR. Hormone replacement therapy and endometrial cancer in Ontario, Canada. J Clin Epidemiol 2000;53:385-91.
14. Lahti E, Blanco G, Kauppila A, Apaja-Sarkkinen M, Taskinen PJ, Laatikainen T. Endometrial changes in postmenopausal breast cancer patients receiving tamoxifen. Obstet Gynecol 1993;81(5 Pt 1):660-64.
15. Fisher B, Costantino JP, Wickerham DL, et al. Tamoxifen for prevention of breast cancer: report of the National Surgical Adjuvant Breast and Bowel Project P-1 Study. J Natl Cancer Inst 1998 Sep 16;90(18):1371-88.
16. Goldstein SR, Scheele WH, Rajagopalan SK, Wilkie JL, Walsh BW, Parsons AK. A 12-month comparative study of raloxifene, estrogen, and placebo on the postmenopausal endometrium. Obstet Gynecol 2000 Jan;95(1):95-103.
17. Barentsen R, Groeneveld FPMJ, Bareman FP, Hoes AW, Dokter HJ, Drogendijk AC. Women's opinion on withdrawal bleeding with hormone replacement therapy. Eur J Obstet Gynecol Reprod Biol 1993;51:203-7.
18. Ferguson KJ, Hoegh C, Johnson S. Estrogen replacement therapy. A survey of women's knowledge and attitudes. Arch Intern Med 1989;149:133-36.
19. Kadri AZ. Perimenopausal women's view on hormone replacement therapy (comment). BMJ 1990;300:1017.
20. Faulkner DL, Young C, Hutchins D, McCollam JS. Patient noncompliance with hormone replacement therapy: A nationwide estimate using a large prescription claims database. Menopause 1998 Winter;5(4):226-29.
21. Berman RS, Epstein RS, Lydick E. Risk factors associated with women's compliance with estrogen replacement therapy. J Womens Health 1997 Apr;6(2):219-26.
22. Gambrell RD Jr, Bagnell CA, Greenblatt RB. Role of estrogens and progesterone in the etiology and prevention of endometrial cancer: Review. Am J Obstet Gynecol 1983;146: 696-707.
23. Staland B. Continuous treatment with natural oestrogens and progestogens. A method to avoid endometrial stimulation. Maturitas 1981;3:145-56.
24. Weinstein L, Bewtra C, Gallagher JC. Evaluation of a continuous combined low-dose regimen of estrogen-progestin for treatment of the menopausal patient. Am J Obstet Gynecol 1990;162:1534-39.
25. Taipale P, Tarjanne H, Heinonen UM. The diagnostic value of transvaginal sonography in the diagnosis of endometrial malignancy in women with peri- and postmenopausal bleeding [published erratum appears in Acta Obstet Gynecol Scand 1995;74:324]. Acta Obstet Gynecol Scand 1994;73:819-23.
26. Fleischer AC, Wheeler JE, Lindsay I, et al. An assessment of the value of ultrasonographic screening for endometrial disease in postmenopausal women without symptoms. Am J Obstet Gynecol 2001 Jan;184(2):70-75.
27. Laifer-Narin SL, Ragavendra N, Lu DS, Sayre J, Perrella RR, Grant EG. Transvaginal saline hysterosonography: characteristics distinguishing malignant and various benign conditions. AJR Am J Roentgenol 1999;172:1513-20.
28. Stenberg A, Heimer G, Ulmsten U, Cnattingius S. Prevalence of genitourinary and other climacteric symptoms in 61-year-old women. Maturitas 1996;24:31-36.
29. Cardozo L, Bachmann G, McClish D, Fonda D, Birgerson L. Meta-analysis of estrogen

therapy in the management of urogenital atrophy in postmenopausal women: second report of the Hormones and Urogenital Therapy Committee. Obstet Gynecol 1998;92(4 Pt 2):722-27.
30. Hextall A, Cardozo L. Managing postmenopausal cystitis. Hosp Pract (Off Ed) 1997;32:191-98.
31. Cardozo L, Benness C, Abbott D. Low dose oestrogen prophylaxis for recurrent urinary tract infections in elderly women. Br J Obstet Gynaecol 1998;105:403-7.
32. Brown JS, Vittinghoff E, Kanaya AM, Agarwal SK, Hulley S, Foxman B; Heart and Estrogen/Progestin Replacement Study Research Group. Urinary tract infections in postmenopausal women: effect of hormone therapy and risk factors. Obstet Gynecol 2001 Dec;98(6):1045-52.
33. Hendrix SL, McNeeley SG. Effect of selective estrogen receptor modulators on reproductive tissues other than endometrium. Ann N Y Acad Sci 2001 Dec;949:243-50.
34. Hendrix SL, Clark AL, Nygaard IE, Aragaki A, Barnabei VM, McTiernan A. Pelvic organ prolapse in the Women's Health Initiative: Gravity and gravidity. Am J Obstet Gynecol In press.
35. Goldstein SR, Neven P, Zhou L, Taylor YL, Ciaccia AV, Plouffe L. Raloxifene effect on frequency of surgery for pelvic floor relaxation. Obstet Gynecol 2001 Jul;98(1):91-96.
36. Abrams P, Blaivas JG, Stanton SL, Andersen JT. The standardisation of terminology of lower urinary tract function. The International Continence Society Committee on Standardization of Terminology. Scand J Urol Nephrol 1988(Suppl.);114:5-19.
37. Bump RC, Friedman CI. Intraluminal urethral pressure measurements in the female baboon: Effects of hormonal manipulation. J Urol 1986 Aug;136(2):508-11.
38. Fantl JA, Bump RC, Robinson D, McClish DK, Wyman JF. Efficacy of estrogen supplementation in the treatment of urinary incontinence. The Continence Program for Women Research Group. Obstet Gynecol 1996 Nov;88(5):745-49.
39. Jackson S, Shepherd A, Brookes S, Abrams P. The effect of oestrogen supplementation on post-menopausal urinary stress incontinence. A double-blind placebo-controlled trial. Br J Obstet Gynaecol 1999 Jul;106(7):711-18.
40. Grady D, Brown JS, Vittinghoff E, Applegate W, Varner E, Snyder T; The HERS Research Group. Postmenopausal hormones and incontinence: the Heart and Estrogen/Progestin Replacement Study. Obstet Gynecol 2001 Jan;97(1):116-20.

Cardiovascular Disease in Women

Jacques E. Rossouw, Peter Collins, Nanette Wenger, and Rodolfo Paoletti

Introduction

Worldwide, cardiovascular disease is the commonest cause of mortality and morbidity in women. This is true in developed countries (where coronary heart disease predominates), and also in developing countries (where stroke and congestive heart failure predominate). In the USA in 1997 there were 230 thousand deaths from coronary heart disease and 89 thousand deaths from stroke, compared to 34 thousand from breast cancer [1]. Thus, death from coronary heart disease was almost 7 times more common than breast cancer, and death from stroke was three times more common.

Risk Factors

The factors (both adverse and protective) contributing to cardiovascular disease in women and men are similar, with the possible exception of sex hormones. The factors for CHD in women include:

- Age
- Personal history of CHD, stroke, TIA, or peripheral vascular disease
- Family history of these conditions
- Dyslipidemia
  - LDL cholesterol
  - HDL cholesterol
  - Triglycerides
- Smoking
- High blood pressure
- Diabetes mellitus
- Obesity, including abdominal obesity
- Lifestyle
  - Diet
  - Physical inactivity
  - Psychosocial factors
  - Alcohol
- Emerging factors

- Homocysteine
- C-reactive protein
- Lp(a)

The relative risks associated with each of these factors are approximately the same or larger in women than in men, but the absolute risks are generally smaller in women [2]. This is because of some unexplained component of femaleness that lowers risk, or of maleness that increases risk. Factors that have a particular impact in women include low HDL cholesterol (in older women), triglycerides, and diabetes mellitus [3-5]. The impact of HDL cholesterol in younger women is about the same as in men, and in older women HDL retains its predictive ability while it weakens or disappears in older men [3]. LDL cholesterol predicts CHD in younger women to a greater extent than in men, but the reverse is true in older persons [3]. Triglycerides are predictive of CHD in younger and older women to a greater extent than in men, even after adjusting for HDL [3,4]. Diabetes mellitus is associated with a high relative risk in women, and in its presence confers a risk of CHD in excess of 20% over 10 years, equivalent to that of a woman or man with pre-existing CHD [5].

Clinical Trials

Randomized controlled clinical trials have demonstrated that aspirin, beta blockers, angiotensin converting enzyme inhibitors, and statins prevent CHD in high-risk women to the same degree as in men [6-9]. In the Antiplatelet Trialists Collaboration summarizing the world literature, in high-risk women 33 cardiovascular events were prevented for every 1,000 persons treated, compared to 37 events in men [6]. In the Beta-blocker Heart Attack Trial of high-risk patients, in women 44 deaths per 1,000 treated were averted, compared to 23 in men [7]. In the Health Outcomes Prevention Evaluation (HOPE) trial, ramipril conferred the same risk reduction for recurrent CVD events in high-risk women as in men [8]. Finally, the statin trials of cholesterol lowering have demonstrated equivalent and significant reduction in CHD events in women and men [9]. There is no reason to believe that the efficacy of any of these interventions will be different in low-risk women (e.g. women without pre-existing CHD), though the cost-effectiveness may decrease in low-risk populations (male or female).

Primary Prevention with Menopausal Hormone Therapy

Although menopausal hormone therapy (MHT) is associated with reduced risk of CHD in observational studies, to date the benefit has not been demonstrated convincingly in clinical trials [10-22]. In the area of primary prevention, the PEPI trial of intermediate outcomes confirmed that that MHT reduces LDL, raises HDL, and raises triglycerides, and has some modest effect on fibrinogen [11]. In healthy women, estradiol reduced carotid intima-media thickness (IMT) compared to placebo [12]. The anticipated lipid effects were found in trials with clinical outcomes, yet a concurrent benefit has not been observed. The large Women s Health Initiative (WHI) includes trials of conjugated equine estrogen (CEE) alone, and in combination with medroxyprogesterone (MPA) [13]. Early in 2000 the investigators notified the 27,000 participants that, during the first two years after randomization, the active treatment groups were showing higher rates of heart attack, stroke, and blood clots in the legs and lungs than the placebo group [14]. Because of uncertainty about the long-term effects and about the overall risk and benefit, the trials are being continued. Final results are expected in late 2005 or early 2006. A similar study in the UK is in the process of recruiting participants [15].

Secondary Prevention with Menopausal Hormone Therapy

More information is available from trials of secondary prevention. The first trial using coronary angiography as the primary outcome showed no benefit for CEE or CEE plus MPA [16]. Similarly, a trial of estradiol did not demonstrate slowing of carotid IMT progression [17]. Three trials with clinical outcomes have reported results [18-20]. In the Heart and Estrogen/progestin Replacement Study (HERS) CEE plus MPA had no effect on CHD over the full 4 years, but there was a significant 52% excess of CHD compared to placebo in the first year [18]. The subsequent trend towards reduced risk needs to be treated with a great deal of caution, because after the first year the analysis no longer deals with a randomized comparison. Also, the significance of the slope depends on the inclusion of the excess in the first year, and finally, for fatal CHD the events by year never entered the zone of apparent benefit. The results from the Women s Estrogen for Stroke Trial (WEST) parallel those for HERS, but with recurrent stroke and all-cause death as the primary outcome [19]. Estradiol had no effect over the full duration of the trial on nonfatal stroke and all-cause death, or on death or nonfatal stroke separately. However, in a post-hoc analysis there was a nonsignificant excess of stroke death (mostly ischemic stroke death) during the first six months in the estradiol group. The Papworth HRT and Survival Enquiry (PHASE) was a small (n = 255) and short (average follow up 11 months) trial of transdermal estradiol with or without norethisterone acetate in women with CHD [20]. The trial was stopped early because of futility and possible harm. At the time of stopping the trial, there had been 52 events (combined unstable angina, MI, and death) in the active treatment group compared to 39 in the control group (not statistically significant).

Future Research Directions

To date, four trials with clinical events as the primary outcome have failed to show benefit in the short term (up to 4 years), and indeed have provided worrisome indications of early harm for arterial (CHD and stroke) as well as venous thrombo-embolic events [12,18-20]. A combined analysis of all the short-term trials of MHT in which clinical outcome data were recorded also suggested an excess of cardiovascular events [21]. Future directions for research on MHT include efforts at identifying the subset(s) of women who are at risk. The working hypothesis of investigators in the field is that there is a subset of women with vulnerable plaques, in whom an interaction of MHT with an underlying susceptibility factor (e.g. a prothrombotic mutation) triggers a clinical event [22]. If such a factor or factors can be identified, these women at high risk could in future be screened out and be advised against MHT. The remaining women without the susceptibility factor would be more likely to benefit from MHT, or at a minimum would not be at increased early risk for cardiovascular events. Studies of the short-term metabolic, gynecologic, and bone effects of lower doses of estrogens are being done, and are predicated on the reasonable notion that the beneficial effects might dominate the adverse effects at lower doses. This will need to be proven with clinical trials of cardiovascular outcomes. Current clinical trials are being continued in order to ascertain the long-term effects of MHT [13,15]. The clinical effects of transdermal MHT need more research, since this route of administration simulates the physiologic situation that might explain the gender difference in CHD onset. More research is also needed on the clinical effects of selective estrogen receptor modulators, androgens, and selective androgen receptor modulators.

Finally, future trials of prevention treatments, and treatments of existing disease, should include sufficient women to allow for the adequate assessment of the effects in women. In the past, women have not been included in sufficient number in individual trials, so that scientists had to make inferences from the results in men, or from meta-analyses combining the effects in women across a number of trials. Fortunately, for most cardiovascular treatments the effects have not been shown to differ by gender; however, there is no guarantee that this will always be the case.

References

1. National Center for Health Statistics: Vital Statistics of the United States, 1997, vol II. Mortality, part A. Washington, DC, Public Health Service, 1997.
2. Expert Panel on Detection, Evaluation, and Treatment of High Blood Cholesterol in Adults. Executive Summary of the Third Report of the National Cholesterol Education Program (NCEP) Expert Panel on Detection, Evaluation, and Treatment of High Blood Cholesterol in Adults (Adult Treatment Panel III). JAMA 2001;285:2486-97.
3. Manolio TA, Pearson TA, Wenger NK, et al. Cholesterol and heart disease in older persons and women: Review of an NHLBI Workshop. Ann Epidemiol 1992;2:161-76.
4. Austin MA, Hokanson E, Edwards KL. Hypertriglyceridemia as a risk factor. Am J Cardiol 1998;81(4A):7B-12B.
5. Haffner SM. Coronary heart disease in patients with diabetes. N Engl J Med. 2000;342: 1040-42.
6. Antiplatelet Trialists' Collaboration. Collaborative overview of randomised trials of antiplatelet therapy--I: Prevention of death, myocardial infarction, and stroke by prolonged antiplatelet therapy in various categories of patients. Br Med J 1994;308:81-106.
7. β-Blocker Heart Attack Trial Research Group (B-HAT). A randomized trial of propranolol in patients with acute myocardial infarction. 1. Mortality results. JAMA 1982;247:1707-14.
8. Yusuf S, Sleight P, Pogue J, Bosch J, Davies R, Dagenais G. Effects of an angiotensin-converting-enzyme inhibitor, ramipril, on cardiovascular events in high-risk patients. The Heart Outcomes Prevention Evaluation Study Investigators. N Engl J Med 2000;342:145-53.

9. LaRosa JC, He J, Vupputuri S. Effect of statins on risk of coronary disease. A meta-analysis of randomized controlled trials. JAMA 1999;282:2340-46.
10. Barrett-Connor E, Grady D. Hormone replacement therapy, heart disease, and other considerations. Annu Rev Public Health 1998;19:55-72.
11. The Writing Group for the PEPI trial. Effects of estrogen or estrogen/progestin regimens on heart disease risk factors in postmenopausal women: The Postmenopausal Estrogen/Progestin Interventions (PEPI) Trial. JAMA 1995;273:199-208.
12. Hodis HN, Mack WJ, Lobo R, et al. Estrogen in the Prevention of Atherosclerosis Trial. Circulation 2000;102(18):II-837 (abstract).
13. The Women's Health Initiative Study Group. Design of the Women's Health Initiative Clinical Trial and Observational Study. Controlled Clinical Trials 1998;19:61-109.
14. http://www.nhlbi.nih.gov/whi/hrt-en.htm
15. Vickers MR, Meade TW, Wilkes HC. Hormone replacement therapy and cardiovascular disease: The case for a randomized controlled trial. Ciba Found Symp 1995;191:150-60.
16. Herrington DM, Reboussin DM, Brosnihan KB, et al. Effects of estrogen replacement therapy on the progression of coronary artery atherosclerosis. N Engl J Med 2000;343:522-29.
17. Angerer P, Stork S, Kothny W, Schmitt P, von Schacky C. Effect of oral postmenopausal hormone replacement on progression of atherosclerosis. Arterioscl Throm Vasc Biol 2001; 21:262-68.
18. Hulley S, Grady D, Bush TL, et al. Randomized trial of estrogen plus progestin for secondary prevention of coronary heart disease in postmenopausal women. JAMA 1998; 280:605-13.
19. Viscoli CM, Brass LM, Kernan WN, Sarrel PM, Horwitz R. Estrogen after ischemic stroke: Effect of estrogen replacement on risk of stroke and death in Women's Estrogen for Stroke Trial (WEST). Stroke 2001;32:329 (abstract).
20. Clarke S, Kelleher J, Lloyd-Jones H, Sharples L, Slack M, Schofield PM. Transdermal hormone replacement therapy for the secondary prevention of coronary artery disease in postmenopausal women. Eur Heart J 200;21:212(abstract).
21. Hemminki E, McPherson K. Impact of postmenopausal hormone therapy on cardiovascular events and cancer: Pooled data from clinical trials. BMJ 1997:315:149-53.
22. Psaty BM, Smith NL, Lemaitre RN, et al. Hormone replacement therapy, prothrombotic mutations, and the risk of incident myocardial infarction in postmenopausal women. JAMA 2001;285:906-13.

MENOPAUSE AND DISORDERS OF NEUROLOGICAL FUNCTION AND MENTAL HEALTH

Victor W. Henderson and Susan M. Resnick

Introduction

An expert panel was assembled under the auspices of the National Heart, Lung, and Blood Institute, the National Institutes of Health Office of Research on Women's Health, and the Giovanni Lorenzini Medical Foundation. The overarching goal was to develop an international position paper on the topic, "Women's Health and Menopause—A Comprehensive Approach." The work of the panel was conducted between the Fall of 1998 and the Summer of 2001. The panel was subdivided by topic areas, and the focus of our particular working group included disorders of neurological function and mental health. Like other working groups, ours was charged with the development of evidence-based practice recommendations. Evidence was resulting primarily from an evaluation of the published literature, and evidence and derived recommendations were categorized according to four levels of certainty: a rich body of data from randomized controlled trials, a limited body of data from randomized controlled trials, evidence from nonrandomized trials or observational studies, and panel consensus. For none of the disorders considered by our working group was there a rich body of clinical trial data, and for many even observational data were sparse.

Menopause is a normal physiological event characterized by the loss of ovarian follicular function, including the loss of ovarian estrogen production. Although the clinical hallmark of the menopause is the permanent cessation of menstruation, the brain is among the many tissues affected by menopausal hormonal changes. In the brain, as in other target organ systems, estrogen effects are multifaceted and occur through both genomic and nongenomic mechanisms of action.

Our working group reviewed evidence on how menopausal estrogen loss as well as menopausal estrogen therapy might affect central nervous system functioning and central nervous system disorders. We did not attempt to summarize evidence or develop practice recommendations for the older women when issues appeared unrelated to menopausal hormonal changes or to menopausal hormone therapy.

The following is a brief summary of our findings. In this summary, cited references are intended as illustrative rather than comprehensive.

Disorders of Neurological Function

Evidence was reviewed regarding age-associated cognitive decline, dementia, and several other select neurological disorders.

Age-Associated Cognitive Decline

Memory and certain other cognitive abilities change between midlife and old age; in most instances changes represent a decline in function. Changes viewed as usual accompaniments of aging are not considered to be pathological. There is little indication that menopause *per se* initiates cognitive deterioration, and serum estrogen concentrations in menopausal women do not appear to be closely related to cognitive skills [1]. Findings from observational studies are not fully congruent. Some indicate that estrogen therapy might help preserve cognitive function [2,3], while others do not [4]. Data from randomized controlled trials are limited. Short-term studies in women who experience the abrupt loss of ovarian function (for example, after oophorectomy) indicate that estrogen may help preserve memory, particularly memory requiring verbal encoding [5]. Most clinical trials of estrogen in older postmenopausal women are less supportive of an estrogen benefit [6-8], although verbal memory is not always specifically assessed in these trials.

In summary, a limited body of data from randomized trials indicates that menopausal estrogen therapy may help preserve specific cognitive skills (for example, verbal memory) immediately after induced menopause, and there is limited, conflicting evidence that estrogen possibly helps preserve cognitive skills during normal aging.

Dementia

In most countries, Alzheimer's disease is the commonest cause of dementia, and there are few data on whether estrogen might influence dementia due to other disorders. A number of observational studies have considered the association between menopausal hormone therapy and Alzheimer's risk. Most [9-12], but not all [13], studies indicate a protective association, with risk reductions of approximately one-third to one-half. No results from randomized controlled trials are available, although such trials are underway.

A few observational studies have implied that women who used estrogen for a number of years and later developed Alzheimer's disease have milder cognitive deficits [14]. Although results of a number of small nonrandomized trials argue for a benefit of estrogen in this disorder, findings from several recent randomized controlled trials failed to confirm a benefit of estrogen for women with mild-to-moderate dementia due to Alzheimer's disease [15,16].

In summary, there is observational evidence that menopausal hormone therapy begun during the menopausal transition or after menopause may reduce risk of Alzheimer's disease. In contrast, limited clinical trial data indicate that estrogen therapy begun after the onset of dementia does not improve Alzheimer symptoms.

OTHER NEUROLOGICAL DISORDERS

Stroke is among the most important disorders that may be affected by menopause or menopausal hormone therapy. For example, favorable effects on serum lipids and vascular endothelial function could indicate a role for estrogen in the prevention of ischemic stroke [17]. However, observational studies have generally failed to show an association between estrogen use and stroke incidence [18,19], and a recent secondary analysis of data from a large randomized controlled trial of estrogen in women with coronary heart disease also uncovered no link between estrogen use and stroke incidence [20].

In younger women, neurological symptoms sometimes vary in association with hormonal changes, such as those occurring during the menstrual cycle or in association with pregnancy. Epilepsy, migraine headache, and multiple sclerosis are three dissimilar disorders that share this common feature. However few data address whether menopause or menopausal hormone therapy is associated with symptomatic change in any of these illnesses.

For Parkinson's disease, very limited clinical trial data raise the possibility that estrogen use might be associated with milder neurological symptoms [21], although estrogen therapy does not appear to be linked to a change in Parkinson risk [22].

During the climacteric, the hot flush is associated with sleep disruption and waking episodes, and these symptoms are reduced by estrogen therapy [23].

In summary, observational studies and limited trial data suggest that menopausal estrogen therapy does not substantially alter stroke risk. For epilepsy, migraine, multiple sclerosis, and Parkinson's disease, no compelling data indicate that estrogen therapy after menopause has substantial effects on symptoms or disability. Some sleep disturbances during the climacteric appear to improve with estrogen therapy, although evidence from randomized clinical trials is lacking.

Disorders of Mental Health

Two important disorders of mental health were considered by the expert panel working group, depression and schizophrenia. Women of all ages have higher rates of depression than men, but the menopausal transition is not observed to represent a time of heightened vulnerability to affective disorders [24]. Estrogen influences noradrenalin and serotonin, neurotransmitter systems implicated in depression. With some exceptions, results from short-term clinical trials indicate that estrogen therapy given during the perimenopausal or menopausal period can enhance mood or enhance subjective sense of well-being [25,26]. However, any potential role of estrogen in major depressive episodes after the menopause is poorly addressed by clinical trial data.

Estrogen effects on dopaminergic and serotonergic systems of the brain could influence schizophrenic symptoms, but menopause does not appear to alter a woman's risk of schizophrenia [27]. Observational and clinical trial data are sparse, and there are no randomized controlled trials of estrogen for schizophrenia symptoms.

References

1. Barrett-Connor E, Goodman-Gruen D. Cognitive function and endogenous sex hormones in older women. J Am Geriatr Soc 1999;47:1289-93.
2. Steffens DC, Norton MC, Plassman BL, et al. Enhanced cognitive performance with estrogen use in nondemented community-dwelling older women. J Am Geriatr Soc 1999; 47:1171-75.
3. Maki PM, Zonderman AB, Resnick SM. Enhanced verbal memory in nondemented elderly women receiving hormone-replacement therapy. Am J Psychiatry 2001;158:227-33.
4. Barrett-Connor E, Kritz-Silverstein D. Estrogen replacement therapy and cognitive function in older women. JAMA 1993;269:2637-41.
5. Phillips SM, Sherwin BB. Effects of estrogen on memory function in surgically menopausal women. Psychoneuroendocrinology 1992;17:485-95.
6. Polo-Kantola P, Portin R, Polo O, et al. The effect of short-term estrogen replacement therapy on cognition: A randomized, double-blind, cross-over trial in postmenopausal women. Obstet Gynecol 1998;91:459-66.
7. Duka T, Tasker R, McGowan JF. The effects of 3-week estrogen hormone replacement on cognition in elderly healthy females. Psychopharmacology 2000;149:129-39.
8. Binder EF, Schechtman KB, Birge SJ, et al. Effects of hormone replacement therapy on cognitive performance in elderly women. Maturitas 2001;38:137-46.
9. Paganini-Hill A, Henderson VW. Estrogen replacement therapy and risk of Alzheimer's disease. Arch Intern Med 1996;156:2213-17.
10. Tang M-X, Jacobs D, Stern Y, et al. Effect of oestrogen during menopause on risk and age at onset of Alzheimer's disease. Lancet 1996;348:429-32.
11. Kawas C, Resnick S, Morrison A, et al. A prospective study of estrogen replacement therapy and the risk of developing Alzheimer's disease: The Baltimore Longitudinal Study of Aging. Neurology 1997;48:1517-21.
12. Slooter AJ, Bronzova J, Witteman JC, et al. Estrogen use and early onset Alzheimer's disease: A population-based study. J Neurol Neurosurg Psychiatry 1999;67:779-81.
13. Brenner DE, Kukull WA, Stergachis A, et al. Postmenopausal estrogen replacement therapy and the risk of Alzheimer's disease: A population-based case-control study. Am J Epidemiol 1994;140:262-67.
14. Henderson VW, Watt L, Buckwalter JG. Cognitive skills associated with estrogen replacement in women with Alzheimer's disease. Psychoneuroendocrinology 1996;21:421-30.
15. Henderson VW, Paganini-Hill A, Miller BL, et al. Estrogen for Alzheimer's disease in women: randomized, double-blind, placebo-controlled trial. Neurology 2000;54:295-301.
16. Mulnard RA, Cotman CW, Kawas C, et al. Estrogen replacement therapy for treatment of mild to moderate Alzheimer disease: A randomized controlled trial. JAMA 2000;283: 1007-15.
17. Mendelsohn ME, Karas RH. The protective effects of estrogen on the cardiovascular system. N Engl J Med 1999;340:1801-11.
18. Grodstein F, Stampfer MJ, Manson JE, et al. Postmenopausal estrogen and progestin use and the risk of cardiovascular disease. N Engl J Med 1996;335:453-61.
19. Petitti DB, Sidney S, Quesenberry CP, Jr., Bernstein A. Ischemic stroke and use of estrogen and estrogen/progestogen as hormone replacement therapy. Stroke 1998;29:23-28.

20. Simon JA, Hsia J, Cauley JA, et al. Postmenopausal hormone therapy and risk of stroke: The Heart and Estrogen/progestin Replacement Study (HERS). Circulation 2001;103:638-42.
21. Tsang K-L, Ho S-L, Lo S-K. Estrogen improves motor disability in parkinsonian postmenopausal women with motor fluctuations. Neurology 2000;54:2292-98.
22. Marder K, Tang M-X, Alfaro B, et al. Postmenopausal estrogen use and Parkinson's disease with and without dementia. Neurology 1998;50:1141-43.
23. Erlik Y, Tataryn IV, Meldrum DR, et al. Association of waking episodes with menopausal hot flushes. JAMA 1981;245:1741-44.
24. Dennerstein L, Lehert P, Burger H, Dudley E. Mood and the menopausal transition. J Nerv Ment Dis 1999;187:685-91.
25. Fedor-Freybergh P. The influence of oestrogens on the wellbeing and mental performance in climacteric and postmenopausal women. Acta Obstet Gynecol Scand 1977;Suppl.64:1-99.
26. Ditkoff EC, Crary WG, Cristo M, Lobo RA. Estrogen improves psychological function in asymptomatic postmenopausal women. Obstet Gynecol 1991;78:991-95.
27. Hafner H, Maurer K, Loffler W, Riecher-Rossler A. The influence of age and sex on the onset and early course of schizophrenia. Br J Psychiatry 1993;262:80-86.

Menopause Hormone Replacement Therapy and Cancer: Epidemiology

Carlo La Vecchia, Louise A. Brinton, and Anne McTiernan

Introduction

Hormone replacement therapy (HRT) reduces climacteric symptoms, has favorable effects on bone metabolism and osteoporosis, and possibly on ischemic heart disease and other cardiovascular diseases [1-3]. It may also reduce the risk of colorectal cancer [4]. Total mortality among women who use postmenopausal hormones is lower than among nonusers, which probably to a large extent reflects favorable health characteristics of women who decide to use HRT [5,6].

HRT, however, has also a number of adverse effects, the main ones being a promotional effect on endometrial cancer, and some elevation in the risk of breast and perhaps ovarian cancer [4,6,7].

Breast Cancer

Most information on HRT and breast cancer comes from a re-analysis of individual data from 51 epidemiological studies, conducted in 21 countries and including 52,705 women with breast cancer and 108,411 controls [8]. This showed a 2.3% (95% confidence interval, CI 1.1-3.6%) increase in the relative risk (RR) of breast cancer for each year of HRT use. This corresponds to a RR of 1.35 (95% CI 1.20-1.49) for current users who had used HRT for 5 years or more, and to a cumulative excess for women who began use of HRT at age 50 of approximately 2 cases/1,000 women for 5-year users, 6 cases/1,000 women for 10-year users, and 12 cases/1,000 women for 15-year users. This increase was comparable with the effect on breast cancer of later menopause, since among never-users of HRT the RR of breast cancer increased by 2.8% (95% CI 2.1- 3.4%) for each increasing year at menopause. This elevated risk, however, leveled off after stopping HRT use, with no material excess risk observed five or more years after stopping, as compared to never-users. The elevated risk associated to late menopause, in contrast, tended to persist for several years [9].

Use of HRT for a short time (i.e. < 5 years) to control menopausal symptoms is not related to any material increase in the risk of breast and perhaps ovarian cancer [8,10,11]. The biologic mechanism underlying this association remains unclear. Changes in the composition of the breast tissue have been documented, with greater mammographic densities having been noted following hormone use [12]. Also of interest is whether genetic factors, including polymorphisms in hormone metabolizing genes, might be etiologically involved.

Another open question is the impact on breast cancer risk of the combination of estrogens and progestins, a therapy effective in reducing the excess endometrial cancer risk associated with estrogen use alone [13]. There are biological reasons to suspect an unfavorable effect of added progestins on breast carcinogenesis, since ovulatory cycles are related to breast cancer risk, and breast mitotic activity is higher during the luteal phase of the cycle [14,15]. An early report of a Swedish cohort study [16] suggested that combined HRT may be more strongly related to breast cancer risk than estrogens alone, with a nonsignificantly elevated relative risk (RR) of 1.2 for ever-use and of 4.4 for more than six-years use, based on 10 cases (hence a wide confidence interval of, CI 0.9- 22.4). An update of the same study [17], confirmed these findings, showing RRs of 1.4 after 1-6 years and 1.7 after more than 6 years of use of combined preparations. The excess risk, however, appeared confined to recent users. Three other studies from Britain [18], Denmark [19], and Sweden [20] showed an association between combined HRT and breast cancer.

A report from the American Nurses Health Study cohort [21] confirmed some excess breast cancer risk among current long-term HRT users: the RRs were 1.3 (95% CI 1.1-1.5) for conjugated estrogen users, 1.3 (95% CI 1.0-1.7) for other estrogen users, and 1.4 (95% CI 1.2-1.7) for estrogen plus progestin. A case-control study in Sweden, involving 3,345 women with breast cancer, found a trend of increasing risk with duration of different types of combined estrogen-progestin use (RR = 2.4 for women treated for at least 10 years) [22].

A report on 46,355 participants followed for a mean of 10.2 years in the Breast Cancer Detection and Demonstration Project showed that women who had used combined estrogen and progesterone had a 40 percent increased incidence rate (RR = 1.4, 95% CI 1.1-1.8) of developing breast cancer compared with never-users [23]. Furthermore, the risk from combined therapy was greater than that observed with unopposed estrogen (20% increase in risk, 95% CI 1.0-1.4). The increased risk was limited to use within the prior four years; women who had used HRT in the past but stopped did not have an increased risk for breast cancer. The increased risk was also largely confined to women with a body mass index of 24.4 or less, which indicates that there could be a threshold effect of HRT, since heavier women are likely to have a higher average level of endogenous estrogen that in itself increases risk.

Likewise, a population-based case-control study of 1,897 postmenopausal cases and 1,637 postmenopausal population controls from Los Angeles County [24] found a RR of 1.06 (95% CI 0.97-1.15) for each 5 years of estrogen replacement therapy use, but of 1.24 (95% CI 1.07-1.45) for combined estrogen-progestin treatment, thus suggesting that addition of a progestin to HRT enhances the risk of breast cancer relative to estrogen use alone. The excess risk for combined therapy may be around 5% per year, as compared with 2.3% for estrogen alone. The data of various studies are inconsistent with reference to sequential versus continuous therapy.

A case-control study from Washington state [25] suggested that combined HRT increases the risk of lobular, but not ductal breast carcinoma, but the findings are inconclusive due to the small number of exposed cases.

Another major issue is the time-risk relation after stopping HRT. The effect of steroid hormones is thought to be on the later stages of carcinogenesis (i.e. they are promoters); consequently, the increased breast cancer risk associated with HRT declines within a few years after stopping use [26].

Although the absence of a long-term cumulative risk is reassuring, a 20 to 30% excess risk of breast cancer in women aged 50 to 65 years (when HRT use is most frequent) has to be weighed against the benefits of HRT on the bone and perhaps on the cardiovascular system, since the incidence of breast cancer in the sixth decade of life is high [27,28].

There are no data from clinical trials on the HRT-breast cancer association, but the Postmenopause Estrogen/Progestin Intervention (PEPI) trial reported that increased mammographic density was observed in 3.5% of the estrogen-only group, but in 16 to 23% of the different estrogen/progestin schedules [29].

Although hormone replacement therapy has been associated with an increased incidence of breast cancer, use appears to lead to lower mortality from breast cancer or improved prognosis in some [11,20,30-32], although not all [4,33], studies. Although some of this effect may be due to increased breast cancer surveillance among hormone users, a favorable biologic effect of hormone use on the biologic characteristics of breast tumors cannot be dismissed [32,34].

In the American Cancer Society Cancer Prevention Study II, breast cancer mortality did not increase with estrogen use overall and no excess risk was observed for thin or heavy women [35].

Although a diagnosis of breast cancer has been conventionally viewed as a contraindication for subsequent HRT use, this notion is being questioned given data showing a favorable effects of HRT on breast cancer prognosis [36]. Although the few studies that have addressed this issue seem to indicate no adverse effects of HRT usage among breast cancer survivors, sample sizes have been limited [37].

Endometrial Cancer

An association of endometrial cancer with HRT was suggested on the basis of a substantial rise in the incidence of endometrial cancer seen in the United States in the early 1970s, following widespread HRT use. Epidemiological evidence confirmed the association between estrogen use and endometrial cancer risk, and the persistence of elevated risk several years after cessation of use [4,6,7,38]. The summary RR for ever versus never estrogen users from a meta-analysis of published studies was 2.3 (95% CI 2.1-2.5) [39]; the RR were similar for cohort (RR 1.7) and case-control studies using hospital or population controls. The risk was related to duration of use: the RR was 1.4 for use < 1 year, 2.8 for 1 to 5 years, 5.9 for 5-9 years and 9.5 for ≥ 10 years [39]. The risk was also inversely related with time since last use [39], suggesting that estrogens have a late-stage effect in endometrial carcinogenesis [26,40].

Estrogen-associated risks for endometrial cancer tend to be higher in leaner than overweight women, who have higher endogenous estrogen levels and availability [41]. Some studies suggested a greater excess risk among smokers [42,43] (who tend to have lower estrogen availability), and a lower excess risk among ex-users of combined oral contraceptives [43,44]

Data on type of estrogen, dose, bioavailability, regimen, or duration of use are inconsistent; overall these variables appear not clearly associated, although users of high-dose preparations tend to have a higher risk [4,38]. In the meta-analysis by Grady et al. [39], the RR was 3.9 for users of 0.3 mg conjugated estrogens, 3.4 for users of 0.625 mg, and 5.8 for users of ≥1.25 mg. As for the type of compound used, the RR was 2.5 for users of conjugated estrogens and 1.3 for users of synthetic estrogens [39]. The cyclic addition of progestins to estrogens for at least 7 days/month protects against endometrial hyperplasia (a supposed precursor of endometrial cancer) [4]. The RR from a meta-analysis of endometrial cancer in women using cyclic combined therapy was 0.8 (95% CI 0.6-2.2) [39]. The number of days/month of progestin addition is an important determinant of risk. In a study from Washington State the RR was reduced from 2.4 to 1.1 for addition of progestins for = 10 days/month [45], and in another from California [46], the RR for ever-users was 3.1 for < 10 days/month of added progestins and 1.3 for 10-21 days. Another study from Los Angeles County [47] showed RRs for 5 year use of 2.2 for unopposed estrogen, 1.9 for estrogens plus progestins for < 10 days/month, and 1.1 (95% CI 0.8-1.4) for progestins added for = 10 days/month. A Swedish study of postmenopausal women confirmed a strong association of endometrial cancer with unopposed estrogen use (RR 6.2 for estradiol and 6.6 for conjugated estrogens for = 5 year use), with a much weaker association for the combination of estrogens and progestins (RR 1.6, 95% CI 1.1-2.4), and an inverse association for continuous use of progestins (RR 0.2, 95% CI 0.1-0.8 for = 5 year use) [48]. A record linkage study, conducted in Sweden on a cohort of 8,438 women at risk of endometrial cancer, found a RR of 4.2 for = 6 year use of unopposed estrogens, and of 1.4 for combined estrogen and progestin therapy [49]. In a Canadian study the RR was 4.1 for use of > 5 year use of unopposed HRT, and around 1.5 for various types of combined therapies [50]. According to a nationwide cohort study from Finland, the long-cycle (3-months) HRT use was associated with a greater endometrial cancer risk (RR 2.0) compared to monthly cycle HRT (RR 1.3) [51].

Ovarian Cancer

Two cohort studies showed no association between use of HRT and ovarian cancer risk, including the Walnut Creek Study on contraception [52], based on 16,638 women followed up for 13 years (RR 1.0), and a Swedish cohort study [53], based on 23,246 women followed up for an average 8.6 years. In contrast, in the American Cancer Society Cancer Prevention Study II [54], based on mortality data of 243,073 women followed up for ≥ 11 years, the RR was 1.71 (95% CI 1.06-2.77); this elevated risk was not explained by other known or likely risk factors for ovarian cancer. The 14-year follow-up of the American Cancer Society's Cancer Prevention Study II [55] confirmed the association between HRT and ovarian cancer risk. The RR was 1.5 (95% CI 1.2-2.0) for ever use, and 2.2 (95% CI

1.5-3.2) for user ≥ 10 years at baseline. Among former users, the RR decreased with time since last use.

A re-analysis of individual data of 12 US case-control studies, based on 2,197 white women with invasive epithelial ovarian cancer [56], found a pooled RR of invasive ovarian cancer for ever-HRT use of 0.9 in hospital-based and 1.1 in population-based studies, with no consistent duration-risk relation. A collaborative re-analysis of 4 European studies from the UK, Italy, and Greece, based on 1,470 women with ovarian cancer, found a RR of 1.71 (95% CI 1.30-2.25) for ever-HRT use, a weak positive association with duration of use, and some indication that the excess risk for ovarian cancer declined with time since last use [57]. The overall RR estimate from a meta-analysis of published data was 1.15 (95% CI 1.0-1.3) for ever use, and 1.27 (95% CI 1.0-1.6) for >10 years use [58].

Colorectal Cancer

Colorectal cancer is the most frequent cancer site in nonsmokers of both sexes combined in western countries. Over the last two decades, mortality rates from colorectal cancer in many developed countries have declined in women but not in men [59] suggesting a role for exogenous female hormones (i.e. oral contraceptives and HRT) on these trends [60].

Eight cohort studies reported information on HRT use and colorectal cancer risk, for a total of over 2,400 cases. Most studies showed RRs around or below unity. A significant inverse association was found in two cohort investigations (including the largest one) focusing on fatal colon cancers. Findings from a recent study suggested that HRT use may improve short-term survival after a diagnosis of colon cancer [61].

Among 12 case-control studies for a total of over 5,000 cases, 5 reported 20-40% significant risk reductions among ever-HRT users [60]. Two additional investigations showed moderate, nonsignificant inverse associations.

Studies showing an inverse association between HRT use and colorectal cancer were among the largest and best controlled ones. The apparent protection tended to be stronger among recent users. Differences in RRs by duration of HRT use and anatomic subsite were not consistent [62].

A meta-analysis of 20 studies published up to December 1996 [63] found an overall RR for ever-HRT use of 0.85 (95% CI 0.7-0.9). The protection was greater for current or recent users (RR 0.69, 95% CI 0.5-0.9) and users of > 5 years (RR 0.73, 95% CI 0.5-1.0).

HRT users may differ from nonusers for colorectal cancer risk factor exposure. Postmenopausal women treated with HRT tend to have higher social class and longer education [64], which may imply a healthier lifestyle (e.g. higher consumption of vegetables, more physical activity, and less being overweight). In addition, long-term HRT users are, by definition, compliant, which is, *per se*, a favorable health indicator [65].

Several biological mechanisms are plausible. Sex hormones modify hepatic cholesterol production and alter bile acid concentration [66]. Secondary bile acids are believed to favor malignant changes in the colonic epithelium, and exogenous estrogens, which decrease secondary bile acid production and can alter intestinal microflora, could, therefore, protect against colorectal cancer.

Issa et al. [67] suggested that methylation-associated inactivation of the estrogen receptor (ER) gene in aging colorectal mucosa could predispose to colorectal tumorigenesis. Exogenous estrogens may counteract the natural decline of circulating estrogens in postmenopausal women. However, data on reproductive and menstrual correlates of colorectal cancer risk are inconclusive [68].

In western countries, the number of deaths from colorectal and breast cancers in women aged 55 or older are similar; thus, a decrease in incidence or mortality from colorectal cancer could greatly affect the balance of risks and benefits associated with the use of HRT.

Selective Estrogen Receptor Modulators

Given the recognized adverse effects of HRT, much recent attention has focused on assessing alternative approaches to treat menopause, including use of tamoxifen and other selective estrogen receptor modulators (SERMs). These agents are recognized anti-estrogens, which presumably will offer many of the same advantages as HRT, while eliminating some of the disadvantages, for instance the HRT-induced (increase in the risk of breast cancer).

In the National Surgical Adjuvant Breast and Colorectal Project (NSABP), a total of 13,388 US ≥ 60 years old women, or with 5 year risk of ≥ 1.66 % of developing breast cancer, or with a history of lobular carcinoma *in situ* were randomly assigned to receive 20 mg daily of tamoxifen or placebo for 5 years [69]. After 69 months of follow-up, women receiving tamoxifen had a 49% lower risk of invasive breast cancer than placebo-treated women. The reduction in risk was limited to estrogen receptor positive tumors. The adverse effects noted in the trial, included excess risks of endometrial cancer, stroke, pulmonary embolism and deep-vein thrombosis, events occurring more frequently in women ≥ 50 years.

Two other clinical trials of tamoxifen in breast cancer prevention have presented *ad interim* results. In a British trial, 2,494 women aged 30-70 years with a family history of breast cancer were randomly assigned to tamoxifen or placebo and followed for up to 8 years [70]. The risk of invasive or *in situ* breast cancer was 1.06 in the group given tamoxifen compared to the group given placebo. In a trial conducted in Italy, 5,408 women who had a hysterectomy were randomized to 5 years of tamoxifen or placebo [71]. After a median of 46 months follow-up, there was no difference in breast cancer incidence by treatment arm. Despite the inconsistent trial results, the U.S. FDA has approved use of tamoxifen for breast cancer risk reduction in high risk women [72].

Less information is available on other SERMs. In the Multiple Outcomes of Raloxifene Evaluation (MORE) trial of 7,705 postmenopausal osteoporotic women under age 81, 60 or 120 mg of raloxifene daily decreased breast cancer risk by 76% (RR 0.24, 95% CI, 0.1-0.4) compared to nonusers [73]. Risk for thromboembolic disease was increased 3-fold, but there was no increased risk for endometrial cancer in raloxifene-treated compared with placebo-treated women. The U.S. National Cancer Institute and the NSABP are now conducting a large, multi-center study to test tamoxifen versus raloxifene.

Research is also beginning to focus on whether more natural approaches to treating the menopause should be recommended. Although there is growing enthusiasm for use of phytoestrogens, considered by some people as "natural" SERMs [74], their effects on cancer risk remain unresolved.

Acknowledgment

This work was conducted with the contribution of the Italian Association for Cancer Research. The authors thank Mrs. M.P. Bonifacino for editorial assistance.

References

1. Brinton LA, Schairer C. Postmenopausal hormone-replacement therapy—Time for a reappraisal? [Editorial]. N Engl J Med 1997;336:1821-22.
2. La Vecchia C. Sex hormones and cardiovascular risk. Hum Reprod 1992;7:162-67.
3. Meade TW, Vickers MR. HRT and cardiovascolar disease. J Epidemiol Biostatistics 1999; 4:165-90.
4. IARC, International Agency for Research on Cancer. IARC Monograph on the Evaluation of Carcinogenic Risks to Humans, Vol.72. Hormonal Contraception and Post-menopausal Hormonal Therapy. IARC, Lyon, 1999.
5. Grodstein F, Stampfer MJ, Colditz GA, et al. Postmenopausal hormone therapy and mortality. N Engl J Med 1997;336:1769-75.
6. Beral V, Banks E, Reeves G, Appleby P. Use of HRT and the subsequent risk of cancer. J Epidemiol Biostatistics 1999;4:191-215.
7. Tavani A, La Vecchia C. The adverse effects of hormone replacement therapy. Drugs Aging 1999;14:347-57.
8. Collaborative Group on Hormonal Factors in Breast Cancer. Breast cancer and hormone replacement therapy: Collaborative reanalysis of data from 51 epidemiological studies of 52,705 women with breast cancer and 108,411 women without breast cancer. Lancet 1997; 350:1047-59.
9. La Vecchia C. Reproductive surgery, menopause and breast cance risk. Eur J Cancer 1999; 35:12-13.
10. Brinton LA, Schairer C. Estrogen replacement therapy and breast cancer risk. Epidemiol Rev 1993;15:66-79.
11. Willis DB, Calle EE, Miracle-McMahill HL, et al. Estrogen replacement therapy and risk of fatal breast cancer in a prospective cohort of postmenopausal women in the United States. Cancer Causes Control 1996;7:449-57.
12. Laya MB, Gallagher JC, Schreiman JS, et al. Effect of postmenopausal hormonal replacement therapy on mammographic density and parenchymal pattern. Radiology 1995; 196:433-37.
13. The Writing Group on the PEPI Trial. Effects of hormone replacement therapy on endometrial histology in postmenopausal women. The Postmenopausal Estrogen/Progestin Intervention (PEPI) Trial. JAMA 1996;275:370-75.
14. Pike MC, Spicer DV, Dahmoush L, et al. Estrogens, progestogens, normal breast cell proliferation, and breast cancer risk. Epidemiol Rev 1993;15:17-35.
15. Stanford JL, Thomas DH. Exogenous progestins and breast cancer. Epidemiol Rev 1993;

15:98-107.
16. Bergkvist L, Adami H-O, Persson I, et al. The risk of breast cancer after estrogen and estrogen-progestin replacement. N Engl J Med 1989;321:293-97.
17. Persson I, Weiderpass E, Bergkvist L, et al. Risks of breast and endometrial cancer after estrogen and estrogen-progestin replacement. Cancer Causes Control 1999;10:253-60.
18. Hunt K, Vessey M, McPherson K, et al. Long-term surveillance of mortality and cancer incidence in women receiving hormone replacement therapy. Br J Obstet Gynaecol 1987; 94:620-35.
19. Ewertz M. Influence of non-contraceptive exogenous and endogenous sex hormones on breast cancer risk in Denmark. Int J Cancer 1988;42:832-38.
20. Persson I, Yuen J, Bergkvist L, et al. Cancer incidence and mortality in women receiving estrogen and estrogen-progestin replacement therapy—long-term follow-up of a Swedish cohort. Int J Cancer 1996;67:327-32.
21. Colditz GA, Hankinson SE, Hunter DJ, et al. The use of estrogens and progestins and the risk of breast cancer in postmenopausal women. N Engl J Med 1995;332:1589-93.
22. Magnusson C, Baron JA, Correia N, et al. Breast-cancer risk following long-term oestrogen- and oestrogen-progestin-replacement therapy. Int J Cancer 1999;81:339-344.
23. Schairer C, Lubin J, Troisi R, et al. Menopausal estrogen and estrogen-progestin replacement therapy and breast cancer risk. JAMA 2000;283:485-91.
24. Ross RK, Paganini-Hill A, Wan PC, Pike MC. Effect of hormone replacement therapy on breast cancer risks: estrogen versus estrogen plus progestin. J Natl Cancer Inst 2000;92: 328-32.
25. Li CI, Weiss NS, Stanford JL, Daling JR. Hormone replacement therapy in relation to risk of lobular and ductal breast carcinoma in middle-aged women. Cancer 2000;88:2570-77.
26. Day NE. Epidemiology: The role of multi-stage models. Cancer Surv 1983;2:579-93.
27. La Vecchia C, Negri E, Franceschi S, et al. Hormone replacement treatment and breast cancer risk: A cooperative Italian study. Br J Cancer 1995;72:244-48.
28. Steinberg KK, Thacker SB, Smith SJ, et al. A meta-analysis of the effect of estrogen replacement therapy on the risk of breast cancer. JAMA 1991;265:1985-90.
29. Greendale GA, Reboussin BA, Sie A, et al. Effects of estrogen and estrogen-progestin on mammographic parenchymal density. Ann Intern Med 1999;130:262-69.
30. Henderson BE, Paganini-Hill A, Ross RK. Decreased mortality in users of estrogen replacement therapy. Arch Intern Med 1991;151:75-78.
31. Hunt K, Vessey M, McPherson K. Mortality in a cohort of long-term users of hormone replacement therapy: an updated analysis. Br J Obstet Gynaecol 1990;97:1080-86.
32. Schairer C, Gail M, Byrne C, et al. Estrogen replacement therapy and breast cancer survival in a large screening study. J Natl Cancer Inst 1999;91:264-70.
33. Ewertz M, Gillanders S, Meyer L, Zedeler K. Survival of breast cancer patients in relation to factors which affect the risk of developing breast cancer. Int J Cancer 1991;49:526-30.
34. Gapstur SM, Morrow M, Sellers TA. Hormone replacement therapy and risk of breast cancer with favorable histology: Results of the Iowa Women's Health Study. JAMA 1999; 281:2091-97.
35. Rodriguez C, Calle EE, Patel AV, et al. Effect of body mass on the association between estrogen replacement therapy and mortality among elderly US women. Am J Epidemiol 2001;153:145-52.
36. Chlebowski RT, McTiernan A. Elements of informed consent for hormone replacement therapy in patients with diagnosed breast cancer. J Clin Oncol 1999;17:130-42.

37. Eden JA, Brush T, Nand S, Wren BG. A case-control study of combined continuous estrogen-progestin replacement therapy among women with a personal history of breast cancer. Menopause: J North Am Menopause Soc 1995;2:67-72.
38. La Vecchia C, Brinton L, McTiernan A. Cancer risk associated with menopausal hormones. In: Menopause and Women's Health: A Comprehensive Approach. Bethesda, Md., US, GPO, 2001, in press.
39. Grady D, Gebretsadik T, Kerlikowske K, et al. Hormone replacement therapy and endometrial cancer risk: A meta-analysis. Obstet Gynecol 1995;85:304-13.
40. Finkle WD, Greenland S, Miettinen OS, et al. Endometrial cancer risk after discontinuing use of unopposed conjugated estrogens (California, United States). Cancer Causes Control 1995;6:99-102.
41. Shields TS, Weiss NS, Voigt LF, et al. The additional risk of endometrial cancer associated with unopposed estrogen use in women with other risk factors. Epidemiology 1999;10:733-38.
42. Baron JA, La Vecchia C, Levi F. The antiestrogenic effect of cigarette smoking in women. Am J Obstet Gynecol 1990;162:502-14.
43. Brinton LA, Hoover RN, for the Endometrial Cancer Collaborative Group. Estrogen replacement therapy and endometrial cancer risk: Unresolved issues. Obstet Gynecol 1993; 81:265-71.
44. Levi F, La Vecchia C, Gulie C, et al. Oestrogen replacement treatment and the risk of endometrial cancer: An assessment of the role of covariates. Eur J Cancer 1993;29A:1445-49.
45. Voigt LF, Weiss NS, Chu J, et al. Progestagen supplementation of exogenous oestrogens and risk of endometrial cancer. Lancet 1991;338:274-77.
46. Beresford SAA, Weiss NS, Voigt LF, et al. Risk of endometrial cancer in relation to use of oestrogen combined with cyclic progestagen therapy in postmenopausal women. Lancet 1997;349:458-61.
47. Pike MC, Peters RK, Cozen W, et al. Estrogen-progestin replacement therapy and endometrial cancer. J Natl Cancer Inst 1997;89:1110-16.
48. Weiderpass E, Adami H-O, Baron JA, et al. Risk of endometrial cancer following estrogen replacement with and without progestins. J Natl Cancer Inst 1999;91:1131-37.
49. Persson I, Thurfjell E, Bergstrom R, Holmberg L. Hormone replacement therapy and the risk of breast cancer Nested case-control study in a cohort of Swedish women attending mammography screening. Int J Cancer 1997;72:758-61.
50. Jain MG, Rhoan TE, Howe GR. Hormonal replacement therapy and endometrial cancer in Ontario, Canada. J Clin Epidemiol 2000;53:385-91.
51. Pukkala E, Tulenheimo-Silfvast A, Leminen A. Incidence of cancer among women using long versus monthly cycle hormonal replacement therapy, Finland 1994-1997. Cancer Causes Control 2001;12:111-15.
52. Petitti, DB, Perlman, JA, Sidney S. Noncontraceptive estrogens and mortality: Long-term follow-up of women in the Walnut Creek Study. Obstet Gynecol 1987;70:289-93.
53. Schairer C, Adami H-O, Hoover R, et al. Causes-specific mortality in women receiving hormone replacement therapy. Epidemiology 1997;8:59-65.
54. Rodriguez C, Calle EE, Coates RJ, et al. Estrogen replacement therapy and fatal ovarian cancer. Am J Epidemiol 1995;141:828-35.
55. Rodriguez C, Patel AV, Calle EE, Jacob EJ, Thun MJ. Estrogen replacement therapy and ovarian cancer mortality in a large prospective study of US women. JAMA 2001;285:

1460-65.
56. Whittemore AS, Harris R, Itnyre J, et al. Characteristics relating to ovarian cancer risk: collaborative analysis of 12 US case-control studies. II. Invasive epithelial ovarian cancers in white women. Am J Epidemiol 1992;136:1184-203.
57. Negri E, Tzonou A, Beral V, et al. Hormonal therapy for menopause and ovarian cancer in a collaborative re-analysis of European studies. Int J Cancer 1999;80:848-51 .
58. Garg PP, Kerlikowske K, Subak L, Grady D. Hormone replacement therapy and the risk of epithelial ovarian carcinoma: A meta-analysis. Obstet Gynecol 1998;92:472-79.
59. La Vecchia C, Negri E, Levi F, et al. Cancer mortality in Europe: Effects of age, cohort of birth and period of death. Eur J Cancer 1998;34:118-41.
60. Franceschi S, La Vecchia C. Colorectal cancer and hormone replacement therapy: An unexpected finding. Eur J Cancer Prev 1998;7:427-38.
61. Slattery ML, Anderson K, Samowitz W, et al. Hormone replacement therapy and improved survival among postmenopausal women diagnosed with colon cancer (USA). Cancer Causes Control 1999;10:467-73.
62. Fernandez E, Franceschi S, La Vecchia C. Colorectal cancer and hormone replaement therapy: A review of epidemiological studies. J Br Menop Soc 2000;6:8-14.
63. Herbert-Croteau N. A meta-analysis of hormone replacement therapy and colon cancer among women. Cancer Epidemiol Biomarkers Prev 1998;7:653-59.
64. Barrett-Connor E. Postmenopausal estrogen and prevention bias. Ann Intern Med 1991; 115:455-56.
65. Parazzini F, La Vecchia C, Negri E, et al. Determinants of estrogen replacement therapy use in northern Italy. Rev Epidem et Santé Publ 1993;41:53-58.
66. McMichael AJ, Potter JD. Host factors in carcinogenesis: Certain bile-acid metabolic profiles that selectively increase the risk of proximal colon cancer. J Natl Cancer Inst 1985;75:185-91.
67. Issa JP, Ottaviano YL, Celano P, et al. Methylation of the oestrogen receptor CpG island links ageing and neoplasia in human colon. Nature Genet 1994;7:536-40.
68. Fernandez E, La Vecchia C, Balducci A, et al. Oral contraceptives and colorectal cancer risk: A meta-analysis. Br J Cancer 2001;84:722-27.
69. Fisher B, Constantino JP, Wickerham DL, et al. Tamoxifen for prevention of breast cancer: Report of the National Surgical Adjuvant Breast and Bowel Project P-1 Study. J Natl Cancer Inst 1998;90:1371-88.
70. Powles T, Eeles R, Ashley S, et al. Interim analysis of the incidence of breast cancer in the Royal Marsden Hospital tamoxifen randomised chemoprevention trial. Lancet 1998;352: 98-101.
71. Veronesi U, Maisonneuve P, Costa A, et al. Prevention of breast cancer with tamoxifen: Preliminary findings from the Italian randomised trial among hysterectomised women. Italian Tamoxifen Prevention Study. Lancet 1998;352:93-97.
72. Gail MH, Constantino JP, Bryant J, et al. Weighing the risks and benefits of tamoxifen treatment for preventing breast cancer. J Natl Cancer Inst 1999;91:1829-46.
73. Cummings SB, Eckert S, Kreuger KA, et al. The effects of raloxifene on risk of breast cancer in postmenopausal women. Results from the MORE randomized trial. JAMA 1999; 281:2189-97.
74. Brzezinski A, Debi A. Phytoestrogens: The "natural" selective estrogen receptor modulators? Eur J Obstet Gynecol Reprod Biol 1999;85:47-51.

Sociocultural Issues in Menopause

Aila Collins

Opposing Models of Menopause

In recent years there has been a dramatic increase in research on women's health in menopause. There is no doubt that biomedical research dominates the field. Since it is ultimately up to women to decide about their own health, it is important to understand the different factors that influence women's experiences in menopause. Psychosocial scientists have pointed out that women's experience of menopause is profoundly influenced by their perception of bodily changes and their perception of how menopause is viewed in their particular society [1-3]. However, controversy and polarization of views still fuel the debate as to how best to conceptualize the menopausal experience of women. The biomedical model of menopause has focused on the biological aspects of declining hormonal levels and on identifying symptoms of the climacteric syndrome. Menopause is thus characterized as a deficiency disease requiring intervention and the treatment is hormone replacement therapy (HRT). It should be emphasized that the only symptoms that have been directly associated with decreasing estrogen levels are night sweats and hot flashes [4]. Management of the menopause is one of the most controversial issues in medical practice today since there are a multitude of different interventions available.

Women increasingly face conflicting images of menopause and thus decisions about treatment in the context of different ideologies [5]. Several critics have emphasized that the biomedical model is negative and may have an influence on how women view themselves and how they are seen in society. This may lead to medicalization lending menopausal women dependent on the medical establishment. Women may feel that they are not in control of their own health and have to seek medical advice in order to be diagnosed as menopausal [6,7]. Media are also portraying the image of menopause as a condition that needs intervention and treatment. Gannon and Stevens [8] found that the portrayal of menopause in the popular media has increased, but the growing attention and the information conveyed is mainly focussed on menopause as a medical condition.

Social scientists on the other hand, have emphasized the social and cultural construct of menopause, describing menopause as a natural event and a life transition requiring adaptation and psychosocial change. Whether climacteric symptoms are experienced and the intensity of these is associated with the meaning attached to menopause in a particular society and the different roles of women. According to the sociocultural model, it is the meaning given to menopause and the perception of older woman in a particular society that will influence women's experience of menopause. The attitudes towards women and the status of women at midlife are critical influences in shaping women's experience of menopause [1,9,10].

More recent trends in epidemiological research have highlighted the need to integrate these two opposing views into a more holistic, interactive model that takes into account more complex and multifaceted aspects of menopause. Flint [11] suggested a psycho-bio-cultural model of menopause for interdisciplinary research and for a better understanding of the different aspects of women's health. Olazabal and his colleagues [5] also have suggested a more holistic approach to menopause, a more balanced view.

Symptom Reporting in a Cross-Cultural Perspective

A challenging question that has been posed is whether menopause is universally associated with the same somatic changes and symptoms, or whether there is cross-cultural variation. In this context cross-cultural comparative studies can help clarify the extent to which the experience of menopause is universal, provide information about symptom variability, and identify important factors influencing the experience of symptoms. Comparison regarding prevalence of symptoms such as hot flushes and psychological symptoms such as depression or sexual interest show considerable variation among countries. One of the best known differences and the one that has received the most attention is the marked contrast between the high prevalence of vasomotor symptoms reported by women in Europe and North America compared with the relatively low prevalence reported by Asian women. Lock's classic studies of Japanese menopausal women [12-14] have been frequently cited. She studied working women and homemakers residing in Kyoto, Nagano, and Kobe by interviewing them and having them fill out symptom ratings. The results showed that the Japanese women experienced a very low frequency of hot flushes: 3% of the homemakers and 10% of the working women reported them although they had a higher incidence of shoulder stiffness and headache. The results also revealed that the Japanese women did not even have a word for hot flushes and the term had to be explained by using different words. Avis et al. remarked on the lack of a word for hot flushes particularly since the Japanese language is generally rather sensitive in describing bodily sensations.

A comparison of U.S., Canadian, and Japanese women by Avis et al. [15] confirmed Lock's results and showed that the symptom profile in Japanese women is quite distinct from their North American counterparts. The Japanese women had the lowest prevalence of hot flushes and depression as well as the lowest intake of medication. The Japanese sample consistently differed from the U.S. and Canadian samples and the rates reported by the Japanese women were generally low. Thirteen of the 16 symptoms studied were rated less than 15% and the highest rate for the Japanese was 27.5% for headaches. In contrast, the symptom rates for the two North American samples were very similar. Comparing the number of core symptoms across the three groups yielded a similar result with Japanese women showing markedly lower rates of multiple symptoms and nearly double the rate for no symptoms compared with the North American women. The use of hormone replacement therapy is also very low in Japan (2.5%). These findings suggest that Asian women do not experience the intense symptoms reported by North American, European, and African women. Lock's interpretation of the results implied that these differences could be explained in terms of the sociocultural meaning of menopause in Japanese society. It is interesting that the Japanese word for midlife transition, "konenki," has social rather than biologic connotations. Another possible explanation is that the observed differences are associated with the diet, which is rich in phytoestrogens, a compound that may have a protective effect [16].

More recent studies of Asian women have shown a more varied picture in that women do report hot flushes but the frequency is generally low and psychological symptoms are rated higher. Boulet and her colleagues [17] in a study of Southeast Asian countries showed that the rate of vasomotor symptoms reported was lower than in western countries and the rate of psychological symptoms was more frequent. Among Chinese women living in Hong Kong about 10% of those who replied to a survey [18] reported hot flushes and again, psychological complaints such as anxiety and nervousness were more prevalent. A study by Hilditch et al. [19] of the frequency and distress experienced by Canadian and Chinese women showed that the women ranked the symptoms very differently. Sixty percent of the Canadian women and 18% of the Chinese women reported hot flushes and the Chinese women ranked other symptoms as more important including poor memory, boredom, numbness in the hands and feet, change in appearance, as well as change in vision, taste, and smell. However, similar rates were reported by the two groups of women for sleep-related symptoms and fatigue. The prevalence of hot flushes thus appears to be lower in Asian women and the types of symptoms are often different. These differences are not readily explained. Vasomotor symptoms such as hot flushes have been directly linked to estrogen deficiency. However, our study [20] and that of Avis et al. [21] showed that hot flushes are modulated by psychosocial factors such as work role, satisfaction with work, and stress at work.

Symptoms across Ethnic and Racial Groups

There are important factors within cultures that may mediate symptom experience. They include differences in attitudes toward aging and menopause as well as socioeconomic factors and women's roles and opportunities in society. An important area of research which has been largely neglected until recently is the study of different ethnic groups within western cultures. In an ongoing population-based study of working women aged 47 to 52 years and residing in the Stockholm area we examined the association between menopause-related symptoms, socioeconomic factors, and quality of work role. The sample reflected a population-based ethnic and socioeconomic diversity and included 950 working women who responded to a health questionnaire. Seventy-nine percent of the women were born in Sweden, 8% were born in another Scandinavian country, and 12% were born outside Scandinavia. Analyses of the data showed that women who were born outside Scandinavia reported more frequent hot flushes compared with Swedish-born women (Collins and Ahs, unpublished data). The women born outside Scandinavia rated more severe symptoms overall and more frequent general health problems than the Swedish-born women after adjusting for education and menopausal status. One possible explanation for these differences may be that immigrant women have a more difficult and more stressful life compared to Swedish-born women. However, their conception of menopause in terms of it being a natural process rather than an illness did not differ significantly from the Scandinavian-born women. We are addressing these issues in depth in the ongoing longitudinal study of women and working life.

Research results from a study of an urban sample of perimenopausal women in the United States [22] found that African-American women were significantly more likely than white women to report menopause-related symptoms. After adjusting for education, income, and body mass index, race remained a significant predictor of hot flushes and other physiological symptoms. Furthermore, the physiological symptom ratings increased with age in African-American women, whereas the reverse was true for white women. The African-American women also reported higher depression scores than the white women. Despite the high prevalence of symptoms few African-American women had discussed treatment of menopausal symptoms with a physician although a relatively large proportion (42%) were motivated to talk to and learn more from a physician about menopause. There may be biases in the prescription of HRT to African-American women. A study by Brown et al. [23] showed that different ethnic groups in the U.S., among them African-Americans, were much less likely to be prescribed HRT as compared with white women. These differences could be associated with problems in communication between patient and doctor. Pham et al. [24] reported that the African-American women tended to see menopause as a natural event and preferred nonprescription remedies for relief of menopausal symptoms. They also relied on family and friends as primary sources of information.

The large-scale, population-based Study of Women's Health Across the Nation (SWAN) in the United States [25] compared symptom reporting among white, African-America, Chinese-American, Japanese-American, and Hispanic women. The Asian-American women had significantly fewer symptoms compared with white women and the African-American women had the highest prevalence of vasomotor symptoms. Comparison of the attitudes of the different groups showed that the African-American women had the most positive attitudes to menopause, whereas the immigrant Asian women had the most negative attitudes.

Conclusions

Attitudes toward and beliefs about menopause vary considerably historically and cross-culturally. Women increasingly face conflicting images of menopause. In the past decade there has been a heated debate among scientists from different disciplines whether menopause should be seen as a deficiency disease or as a natural stage of life. A central issue concerns whether menopause is characterized by similar symptoms in different countries or whether there is cultural variation in symptom reporting. Cross-cultural comparisons have demonstrated that there are distinct differences in pattern and prevalence of symptoms between women from different cultures and ethnic background. Thus, the data derived from such studies do not support a universal menopausal deficiency syndrome, instead symptoms seem to be modulated by cultural norms, beliefs, and traditions. Sociocultural factors should be recognized as important in mediating women's experience of menopause. However, methodological flaws have hampered research in this area making it difficult to compare study results. Future research should use more well-controlled designs and more sophisticated instruments adapted to each culture. A better appreciation of cross-cultural differences may be derived from an emerging interdisciplinary model in which symptoms are seen as the result of increased vulnerability due to biological changes in interaction with psychosocial and cultural influences.

References

1. Gannon K, Ekstrom B. Attitudes towards menopause. The influence of sociocultural paradigms. Psychol Women Q 1993;17:275-88.
2. Bell S. Sociological perspectives on the medicalization of menopause. In: Flint M, Kronenberg F, Utian W, editors. Multidisciplinary perspectives on menopause. New York: The New York Academy of Sciences, 1990:173-78.
3. Kaufert PA, Locke M. Medicalization of women's third age. J Psychosom Obstet Gynecol 1997;18:81-86.
4. Khan SA, Pace JE, Cox L, Gau DW, Hodkinson H. Climacteric symptoms in healthy middle-aged women. B J Clin Pract 1994;48(5):240-42.
5. Olazabal Ulacia JC, Garcia Paniagua R, Montero Luengo J, et al. Models of intervention in menopause: Proposal of a holistic or integral model. Menopause 1999;6(3):264-72.
6. Hovelius B, Ekstrom H, Landgren BM, Vinge E. Climacteric-medicalization, minimalization or normalization. Läkartidningen 2000;13;97(50):5927-30.
7. Kaufert PA. The social and cultural context of menopause (review). Maturitas 1996;23: 169-80.
8. Gannon L, Stevens J. Portraits of menopause in the media. Women Health 1998;27(3):1-15.
9. Collins A. Sociocultural issues in menopause. In: Paoletti R, Wenger N, editors. International position paper on women's health and menopause: A comprehensive approach. Bethesda, Maryland:National Institutes of Health (in press).
10. Barth Olofsson A, Collins A. Psychosocial factors, attitude to menopause and symptoms in Swedish perimenopausal women. Climacteric 2000;3:33-42.
11. Flint S, Samil RS. Cultural and subcultural meanings of menopause (review). Ann NY Acad Sci 1990;592:134-48.
12. Lock MM. Ambiguities of aging: Japanese experience and perceptions of menopause. Cult Med Psychiatry 1986;10:23-46.
13. Lock MM. Menopause: Lessons from anthropology (review). Psychosom Med 1998;60: 410-19.
14. Lock MM. Encounters with aging: Mythologies of menopause in Japan and North America. Berkeley: University of California Press, 1993.
15. Avis NE, Kaufert PA, Lock MM, McKinlay SM, Vass K. The evolution of menopausal symptoms. Ballieres Clin Endocrinol Metab 1993;7:17-32.

16. Eden J. Phytoestrogens and the menopause (review). Baillieres Clin Endocrinol Metab 1998;12:581-87.
17. Boulet MJ, Oddens BJ, Lehert P, Vemer HM, Visser A. Climacteric and menopause in seven South-east Asian countries. Maturitas 1994;14:157-76.
18. Tang GWK. Menopausal symptoms. Journal of the Hong Kong Medical Association 1993; 45:249-54.
19. Hilditch RJ, Chen S, Norton PG, Lewis J. Experience of menopausal symptoms by Chinese and Canadian women. Climacteric 1999;2:164-73.
20. Collins A. Psychological aspects of the transition to menopause. In: Aso T, editor. The menopause in the new millennium. Lancaster, United Kingdom: Parthenon, 2000: 526-30.
21. Avis NE, Crawford SL, MCKinlay SM. Psychosocial, behavioral and health factors related to menopause symptomatology. Women's Health 1997;3:103-20.
22. Freeman EW, Grisso JA, Berlin J, Sammel M, Garcia-Espana B, Hollander L. Symptom reports from a cohort of African American and white women in the late reproductive years. Menopause 2001;8(1):33-42.
23. Brown AF, Perez-Stable EJ, Whitaker EE, Washington AE. Ethnic differences in hormone replacement prescribing patterns. J Gen Intern Med 1999;14:663-69.
24. Pham KT, Freeman EW, Grisso JA. Menopause and hormone replacement therapy: Focus groups of African-American and Caucasian women. Menopause 1997;4(2):71-79.
25. Avis NE, Stellato R, Crawford S, et al. Is there a menopausal syndrome? Menopausal symptoms across racial/ethnic groups. Soc Sci Med 2001;52:345-56.

Exercise Effect on Body Weight in Postmenopausal Women: The Physical Activity for Total Health Study

Melinda L. Irwin and Anne McTiernan

Introduction

The prevalence of overweight and obesity is alarmingly high and is increasing in the United States and many other nations [1,2]. Currently, 55% of the adult American population is considered overweight or obese [1] and the prevalence is even higher in older persons. Obesity comorbidities include cardiovascular disease, diabetes, hypertension, stroke, and certain cancers [3]. One fundamental cause of obesity is a sedentary lifestyle or low physical activity levels [4].

There has been considerable debate on whether exercise alone is a plausible weight loss aid [5]. In a recent review of randomized controlled trials of exercise versus no treatment on weight loss, Wing [5] concluded that exercise alone produces modest weight losses averaging 1 to 2 kg. The modest effects may result from small sample sizes, short study duration, and poor adherence to the exercise prescriptions. Consequently, it is not clear how effective exercise training is in reducing body weight. In contrast, large observational studies have found that increased physical activity is associated with less weight gain in adult years [6]. Furthermore, increased physical activity after weight loss has been found to aid in maintenance of weight loss in obese men and women [6].

In 1999, the American College of Sports Medicine sponsored a scientific roundtable on the role of physical activity in the prevention and treatment of obesity and its comorbidities [7]. A major conclusion of this meeting was the need for more and better-designed randomized controlled trials of physical activity in overweight and obese groups, specifically among women since many previous trials appear to have been lacking in women as subjects.

Funded in 1998, the Physical Activity for Total Health Study is a randomized, controlled, year-long clinical trial designed to examine the effects of aerobic exercise versus control on body fat and circulating sex hormone concentrations among postmenopausal women [8].

The primary purpose of the present study was to examine the effects of this moderate-intensity aerobic exercise intervention versus control on body weight changes. A secondary purpose was to further explore the exercise effect on body weight by age, body mass index (BMI) at baseline, cardiorespiratory fitness level at baseline, and adherence to the exercise intervention. We hypothesized that better adherence to the exercise intervention would result in greater weight loss.

Methods

PARTICIPANTS

Details of the aims, experimental design, inclusion and exclusion criteria, and measurement protocols of the study were presented in detail in a previous publication [8]. Participants were postmenopausal women from the greater Seattle area, aged 50 to 75 years at entry, sedentary at baseline (< 60 minutes/week of moderate- and vigorous-intensity recreational activity), with a BMI ≥ 25.0 (or 24.0-24.9 and body fat > 33% measured by bioelectrical impedance), not taking hormone replacement therapy, nondiabetic, nonsmoker, and not drinking more than two alcohol drinks per day.

Women were recruited through a combination of mass mailings and media placements. After careful and extensive screening, 173 women were randomly assigned to the aerobic exercise intervention group (n = 87) or the stretching (control) group (n = 86). Randomization was blocked on BMI < 27.5 versus ≥ 27.5 to ensure equal numbers of heavier and lighter women in each study arm. Of this total, 173 had complete data at 3 months and 142 have had complete data as of this analysis at 12 months and constitute the sample of this study.

BASELINE, 3-MONTH, AND 12-MONTH MEASURES

Demographic and health history information was collected via questionnaires at a baseline clinic visit. Baseline, 3-month, and 12-month height and body weight were measured to the nearest 0.1 cm and 0.1 kg, respectively, by using a stadiometer and balance-beam scale. Both measurements were taken in duplicate and then averaged.

All participants completed a baseline and 12-month maximal-graded treadmill test, with heart rate and oxygen uptake monitored by a Medgraphics automated metabolic cart (Medgraphics, MN). The grade or speed of the treadmill was increased every 2 minutes until the participant reached volitional fatigue.

Total caloric intake was measured at baseline, 3 months, and 12 months via a 120-item self-administered food frequency questionnaire [9].

EXERCISE INTERVENTION

The exercise prescription consisted of at least 45 minutes of moderate-intensity aerobic exercise 5 days per week for 12 months. A combined facility and home exercise program was offered. Participants were required to attend 3 sessions per week at the facility during months 1, 2, and 3, and to exercise 2 days per week at home. For months 4 through 12, participants were required to attend at least 1 session/week at the facility while exercising the remaining days on their own to total 5 days per week. The training program started at

40% of maximal oxygen consumption for 16 minutes per session and gradually increased to 60-75% of maximal oxygen consumption for 45 minutes per session by week 8, where it was maintained for the duration of the study. Facility sessions consisted of treadmill walking and stationary bicycling. Participants also did approximately 10 minutes of weight training 3 days per week, to strengthen muscles around joints to help reduce risk of injury and to improve adherence to the aerobic exercise intervention. The majority of home exercise consisted of outdoor walking. Participants wore heart rate monitors during their exercise sessions.

Several techniques for promoting adherence were used including: 1) individualized attention in facility classes; 2) individual and group exercise behavior change education classes; 3) weekly phone calls to promote adherence; 4) individual meetings at baseline and every 3 months to outline goals and provide feedback on progress; 5) incentives; 6) quarterly newsletters; and 7) tri-annual group activities such as hikes.

Women randomized to the control group attended weekly 45-minute stretching sessions, and were asked not to change their other exercise habits during the study. All exercisers and stretching control participants were asked not to change their diet during the 1-year study.

MEASURE OF EXERCISE ADHERENCE

Women randomized to the exercise group recorded their daily exercise in an exercise log designed for this study. Participants recorded the type of exercise, their peak heart rate, rating of perceived exertion (scale 6 to 20), and duration of exercise. Daily activity logs were completed every day by participants and turned in weekly to the exercise trainer. The trainer then assigned a metabolic equivalent (MET) level to each activity (based on the Compendium of Physical Activities, [10].

STATISTICAL ANALYSES

Exercise data were summed as minutes per week and MET-minutes (the product of the minutes for each activity times the MET intensity level) per week. One MET-minute is roughly equivalent to 1 kcal/min for a 60-kg person. Only activities that were sports or recreational activities at a moderate- or vigorous-intensity (> 3 METs) were included in the data analysis. BMI was calculated as kg/m^2. Baseline height was used for both baseline and follow-up BMI calculations.

Means and SDs of physiological and demographic characteristics were determined by study arm. General linear modeling was conducted with least square means to determine significant differences in 3- and 12-month mean weight changes by intervention group. Among exercisers, general linear modeling was also conducted with least square means to determine significant differences in 3- and 12-month mean weight changes by BMI, cardiorespiratory fitness level, and measures of adherence.

Results

Baseline physiologic and demographic data for exercisers and controls are presented in Table 1. No statistically significant differences in any of the variables were observed between exercisers and controls at baseline ($p > .05$). The mean age (60.7 ± 6.7) was similar for intervention and control participants. Similarly, baseline body weight and BMI were virtually identical for intervention and control participants. After 3 months of exercise, 91 % of the participants adhered to 80% of the exercise prescription (45 minutes, 5 days per week of moderate- to vigorous-intensity exercise). By 12 months, 81% of the participants adhered to 80% of the exercise prescription. On average, the exercisers participated in moderate- to vigorous-intensity physical activity on 3.5 days per week and 174 minutes per week. Only 6 (8%) exercisers dropped the exercise intervention (all after 3 months). However, only 2 women (1 exerciser and 1 control) out of 142 women have declined a 12-month follow-up visit.

Table 1. Baseline characteristics[1] of randomized participants in The Physical Activity for Total Health Study (N = 173)

	Exercisers	Controls
	Mean ± SD	Mean ± SD
N	87	86
Age (years)	60.7 ± 6.7	60.6 ± 6.8
Ethnicity (% Non-Hispanic White)	85%	87%
Education (% High School graduate)	98%	100%
Employment (% Full-Time Employed)	29%	29%
Weight (kg)	81.4 ± 14.1	81.7 ± 12.1
BMI (kg/m^2)	30.8 ± 5.4	30.6 ± 3.8
Cardiorespiratory Fitness (ml/kg/min)	20.1 ± 3.5	20.5 ± 3.0
Total Caloric Intake (kcals/day)[2]	1635 ± 792	1722 ± 672

[1] No statistically significant differences between exercisers and controls for any of the baseline characteristics ($p > .05$)

[2] Measured by food frequency questionnaire

The age-adjusted mean weight change at 3 and 12 months from baseline among exercisers and controls is presented in Table 2. A statistically significant difference in weight change at 12 months was observed between the exercisers and controls ($p < .05$).

Exercisers lost 1.4 kg at 12 months compared to a 0.1 kg weight gain among the controls. Older exercisers (60 years and older) lost significantly more body weight at 12 months (2.5 kg weight loss) as compared to younger exercisers (50-59 years old, 0.2 kg weight loss).

Table 2. Adjusted[1] mean weight change at 3 and 12 months from baseline among exercisers and controls in The Physical Activity for Total Health Study

	Weight Change at 3 months		Weight Change at 12 months	
	N	Mean ± SE	N	Mean ± SE
Group				
Exercisers	87	-0.5 ± 0.3	70	-1.4 ± 0.4*
Controls	86	0.0 ± 0.3	72	0.1 ± 0.4
Age at Baseline				
50 – 59 years				
Exercisers	47	-0.5 ± 0.4	33	-0.2 ± 0.6
Controls	45	-0.3 ± 0.4	33	0.7 ± 0.5
60 – 69 years				
Exercisers	27	-0.2 ± 0.5	25	-2.5 ± 0.5*Φ
Controls	29	-0.1 ± 0.4	27	-0.5 ± 0.6
70 – 75 years				
Exercisers	13	-1.2 ± 0.8*	12	-2.3 ± 1.0Φ
Controls	12	1.3 ± 0.7	12	-0.5 ± 0.9

1 Adjusted for age and total caloric intake measured by food frequency questionnaire
*statistically significant difference from controls
Φstatistically significant difference from age group 50-59 years

The mean weight change at 3 and 12 months from baseline for exercisers by BMI, cardiorespiratory fitness level, and measures of adherence adjusted for potential confounders is presented in Table 3. Women who exercised at least 4 days per week on average over 12 months lost significantly more body weight (-3.4 kg) than women who exercised less than 3 days per week (these latter women gained an average of 1.6 kg during the 12-month follow-up).

Table 3. Adjusted[1] mean weight change at 3 and 12 months from baseline among exercisers in The Physical Activity for Total Health Study (n = 70)

	Weight Change at 3 months		Weight Change at 12 months	
	N	Mean ± SE	N	Mean ± SE
BMI at Baseline				
24.1 - 27.5	24	0.4 ± 0.6	18	-0.1 ± 1.2
27.6 - 29.9	21	-0.1 ± 0.6	20	-2.0 ± 0.9
30.0 - 62.4	42	-1.1 ± 0.5	32	-0.6 ± 0.9
Cardiorespiratory Fitness At Baseline (ml/kg/min)				
13.4 - 17.9	23	-0.2 ± 0.6	20	0.0 ± 1.0
18.0 - 21.9	38	-1.0 ± 0.4	32	-1.3 ± 0.7
22.0 - 32.5	26	0.0 ± 0.6	18	-1.3 ± 1.0
Days Exercised / Week				
1.0 - 2.9	22	0.8 ± 1.1	23	1.6 ± 1.5
3.0 - 3.9	31	-0.5 ± 0.5	22	-0.8 ± 0.8
4.0 - 6.0	34	-0.2 ± 0.8	23	-3.4 ± 1.5*
Minutes Exercised / Week				
22 - 149	37	-0.1 ± 0.7	23	-0.8 ± 1.4
150 - 539	37	-0.4 ± 0.5	23	-0.2 ± 0.9
180 - 400	13	-1.7 ± 1.3	24	-1.7 ± 1.2
MET-mins Exercised / Week[2]				
100 - 449	37	-0.3 ± 0.6	23	-0.5 ± 1.4
450 - 539	34	-0.3 ± 0.5	23	-0.8 ± 1.0
540 - 1620	16	-1.3 ± 1.0	24	-1.4 ± 1.2
Increase in cardiorespiratory fitness (%)				
-10.0 - 4.9	—	—	34	0.3 ± 1.2
5.0 - 14.9	—	—	18	-0.8 ± 0.9

[1] Adjusted for baseline age, baseline BMI, baseline cardiorespiratory fitness level, days exercised per week, minutes exercised per week, MET-mins exercised per week, increase in cardiorespiratory fitness at 12 months, and change in total caloric intake at 12 months from baseline.

[2] MET intensity reflects the associated metabolic rate for an activity divided by the standard resting metabolic rate.

* statistically significant test for trend, $p < .05$

Discussion

A significant difference in body weight change at 12 months from baseline was observed between women randomized to an aerobic exercise group versus women randomized to a control group, although the overall weight loss was modest. Older participants (age 60 and older) experienced greater weight losses compared with women under age 60.

Whether BMI and cardiorespiratory fitness levels at baseline modify the exercise effect on weight loss is not well understood. In the present study, a nonsignificant trend towards greater weight loss at 3 months was observed among exercisers with a higher BMI, but this trend was not observed at 12 months. A nonsignificant trend towards greater weight loss at 12 months was observed among the more fit exercisers. Cardiorespiratory fitness is an objective, indirect measure of vigorous-intensity physical activity [11]. A higher fitness level at baseline may be a predictor of better adherence to an exercise intervention and thus greater weight loss.

However, women who exercised at least 4 days per week on average over 12 months lost significantly more body weight (-3.4 kg) than women who exercised less than 3 days per week (+1.6 kg) adjusted for cardiorespiratory fitness levels, age, BMI, and duration and intensity of activity. Similar trends of greater weight loss with increasing minutes and MET-minutes per week of moderate- and vigorous-intensity physical activity were also observed. A nonsignificant trend towards greater weight loss with increases in cardiorespiratory fitness at 12 months was also observed. Women who had a 15% increase in cardiorespiratory fitness lost on average 2.2 kg of body weight as compared to women who had a less than 5% increase in fitness (0.3 kg weight gain).

Results from our study support Wing's [5] conclusion of a 1 to 2 kg weight loss observed in her review of randomized controlled trials of exercise versus no treatment on weight loss. However, our results also show a significantly greater weight loss with exercise among older women and women with a better adherence to the exercise prescription. Many of the studies that have examined the exercise effect on weight loss did not control for potential confounding variables [12,13]. Some studies randomized individuals who were moderately active at baseline; thus the dose of exercise needed to observe a decrease in body weight would need to be even greater than with a sedentary population. Most studies had a small sample size (< 50 subjects) and large individual variability in response to exercise training [12-14]. In addition, most studies did not report adherence to the exercise prescription or changes in body weight by dose of exercise [5]. The net result is a general lack of a solid research database regarding the role of physical activity in the treatment of overweight and obesity as well as their comorbidities.

In conclusion, weight loss was greater in women who exercised more days per week and at higher intensities. Weight lost through exercise may be limited to certain subgroups of postmenopausal women. Attention needs to be paid to exercise adherence and lifestyle issues in women taking up exercise programs for weight loss.

Acknowledgments

The PATH Study was funded by the National Institutes of Health. We would like to thank Erin Akard, Marcelle Aquino, Jim Brockmeyer, Patricia Cheyne, Claudia Kumai, Kristin LaCroix, Lynda McVarish, Heather Nakamura, Judy Schramm, Shelley Tworoger, Cornelia Ulrich, and Danielle Yancey for their contributions to the study.

References

1. Flegal KM, Carroll MK, Kuczmarski RJ, and Johnson CL. Overweight and obesity in the United States: Prevalence and trends, 1960-1994. Int J Obes 1998;22:39-47.
2. World Health Organization. Obesity: Peventing and managing the global epidemic. Report of a WHO consultation on obesity. Geneva: World Health Organization, 1998.
3. Pi-Sunyer FX. Comorbidities of overweight and obesity: Current evidence and research issues. Med Sci Sports Exer 1999;31(11):S602-608.
4. Jebb SA, Moore MS. Contribution of a sedentary lifestyle and inactivity to the etiology of overweight and obesity: Current evidence and research issues. Med Sci Sports Exer 1999;31(11):S534-S541.
5. Wing RR. Physical activity in the treatment of the adulthood overweight and obesity: current evidence and research issues. Med Sci Sports Exer 1999;31(11): 547-S552.
6. Fogelholm M, Kukkonen-Harjula K. Does physical activity prevent weight gain? A systematic review. Obesity Reviews 2000;1:95-111.
7. Blair SN, Bouchard C. Physical activity and obesity: American College of Sports Medicine Consensus Conference. Med Sci Sports Exer 1999;31(11):S497.
8. McTiernan A, Ulrich CM, Yancey D, et al. The Physical Activity for Total Health (PATH) Study: Rationale and design. Med Sci Sports Exer 1999;31:1307-12.
9. Patterson RE, Kristal AR, Tinker LF, Carter RA, Bolton MP, Agurs-Collins T. Measurement characteristics of the Women's Health Initiative food frequency questionnaire. Ann Epidemiol 1999;9(3):178-87.
10. Ainsworth BE, Haskell WL, Whitt MC, et al. Compendium of physical activities: an update of activity codes and MET intensities. Med Sci Sports Exer 2000;32(9): 498-S516.
11. Montoye HJ, Kemper H, Saris W, Washburn R. Measuring physical activity and energy expenditure. Human Kinetics 1996:6-10.
12. Verity LS, Ismail AH. Effects of exercise on cardiovascular disease risk in women with NIDDM. Diabetes Res Clin Pract 1989;6:27-35.
13. Ronnemaa T, Marniemi J, Puukka P, Kuusi T. Effects of long-term physical exercise on serum lipids, lipoproteins, and lipid metabolizing enzymes in type 2 diabetic patients. Diabetes Res 1988;7:79-84.
14. Hammer RL, Barrier CA, Roundy ES, Bradford JM, Fisher AG. Calorie-restricted and low-fat diet and exercise in obese women. Am J Clin Nutr 1989;49:77-85.

QUALITY OF LIFE: ASIAN WOMEN AND THE MENOPAUSE

Takeshi Aso

The Significance of Menopause in Women's Life

In the process of aging, women proceed a sequence of stages including puberty, reproductive age, menopause and finally reach to senium. Among them, menopause not only signals the end of a woman's reproductive function but also the start of a new phase in which she has the freedom to appreciate the quality of her own life. It is obvious that physical and mental conditions during this stage of life are the consequence of events in previous stages, and at the same time, they have a significant influence on her later years. Thus, the quality of life (QOL) in menopause should be discussed viewing total women's life stages.

QOL and Relating Domains

Quality of life is defined as the individual's perception of the position in life in the context of the culture and value system in which they live and in relation to their goals, expectations, standards, and concerns [1]. In this definition, physical and psychological conditions (physical and mental health), level of independence, social relationships, environment (functions in daily and social life), and spirituality/religion/personal beliefs are included as the domain relating to QOL. The relative significance of domains is different from person to person who has various backgrounds built up on the personal and environmental basis. Therefore, QOL, in other words, the aims of living and satisfaction of life, is to be evaluated on basis of total sum of these domains (Figure 1) [2].

Health-Related QOL in Menopause

CHANGES OF PHYSICAL FUNCTIONS IN MENOPAUSE

In order to discuss the QOL in menopause, it is of importance to understand the specific aspects of physical functions of menopausal women. In adult women at the beginning of the transition from reproductive to nonreproductive stages, the diminishing ovarian secretions induce a functional imbalance in the hypothalamic-pituitary-ovarian axis. The sustained estrogen deficiency after menopause increases the risk of a variety of disorders for them. Although, obviously, the biologically programmed processes of this period have a great impact on women's mental and physical functions, many of these effects at this early stage may not be subjectively recognized and the overt clinical manifestations usually appear much later, in the elderly. The common diseases such as osteoporosis/fractures, hyperlipidemia/ischemic heart disease, dementia/Alzheimer's disease, etc. may develop into life-threatening conditions that frequently can not be normalized again, not even by intensive interventions in the elderly.

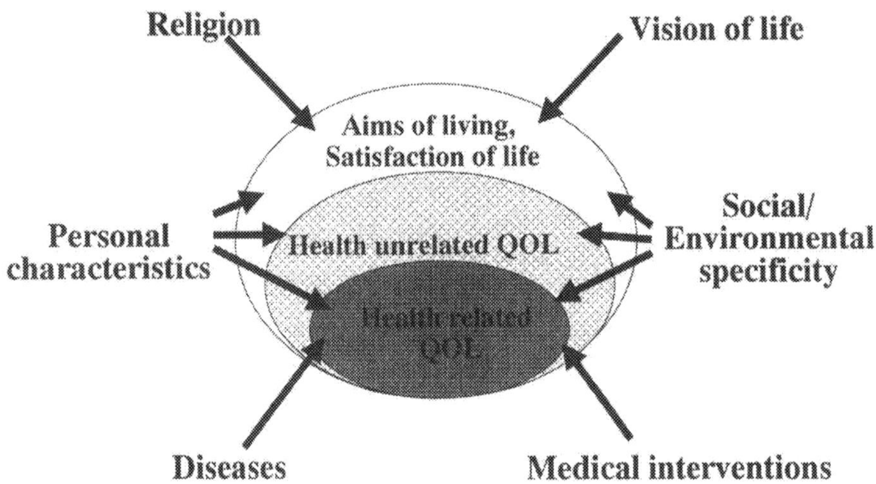

Figure 1. The concept of quality of life (modified from reference 2).

COMMON DISEASES AND CLIMACTERIC SYMPTOMS OF ASIAN WOMEN

It is apparent that the increased risk of diseases common for menopausal women have a serious negative impact on their QOL, but the death rates from particular diseases in a specific part of the world may be significantly different from that of other parts. For instance, the age-standardized death rates from heart disease and breast cancer in the U.S. were 4 and 3 times greater those in Japan, respectively. On the contrary, the age-standardized death rates from cerebrovascular disease in Japan was approximately 1.5 times greater than that in the U.S. It has been reported that the majority of Asian countries showed the same pattern as that of Japan.

It was once assumed that menopause was not only a universal event but that it's timing and physiological implications were universally the same. However, the accumulation of the global information concerning the status of women in menopause from different parts of the world raised questions whether women experience menopause at the same age, with the same complains, and the same mortality irrespective the place they live. It was concluded that menopause seems to be associated with fewer and less severe symptoms in Asia than in the West. Even so, it is clear that Asian menopausal woman also experience psychological complaints such as anxiety, irritability, headache, depression, and insomnia, in addition to vasomotor complaints including hot flashes, sweating, palpitation, and dizziness. Some of these symptoms are severe enough to disturb the daily life of a certain number of women. Although there is a great heterogeneity in socioeconomic and cultural backgrounds among women living in the Asian region, some similar and some differing aspects in the status of the menopausal women have been identified. A recent survey conducted by our group covering more than 3,200 healthy Japanese women between the age of 45-60 revealed that shoulder stiffness is the most common complaint (45%). Fatigue sensation and headache followed it, and the percentage of women who were disturbed by severe vasomotor symptoms was approximately 25% (Figure 2) [3]. In contrast, it has been reported that approximately 40% of women in Canada and USA complained hot flashes throughout the period of menopause [4]. Thus, it seems that the major complaints of Japanese menopausal women are not directly related to estrogen deficiency.

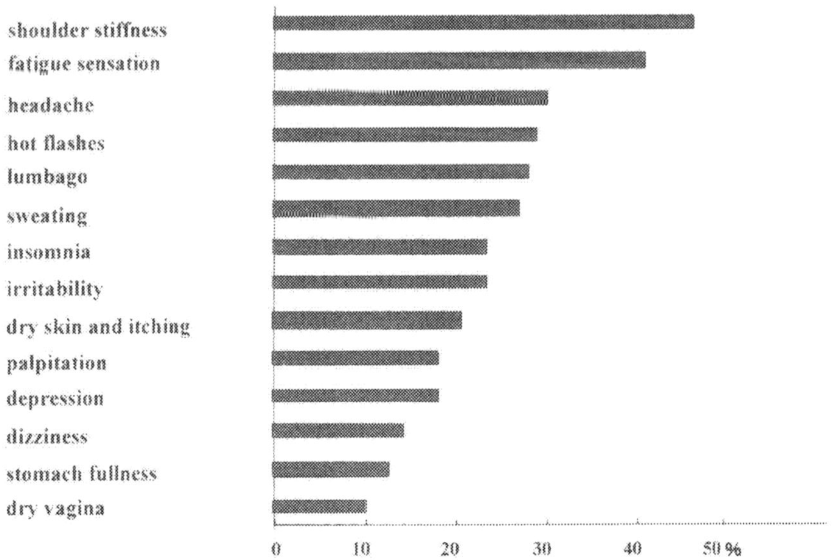

Figure 2. The incidence of climacteric symptoms in Japanese women during perimenopause.

Several factors have been postulated to influence the regional difference in climacteric symptoms. In particular, the life-style including dietary habits has been considered as an important factor. One of the possible factors, the intake of soy products, has been indicated to relate to the incidence and severity of climacteric symptoms. It has been reported that the daily intake of genistein, one of the potent components of isoflavone, taken by Asian people is 20 to 80mg/day. On the contrary, the amount taken by people in the U.S. is less than 2 mg/day. It was also revealed that bone mineral density (BMD) of early menopausal women whose intake of soy products is higher showed greater BMD than did the lowest intake group [5]. It is suggested that the traditional dietary habits have an influence on the pattern of climacteric symptoms and bone metabolism, and eventually affect health-related QOL of Asian women.

Psychosomatic Symptoms and QOL

It has been estimated that the proportion of women who want medical treatment for climacteric symptoms is approximately 5% of total number of women in menopause in Japan. However, the influence of the symptoms on QOL needs to be clarified. The results of a study analyzing the relationship between common psychosomatic symptoms and QOL of Japanese menopausal women are shown in Table 1. In this study [6], QOL of 676 menopausal women were assessed by the factors concerning their impact on feelings and behaviors, such as loss of wellness, limited daily activities, limited minimal daily activities, loss of present conversation, and loss of being fulfilled. More than 95% of the women complained of a loss of wellness as indicated by sleep disturbance, fatigue sensation, depression, and loss of desire. It is clear that most of the common symptoms seriously affect QOL but they are managed mainly by patients' control. The general and traditional attitude towards such symptoms of women in Japan and most of the other regions in Asia has been to accept them as natural events to be tolerated and ignored. Awareness and support in such situations by partners, family, and the general public are important to improve the QOL of menopausal women.

As discussed above, the establishment of health care and promotion systems is urgently needed for the improvement of health-related QOL in the Asian region based on ethnic and racial specificity.

QOL and Sociocultural/environmental Domains

It is obvious that the health-related QOL is greatly influenced by sociocultural/ environmental domains. Since various factors are included in these domains and the response to the factors are inconsistent individually, it is not always possible to analyze their effects on QOL objectively.

The life style and involvement in social activities of Asian women

Although the contribution of women in social activities has been promoted in current Asian societies, the proportion of middle-aged women having regular occupations is still limited. The roles expected of them by society and the major interest in their daily lives have been focused on domestic matters, specifically housekeeping and childcare. In most families, children live with their parents until the time of marriage, especially daughters. Needless to say, actual support by the family, especially by husbands, is the prerequisite to the possibility of women joining any social activities. But, husbands' roles in housekeeping in Japanese families are markedly different from those of Western countries. It was reported that the average time spent on housekeeping jobs by husbands was not more than 10% of those of their wives. The chief factors causing stress for men and women are shown in Figure 3. For women, the stress from childcare and education is the main factor up to the age of 40 years, and stress from family health and their own health and sickness obviously increase as they get closer to the age of menopause. These situations are not favorable for middle-aged women who want to be involved actively in social activities. More or less, the same pattern can be seen in Asian countries. Although the traditional attitude and behavior of these regions have seen gradual changes in the younger generation, one can hardly expect a general drastic positive alteration in the situation of the menopausal women in the near future. As active participation in social activities which enhances the level of independence and advances social relationships of women is one of the important factors in sociocultural/environmental domain of QOL, further efforts should be made to improve domestic conditions.

Table 1. Table 1. Relationship between Psychosomatic Symptoms and QOL in Japanese Menopausal Women

	No.	Loss of wellness	Limited daily activities	Limited minimal daily activities	Loss of present conversation	Loss of being fulfilled
Sleep disturbance	142	92.3%	88.0%	83.1%	50.0%	95.8%
Fatigue sensation	237	96.2%	84.8%	77.2%	75.9%	96.1%
Depression, loss of desire	205	91.7%	79.5%	67.3%	76.6%	95.6%
Vertigo	189	87.8%	79.9%	67.7%	55.0%	85.7%
Palpitation	95	85.3%	74.7%	61.1%	34.7%	85.3%
Hot flashes	243	80.7%	58.8%	48.1%	35.4%	74.1%
Shoulder stiffness	439	80.4%	70.8%	50.8%	35.3%	74.0%
Cold extremities	166	83.5%	57.8%	44.6%	31.9%	84.9%

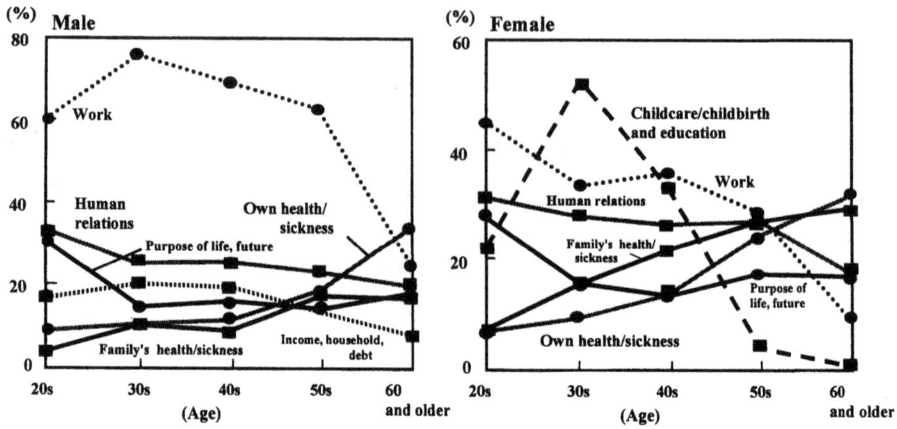

Figure 3. The factors causing stress in male and female in different age groups.

Based on such sociocultural and domestic backgrounds, the position and situations of menopausal women are summarized as followings:

1) Empty nest (end of maternal role, release from worrying about children's cares, and separation from children. The positive response of menopausal women to these changes is unloading of goods, but at the same time they feel a mental vacancy).
2) Instability due to economical problems (partner's retirement)
3) Loneliness and solitariness (deaths of parents, relatives, and intimate friends)
4) Mid-life crisis (fear of cancer and life-style related diseases)
5) Generation gaps (conflicts between younger and elderly generations)
6) Manager syndrome (frustration caused by managing the problems in neighboring society)
7) Sandwich syndrome (problems in dealing with disagreements between junior and senior staffs of a company)

Influence of Aging Society on QOL

As aggregate statistics strongly indicate, the number of postmenopausal women is sharply increasing globally, including in the Asian region. In Japan, the average life expectancy increased gradually in recent years, and the figures for men and women in 1999 were 77.1 and 83.9 years, respectively. The aging society we are facing is creating various problems [7]. The analysis of the health conditions of elderly people 65 years of age and over indicated that approximately 25% of them needed support, but the proportion of elderly who need care at nursing institutions was 5%. At the same time, it is also true that about

80% of them can live at home. Hence, the aging society has to arrange a system to accommodate them as active members and respect their right of living with dignity, which are essential domains of QOL. As an approach to establishing a social system to support QOL of the elderly, a long-term care-providing project named "CARE plan '97" was developed in Japan. The concept of plan is expressed by four key words, namely, "Communication, Affection, Reliability, and Efficiency." Although such project is in progress, 70% of actual long-term care for the elderly is provided by family relationship, mainly by daughters and daughters-in-law. It should be emphasized that these care providers are in the life stage of menopause in which they are exposed various risk factors disturbing their physical and mental functions. Thus, the aging society is facing complicated problems not only for the elderly but also for the generation supporting them, especially for menopausal women.

Summary

The general basic attitude of Asian menopausal women to the aging process is passive, and they are willing to accept the mental, physical, and social changes of the postmenopause period as a natural consequence of aging. Additionally, they used to complain rarely of the climacteric symptoms. But, longevity and increasing life span after reproductive age in recent years have made dramatic changes in the life-style and the role of the elderly in the society. The current situation has provoked great interest on QOL of the postmenopausal women. The specific features of postmenopausal women should be clarified on the national level in Asian countries, those which have heterogeneous properties, in order to evaluate and improve their QOL.

References

1. World Health Organization. World Health Organization Report of the WHO Meeting on the Assessment of Quality of Life in Health Care. (MNH/PSF-91.4). Geneva: WHO, 1994.
2. Ikegami N, Fukuhara S, Shimotsuma A, Ikeda T. Clinical handbook for QOL evaluation. Tokyo, Igakushoin, 2001: 2-7.
3. Aso T. Demography of the menopause and pattern of climacteric symptoms in the East Asian region. Proceedings of the First Concensus Meeting on Menopause in the East Asian Region. Ratnam SS, Campana A, editors. 1997 May 26-30 Geneva. Zeist, The Netherlands: Medical Forum International 1998: 24-32.
4. Lock M. Encounters with aging: Mythologies of menopause in Japan and North America. Berkeley, CA: University of California Press; 1993.
5. Somekawa y, Chiguchi M, Oshibashi T, Aso T. Soy intake related to menopausal symptoms, serum lipids, and bone mineral density in postmenopausal Japanese women. Obstet Gynecol 2001;97:109-15.
6. Ushiroyama N. Establishment of QOL for menopausal women in total women health care. J Japanese Society of Psychosomatic Obstetrics and Gynecology 2000;5:123-32.
7. Aso T. The significance of the menopause in human life in the present and next centuries. The menopause at the new millennium. Proceedings of the 9th International Menopause

Society World Congress on the Menopause. Aso T, Yanaihara T, Fujimoto S, editors. 1999 October 17-21. Yokohama. London: Parthenon 1999: 88-94.

SEXUALITY, MIDLIFE, AND MENOPAUSE

Lorraine Dennerstein, Philippe Lehert, and Henry Burger

Introduction

Women attending menopause clinics often complain of increasing sexual problems [1]. But clinical experience is known to be based on a small proportion of self-selecting, predominantly ill women and may not be representative of most women's experience [2,3]. Population-based surveys can help address the question of a link between aging, menopause, and sexuality. Aging and length of the relationship are known to affect sexual functioning of both men and women. For example, James [4] used cross-sectional and longitudinal data to show that coital rate halved over the first year of marriage and then took another 20 years to halve again. Studies that have included women of disparate ages have found a pattern of an incremental increase in the decline in sexual functioning in midlife [5-9].

An attempt has been made by some studies to disentangle the age effect from the effect of menopausal status, with which it is confounded. The Gothenburg studies of Hallstrom [6,7] were seemingly in a better position than most cross-sectional studies to address this issue, as it was age stratified instead of having age groups. Within each age group of women aged 38, 46, 50, and 54 were pre, peri and postmenopausal women. When age was controlled the relationship between menopausal status and decreased sexual functioning remained highly significant but when menopausal phase was held constant the relationship between age and sexual functioning was not significant, indicating a significant independent contribution from the menopause. Other cross-sectional studies have found a significant independent effect of menopausal status on sexual functioning [5,10,11]. Conflicting findings were reported by Oxford [8,9] and Danish studies [12].

Population-based surveys have found many psychosocial and health status factors are associated with female sexual functioning in midlife [5-9,11,12]. These include presence of a sexual partner, partner's age and health, length of the relationship, feelings towards the partner, level of past sexual functioning, social class, educational level, stressors, employment, personality factors, negative attitudes towards the menopause, and experience of physical or psychological ill-health.

The menopausal transition is a time of psychosocial as well as biologic change. Clearly many of these variables interact. A major problem is the need for appropriate data analysis techniques, which will disentangle the effect of aging from that of the menopausal transition and also depict how different factors interact with each other to affect sexual functioning. This paper utilizes summary statistics to illustrate changes in different domains of sexual functioning with the menopausal transition and structural global modeling to illustrate how biological, psychological, and social factors interact to affect different aspects of female sexual functioning during the menopausal transition.

The Melbourne Women's Midlife Health Project

The Melbourne Women's Midlife Health Project is one of the few longitudinal population based studies to have measured the relationship between sexuality, mood, menopausal status and a range of other variables including hormone levels, and psychosocial factors.

Cross-sectional data was reported from the initial baseline telephone interview of a population sample of 2,001 randomly selected Australian born women aged between 45 and 55 years [11]. The major outcome variables (obtained in a telephone interview) were: responses to questions relating to changes in sexual interest over the prior 12 months, reasons for any changes, occurrence of sexual intercourse, and of unusual pain on intercourse. Although the majority of women (62%) reported no change in sexual interest, 31% reported a decrease. Reduction in sexual interest was significantly associated with natural menopause rather than age, decreased wellbeing, lower education, lack of paid employment, and increased symptomatology. This initial study was limited by using only four questions about sexual functioning rather than a valid, reliable measure of sexual functioning. Hormone levels were not assessed at baseline but were introduced into the longitudinal study described below.

A later paper reported the internal validity, reliability, and utility of a detailed questionnaire, the Personal Experiences Questionnaire, using cross-sectional analysis of data from the fourth year of the longitudinal study [13]. Internal consistency as measured by Cronbach's alpha, was 0.71. Six factors were found on principal components factor analysis. Of the six factors, two are considered as determinants of sexual functioning (Factor 1 Feelings for Partner; and Factor 5 Partner Problems). The remaining four factors are considered as dependent or outcome variables: Factor 2 Sexual Responsivity, Factor 3 Frequency of Sexual Activities, Factor 4 Libido, and Factor 6 Vaginal Dryness/ Dyspareunia. Linear modeling of these factors to age, menopausal status, and hormone levels found that most aspects of sexuality were not affected by age, menopausal status, or hormone levels. Sexual Responsivity decreased significantly with age while Vaginal Dryness/Dyspareunia decreased with log oestradiol. Only a small number of variables were included in this analysis.

Preliminary longitudinal analysis [14] tested the effects on Libido (Factor 4) of aging, menopausal status, hormone levels, and Feelings for Partner (Factor 1). Multivariate analysis of variance found significant effects on Libido of "ovarian functioning" (a latent variable defined by the first factor in an exploratory factor analysis on FSH, E^2, and Inhibin) ($p = 0.02$). The effects of menopausal status and age were then no longer significant. Feelings for Partner (Factor 1) had an even more powerful effect on Libido ($p = 0.003$) [14]. This type of analysis was unable to handle all the possible biological, psychosocial, and lifestyle factors which may affect sexual functioning and their interactions.

The present analysis utilizes data drawn from baseline and the subsequent eight annual follow-up interviews to model changes in different domains of sexual functioning during menopausal transition and the interaction of physical and psychosocial factors on sexuality.

Methods

SUBJECTS

The study began in 1991 with population sampling by random telephone digital dialling and baseline interview of 2,001 Australian-born women aged between 45 and 55 years and residing in Melbourne (71% response rate) [15]. All those women at baseline who had experienced menses in the prior 3 months, and who were not taking the oral contraceptive pill or hormone therapy, were invited to participate in a longitudinal study. Of those eligible, only 56% chose to do so (n = 438). Volunteers for the longitudinal study were more likely than nonparticipants to report: better self-rated health, paid employment, more than 12 years of education, having ever had a pap smear, exercising at least once a week, and having undergone dilatation and curettage [16].

The retention rate by year 8 of follow-up was 88%. Women were excluded from the present analysis for the following reasons: dropouts, surgical menopause during the study, oral contraceptive use at any year. This left a sample size of 354 women of whom 197 provided data from passage through the natural menopausal transition.

MEASURES AND PROCEDURES

The study was approved by the Human Research Ethics Committee of the University of Melbourne and the procedures followed were in accordance with the ethical standards of the National Health & Medical Research Council. All subjects provided written informed consent for their participation in the study.

The longitudinal study involves annual face-to-face assessments in the women's own homes, with interviews and physical measures. Eight years of follow-up data were used in the present analysis.

The Melbourne research team was allowed access to questionnaires carefully constructed by Kaufert and McKinlay and used in cross-sectional and longitudinal studies in North America [2,17]. The core questionnaire was modified for use in Australia after advice from co-investigators and a community advisory committee. Additional references are given below for specific variables and for those questions or instruments, which supplemented the core questionnaire. Measures were selected for inclusion in this analysis based on significant relationships with sexual interest in the baseline cross-sectional study [11] and review of the literature [18]. Interview information was collected annually on the following variables: menstrual status; sociodemographic factors (age, marital status, paid work status); symptoms (total score used) [15]; daily hassles [19,20]; stress [21]; wellbeing

[21,22], and use of hormone replacement therapy (HRT). The number of years spent in education was obtained at baseline.

The Personal Experiences Questionnaire was based on the McCoy Female Sexuality Questionnaire [23] with modifications as already described [13]. The questionnaire is handed to each woman annually at the time of interview. The woman completes the questionnaire and hands it back to the fieldworker. The means of the short form of the questionnaire [24] (SPEQ) are used in summary statistics. Table 1 lists the items retained in the factors in both short and long versions of the scale. Items are meaned within each PEQ and SPEQ factor, and a Total Score is calculated as the sum of SPEQ Factor2 (Sexual Responsivity), SPEQ Factor3 (Frequency of Sexual Activities), and SPEQ Factor 4 (Libido).

Table 1. The Personal Experiences Questionnaire (PEQ)

PEQ Factors	Items	
	PEQ	SPEQ
Factor 1: Feelings for partner		
	Companionable love for partner	
	Satisfied with partner as friend	
	Passionate love for partner	Passionate love for partner
	Satisfied with partner as lover	Satisfied with partner as lover
	Resentment towards partner	
	Hostility towards partner	
Factor 2: Sexual Responsivity		
	Arousal during sexual activities	Arousal during sexual activities
	Orgasm during sexual activities	Orgasm during sexual activities
	Enjoyment of sexual activities	Enjoyment of sexual activities
Factor 3: Frequency of Sexual Activities		
	Sexual intercourse in last month (frequency)	
	Sexual activities in the last two weeks (frequency)	Sexual activities in the last two weeks (frequency)
	Satisfied with frequency of sexual activity	
Factor 4: Libido		
	Sexual thoughts/fantasies in last month (frequency)	Sexual thoughts/fantasies in last month (frequency)
	Masturbation (frequency)	
Factor 5: Partner Problems		
	Partner difficulties in sexual performance	Partner difficulties in sexual performance
Factor 6: Vaginal Dryness/ Dyspareunia		
	Lack vaginal wetness during sexual activity	
	Pain during intercourse	Pain during intercourse

Fasting morning blood samples for hormone radioimmunoassays were taken between days 4 and 8 of the menstrual cycle for those still cycling, or after 3 months of amenorrhoea as previously described [16].

Menopausal status was determined from change in menstrual status asked at each annual interview for those women who were not taking HRT. Premenopausal status was assigned to women who reported no change in menstrual frequency. Early perimenopausal status was used when women reported change in menstrual frequency. Late perimenopausal status was assigned when women reported at least 3 months of amenorrhea but less than 12 months amenorrhea. Women were deemed to be postmenopausal when there had been amenorrhea for at least 12 months.

Statistical Analysis

All hormones were log transformed to normalise the distributions. The summary statistics method used calculated the arithmetic mean of SPEQ domains, for each of the following menopausal states: PRE (Pre- and Early Perimenopause combined), LPERI (Late Perimenopause), and POST (Postmenopause). We chose to compare these three states as we have previously shown that hormonal change of FSH and estradiol are maximal at the late perimenopause [25] and this is also the phase at which there is a significant increase in the reporting of vasomotor symptoms [26]. Study years on HRT or after surgical menopause were excluded from the calculation of summary means. Changes between menopausal states (a) PRE to LPERI and (b) LPERI to POST were then calculated and compared with the null hypothesis of zero change using one-sample t-tests. Mean changes are presented for those who passed through the natural menopause transition (Group M) with 95% confidence intervals and nominal p-values. Two control groups were selected from the subjects not included in the summary statistics analysis. These control groups provide information about change in sexual functioning with time when menopausal status was unchanged. Control Group A stayed PRE between years 1 and 7 ($n = 35$) and Control Group B stayed POST between years 3 and 8 ($n = 33$).

Structural equation modelling (SEM) [27,28] was used on 6 years of data to model the interaction of the various possible determinants with the different aspects of sexuality studied. SEM combines Path Analysis and Regression, allowing the researcher to formulate a model which fixes a priori sets of causal paths between certain pairs of variables and bidirectional correlations between other pairs. SEM is able to manage latent concepts [29,30]. For example in this particular exercise, ovarian functioning is a complex phenomenon not directly measurable, and thus latent, for which hormone measurements can be considered as indicators. SEM has the essential ability to assess the whole model by means of a unique global goodness of fit test, compared to separate regressions. In addition to the global goodness of fit test, other association coefficients allow the measurement of the strength of a model. In order to reduce the multiplicity of tests, only a few models were *a priori* selected for assessment. These were based on the literature review reported above. Statistical modelling was carried out, in part, using the SAS under Windows (Version 3-06, Kallis procedure) and AMOS (Version 3.61). For SEM modelling the early and late menopausal transition results were combined and compared with results from premenopause and postmenopause.

POWER ANALYSIS

Using the summary statistics technique and a sample size of 197, the one-sample t-test is able to detect with less than 5% alpha error, and greater than 90% power, a decline as large as 0.4 on the SPEQ total score. The range of possible values for the SPEQ total score is 1 to 25.

For SEM we provide, for each comparison, a guarantee that there is sufficient power given the actual sample size. Alternative models are compared when the power to reject this model, on the basis of the best model, is at least 75%. Finally, when two models cannot be differentiated, priority is given to the one which is the most simple and which gives the best goodness of fit.

Results

SAMPLE PROFILE

The women had a mean age of 48.1 years (SD ± 2.5) at baseline. Thirty-six percent had more than 12 years education. The median parity was 3, range 0 to 9. Eighty-two percent of women were married or living with a partner in year 1 and 79% of women were married or living with a partner by year 6 of follow-up.

CHANGE IN DOMAINS OF SEXUAL FUNCTIONING WITH THE MENOPAUSAL TRANSITION [31]

When data from Group M was analyzed, summary statistics found a significant decline in sexual functioning. The various domains of sexual functioning were differentially affected by the menopausal transition. The total score of sexual functioning fell dramatically from early in the menopausal transition to the late perimenopause ($p < 0.001$). Sexual Responsivity was the only domain of female sexual functioning to decline significantly from early in the transition to late perimenopause ($p < 0.0001$). During the same phase, Partner's Problems with sexual performance increased significantly ($p < 0.001$) and the woman's positive Feelings for Partner declined significantly ($p < 0.05$). From late perimenopause to postmenopause there were further but less dramatic declines in the total score of female sexual functioning ($p < 0.01$), Sexual Responsivity ($p < 0.01$), and significant declines in Libido ($p < 0.01$), and Frequency of Sexual Activities ($p < 0.05$), a significant increase in Vaginal Dyspareunia ($p < 0.01$) and a further significant increase in Partner's Problems in sexual performance ($p < 0.05$) [31].

CHANGE IN DOMAINS OF SEXUAL FUNCTIONING WITH TIME [31]

Data from Control Group A (n = 35) were available for 7 years during which time they remained pre- or early perimenopausal. The only parameter to show any significant change over 7 years in this group was Sexual Responsivity (mean change = -0.78, confidence interval -1.16, -0.41, $p = 0.0002$). Although women who remained in this group appeared to be in the earlier part of the menopausal transition in that they had not reported 3 months of amenorrhea, their FSH levels were significantly raised from the first to the seventh year ($p = 0.0001$) [31].

Data from Control group B ($n = 33$) were analyzed for 5 years during which they remained postmenopausal. The only parameter of sexual functioning to show any change was again Sexual Responsivity (mean change = -0.51, confidence interval -0.99, -0.02, $p = 0.04$). There were no significant changes in hormone levels of FSH or estradiol during these 5 postmenopausal years [31].

STRUCTURAL MODELING

Using the set of 354 women, we tried to fit in one global model the sexual outcome factors measured by the PEQ, and possible determinants: menopausal status, HRT use, symptoms, hormone levels, social factors (education, paid work, stress, daily hassles), wellbeing, Feelings about Partner and Partner Problems [32]. The aim of this analysis is to depict in a systematic analysis, all the interrelationships. Before applying SEM, the multivariate distribution of the Clau-S dimensions was tested (Wagle multivariate normality goodness of fit test, $p = 0.46$) [33].

The best fit model is shown in Figure 1. The goodness of fit test did not reject this model ($p = 0.06$), and the Normal Fit Index was 0.92, which means that the fit was not too far from the perfect fit, taking the independence model as the zero fit. Rectangles represent the measured variables. The circle denotes the latent variable (ovarian functioning) and arrows designate a causal path and its direction. Two directional arrows indicate covariance between two variables. In this study, as variables do not have the same unit, we used standardized path coefficients. Thus each directional path weight is the standardized regression (Beta) weight, measuring the strength of each path and enabling comparison among the paths. Menopausal status has its most pronounced effects on Vaginal Dryness/ Dyspareunia. Social factors such as stress, daily hassles, educational level, and paid work have only indirect effects on sexual functioning, through effects on wellbeing and experience of problematic symptoms, both of which affect parameters of sexual functioning. Women's increasing positive Feelings for Partner have significant and powerful positive effects on their Libido, Sexual Responsivity, and wellbeing and protect against experience of symptoms. The covariance between Feelings for Partner and menopausal status may indicate a vulnerability during the menopausal transition. This close relationship during the menopausal transition is also evident for experience of stress. Similarly covariance is evident between stress and daily hassles, stress and paid work, and paid work and educational status. Decreasing Sexual Responsivity and increasing Vaginal Dryness/Dyspareunia increase partner problems. The presence of Partner Problems leads to lower Frequency of Sexual Activities but increased Libido (a measure of autoeroticism). Increasing Vaginal Dryness/Dyspareunia has a significant negative effect on Sexual Responsivity, Libido, and Frequency of Sexual Activities.

Discussion

The longitudinal analysis confirms previous studies which show a decline in aspects of female sexual functioning with both age and the menopausal transition. The use of comparison groups chosen from the same sample so that the effect of time could be studied while menopausal status remained stable demonstrated that Sexual Responsivity decreased with time. The other domains studied were not significantly affected by time. Frequency of Sexual Activities and Libido are decreased most in the postmenopause and may relate to the significant increase in Vaginal Dyspareunia in the postmenopause. The occurrence of bothersome hot flushes i also increasing in the late perimenopause [26], and the occurrence of such symptoms may impact on other areas of quality of life including sexual functioning.

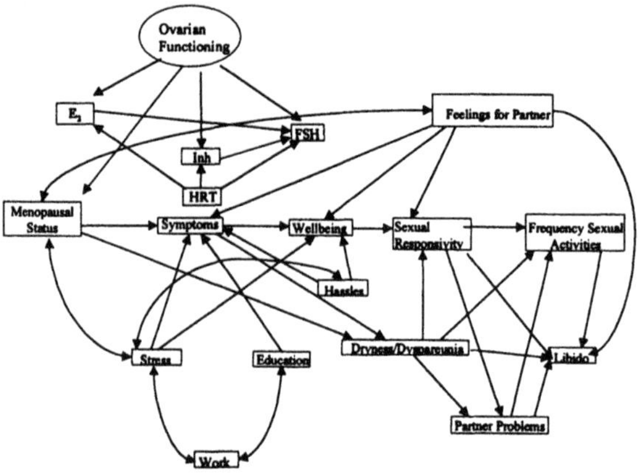

Figure 1. Global model of factors affecting sexual functioning (reprinted with permission from [32])

The structural equation modeling [32] sets out to depict the inter-relationships between different domains of women's sexual functioning and a number of possible determinants. The SEM model provides an adequate way of controlling confounding, concomitant factors which may affect separate linear regressions. Some effects of hormone levels are present (indicated through a significant effect of menopausal status on Vaginal Dyspareunia and direct effects of menopausal status on the number of bothersome symptoms). The number of symptoms then effects wellbeing which influences Sexual Responsivity, which in turn influences Frequency of Sexual Activities and Libido. This highlights the need of analytic models to include most of the variables rather than just a few. A powerful effect of Feelings for Partner on Libido was found, confirming our preliminary analysis which found that the effect of Feelings about Partner on Libido was much more significant ($p = 0.003$) than that of hormones ($p = 0.02$) [14]. Other social factors such as educational level, experience of interpersonal stress, and daily hassles affect sexual functioning indirectly by influencing symptoms and/or wellbeing. The structural equation modeling was essentially a pooled analysis based on only 6 years of follow-up and less women had transited the later phases of the menopausal transition at this phase. As well the data from early and late perimenopause were combined and compared with premenopause and postmenopause. This may have obscured the effects of the menopausal transition on sexual functioning. These effects were better revealed by the longitudinal analysis carried out using the summary statistics on 8 years of follow-up.

Conclusion

Sexual Responsivity declines significantly with time. Other parameters of female sexual functioning are differentially affected by the menopausal transition. Detrimental effects on Libido, Frequency of Sexual Activities, and Vaginal Dyspareunia become more pronounced as women become postmenopausal. Both biologic and psychosocial factors affect women's sexual functioning during the midlife years, with particularly powerful effects of feelings for partner.

Acknowledgment

This study was supported by grants from the Public Health & Research Development Committee of the National Health & Medical Research Council and the Victorian Health Promotion Foundation, the ANZ Trustees and Pharmacia & Upjohn. Prince Henry's Institute of Medical Research, Monash Medical Centre, received grants from Organon Pty Ltd. Ms Emma Dudley carried out the summary statistics analysis using the method of Prof. P. Lehert.

References

1. Sarrel P, Whitehead M. Sex and menopause: Defining the issues. Maturitas 1985;7(3):217-24.
2. McKinlay J, McKinlay S, Brambilla D. Health status and utilization behavior associated with menopause. Am J Epidemiol 1987;125(1):110-21.
3. Morse C, Smith A, Dennerstein L, Green A, Hopper J, Burger H. The treatment-seeking woman at menopause. Maturitas 1994;18(3):161-73.
4. James W. Decline in coital rates with spouses' ages in duration of marriage. J Biosoc Sci 1983;15:83-87.
5. Pfeiffer E, Davis G. Determinants of sexual behavior in middle and old age. J Am Geriatr Soc 1972;20(4):151-58.
6. Hallstrom T. Sexuality in the climacteric. Clin Obstet Gynecol 1977;4(1):227-39.
7. Hallstrom T, Samuelsson S. Changes in women's sexual desire in middle life: The

longitudinal study of women in Gothenburg. Arch Sex Behav 1990;19(3):259-68.
8. Hawton K, Gath D, Day A. Sexual function in a community sample of middle-aged women with partners: Effects of age, marital, socioeconomic, psychiatric, gynecological, and menopausal factors. Arch Sex Behav 1994;23:4:375-95.
9. Osborn M, Hawton K, Gath D. Sexual dysfunction among middle aged women in the community. BMJ 1988;296:959-62.
10. Hunter M, Battersby R, Whitehead M. Sexual dysfunction among middle aged women in the community. Maturitas 1986;8:217-28.
11. Dennerstein L, Smith A, Morse C, Burger H. Sexuality and the menopause. J Psychosom Obstet Gynaecol 1994;15:59-66.
12. Koste A, Garde K. Sexual desire and menopausal development. A prospective study of Danish women born in 1936. Maturitas 1993;16:49-60.
13. Dennerstein L, Dudley E, Hopper J, Burger H. Sexuality, hormones and the menopausal transition. Maturitas 1997;26:83-93.
14. Dennerstein L, Lehert P, Burger H, Dudley E. Biological and psychosocial factors affecting sexual functioning during the menopausal transition. In: Bellino F, editor. Biology of menopause. Part II. New York: Springer-Verlag, 2000: 211-22.
15. Dennerstein L, Smith A, Morse C et al. Menopausal symptoms in Australian women. Med J Aust 1993;159:232-36.
16. Burger H, Dudley M, Hopper J, et al. The endocrinology of the menopausal transition: A cross-sectional study of a population-base sample. J Clin Endocrinol Metab 1995;80(12): 3537-45.
17. Kaufert P, Syrotuik J. Symptom reporting at the menopause. Soc Sci Med 1981;15(3):173-84.
18. Dennerstein L. Menopause and sexuality. In: Ussher JM, editor. Women's health: Contemporary international perspectives. Leicester: British Psychological Society Books, 1999:190-96.
19. Kanner A, Coyne J, Schaefer C, Lazarus R. Comparison of two modes of stress measurement: Daily hassles and uplifts versus major life events. J Behav Med 1981;4:1-39.
20. Dennerstein L, Lehert P, Burger H, Dudley E.. Mood and the menopausal transition. J Nerv Mental Dis 1999;187:685-91.
21. Dennerstein L, Dudley E, Burger H. Wellbeing and the menopausal transition. J Psychosom Obstet Gynaecol 1994;18:95-101.
22. Kammann R, Flett R. Affectometer 2: A scale to measure current level of general happiness. Aust J Psych 1983;35:2:259-65.
23. McCoy N, Matyas J. Oral contraceptives and sexuality in university women. Arch Sex Behav 1996;25:73-79.
24. Dennerstein L, Lehert P, Dudley E. Short scale to measure female sexuality: Adapted from McCoy Female Sexuality questionnaire. J Sex Marital Ther 2001;27(4):339-51.
25. Burger H, Dudley E, Hopper J, et al. Prospectively measured levels of serum FSH, estradiol and the dimeric inhibins during the menopausal transition in a population-based cohort of women. J Clin Endocrinol Metab 1999:84;4025-30.
26. Dennerstein L, Dudley EC, Hopper JL, Guthrie JR, Burger HG. A prospective population-based study of menopausal symptoms. Obstet Gynecol 2000;96:351-58
27. Bentler PM, Stein JA. Structural equation models in medical research. Stat Methods Med Res 1992;1:159-81.

28. Hoyle R. Introduction to special section: Structural equation modelling in clinical research. J Consult Clin Psychol 1994,62:427-28.
29. Bollen KA. Structural equations with latent variables. New York: J. Wiley, 1989.
30. Loehlin JC. Latent variable model, 2d edition. Hillsdale, NJ: Lawrence Erlbaum Associates, 1992.
31. Dennerstein L, Dudley E, Burger H. Are changes in sexual functioning during midlife due to aging or menopause? Fertil Steril 2001;76(3):456-60.
32. Dennerstein L, Lehert P, Burger H, Dudley E. Factors affecting sexual functioning of women in the midlife years. Climacteric 1999;2:254-62.
33. Wagle G. Multivariate beta distribution and a test of multivariate normality. J R Stat Soc Ser B 1968;30:511-16.

WOMEN'S HEALTH AND MENOPAUSE IN RESEARCH AND CLINICAL PRACTICE: SESSION SUMMARY

Vivian W. Pinn, Marianne J. Legato, JoAnn E. Manson, Christine Goertz

Introduction

V.W. Pinn

Many of the questions most commonly asked by women as they approach menopause concern the risks and benefits of hormone replacement therapy (HRT), and/or about alternative therapies to HRT. Research continues to yield new information about the risks and benefits of HRT, as well as other therapies and interventions that can improve or preserve the health of menopausal and postmenopausal women. Nevertheless, studies conducted to date have sometimes generated as much controversy as they have irrefutable conclusions. Long-term, randomized prospective clinical trials to scientifically document the effects of HRT and other interventions on women's health are now underway.

The participants in the panel on "Women's Health and Menopause in Research and Clinical Practice" described the state-of-the-science in three important and controversial areas related to the clinical treatment of women patients during the menopausal transition. The evaluation of patients for hormone replacement therapy was discussed by Dr. Legato, based on recent data concerning HRT's potential to prevent or ameliorate coronary artery disease, Alzheimer's disease, and osteoporosis. Dr. Manson concentrated on the modification of traditional risk factors for coronary artery disease and the promulgation by physicians and other health care providers of guidelines on exercise and the adoption of other behavior-based modifications by women as they transition through menopause. The use of alternative or complementary therapies by women as they experience the symptoms of menopause was discussed by Dr. Goertz, who cited the use of such specific complementary medicinals as soy phytoestrogens and Black Cohosh by women in the United States.

Evaluating the Office Patient for Hormonal Replacement Therapy

M.J. Legato

Physician's enthusiasm for hormonal replacement therapy (HRT) for the female patient has diminished since the publication of recent data which indicate that estrogen is not unequivocally proven to prevent or ameliorate coronary artery disease (CAD) and in fact may be damaging, even lethal, for women with established illness. For example, participants in the Women's Health Initiative have been asked to sign new consent forms because of a trend (albeit not yet significant) to untoward events in the group taking estrogen compared with controls. Other recent work in elderly women with well established Alzheimer's disease showed no benefit from a year of estrogen therapy. Finally, the controversy over the role of estrogen in inducing or promoting breast cancer continues. Given these reservations about HRT, physicians are turning to other therapeutic options for the prevention and treatment of CAD (particularly the statins, which may be even more effective in women than in men) and of osteoporosis (specifically, the bisphosphonates and calcitonin, both shown to replace lost bone and reduce fracture rate). Patients themselves are aggressively seeking alternative therapies for both menopausal symptoms and for improved intellectual performance; these are gaining increasing acceptance among the professional community.

Primary Prevention of Cardiovascular Disease in Women
J.E. Manson

Coronary heart disease (CHD) remains the leading cause of death among U.S. women, but several lifestyle modifications and pharmacologic interventions hold promise in reducing CHD incidence and mortality. A major focus of current research includes the potential roles of low-dose aspirin prophylaxis, postmenopausal hormone replacement therapy, antioxidant vitamins, and homocysteine lowering through folic acid/B6 supplementation. Modification of traditional risk factors, however, including cigarette smoking, dyslipidemia, hypertension (including isolated systolic hypertension), diabetes mellitus, obesity, sedentary lifestyle, and poor nutrition, remain the cornerstone of CHD prevention. Although most risk factors for CHD are similar in women and men, gender differences have been documented for some, particularly diabetes and dyslipidemia. Secular trends indicate that although most risk factors have been declining (through prevention and improved detection and treatment), some risk factors such as obesity, sedentary lifestyle, and type 2 diabetes have been increasing in prevalence. Recent Federal exercise guidelines endorse at least 30 minutes of exercise per day. Evidence is mounting that moderate-intensity activity such as brisk walking is cardioprotective. Physicians and other health practitioners need to become more actively involved in promulgating these guidelines. Dietary modifications are also of tremendous importance, including increasing intake of vegetables, fruits, whole grains, fiber, fish, and reducing saturated fat, trans fatty acids, and total calories. The increasing importance of traditional risk factor modification, including the estrogen/CHD controversy, was emphasized. Research on micronutrient and pharmacologic interventions offers great promise for the future.

The Use of Complementary and Alternative Therapies for Menopause - An Overview
C. Goertz

The use of complementary or alternative medicine (CAM), is common both within the

United States (40%) and worldwide (66%) and appears to be increasing. CAM use in the United States rose from just over 30% in 1990 to 40% in 1997. Studies consistently show that women are more likely to use CAM therapies than men and, while the number of women turning to CAM therapies for relief from menopause symptoms is currently unknown, it has been estimated that women spent $600 million on CAM for menopausal symptoms in 1999. Common CAM therapies used for menopause are dietary phytoestrogens, vitamin E and herbs such as Black Cohosh, Dong Quai, and ginseng. Dietary phytoestrogens, such as those found in soy, are natural plant sterols which demonstrate activity similar to that of estrogen. Epidemiological studies report that populations with high soy consumption (Indonesia, Japan) report fewer cardiac events and less difficulty with hot flashes in postmenopausal women. In addition, clinical studies show decreases in cholesterol and blood pressure with increased soy intake (25 g soy protein/day). Equivocal results regarding effect on the frequency or severity of hot flashes have been found. Soy consumption is generally believed to be safe, although current research is underway to study the effects of soy in women at risk for breast cancer. Vitamin E is an antioxidant found in vegetable oils (soybean, olive, safflower). Intake may reduce risk of coronary heart disease in post-menopausal women. However, anecdotal reports of beneficial effects on menopausal symptoms are not strongly supported by the literature. Vitamin E is generally safe at therapeutic does of 200-2000 IU/day. Side effects can include gastric upset, fatigue, decreased iron absorption, and decreased thyroid activity. The most widely used herb for the treatment of menopause is Black Cohosh (*Actaea racemosa*), a large woodland perennial herb found in eastern North America. There is a long tradition for the use of Black Cohosh in the United States, starting with indigenous Native American cultures and persisting to this day. Active constituents are thought to be triterpene glycosides. Several clinical studies have shown that Black Cohosh decreases menopausal symptoms, including hot flashes. Transient gastrointestinal disturbances have been reported and current contraindications include pregnancy and lactation. Other herbs such as Dong Quai (*Angelica sinensis*) and ginseng (*panex ginseng*) are also popular. However, use for relief of menopausal symptoms has not yet been established by the scientific literature. In summary, the use of CAM for menopausal symptoms is popular in the United States. Studies indicate that soy phytoestrogens and Black Cohosh may be of some benefit. However, more research on these and other CAM interventions is needed.

Conclusion
V.W. Pinn

It is clear that, before we can provide scientifically sound answers concerning any form of HRT or alternative and/or complementary therapies, we must be sure that we have enough data from both basic science and clinical studies on which to base guidance for clinicians and their patients. At present, current data from scientific studies, weighed against a patient's individual health history and health needs, can provide physicians and their patients with the most reliable guideposts for decision-making related to preservation of health in the postmenopausal years.

WOMEN AND CHD: THE CASE FOR PREVENTION

David J. Gordon

Introduction

Because of the widespread perception that atherosclerotic coronary heart disease (CHD) is primarily a disease of middle-aged men, clinical trials of the prevention and treatment of CHD have until recently focused primarily in this patient population. However, the realization that CHD events are also potentially preventable in older patients and that CHD is the leading killer of women as well as men after age 65 has prompted increased attention in the past decade to the study of interventions that might reduce CHD morbidity in women as well as men.

Because of the relatively low CHD rates among premenopausal women and because of the presumptive beneficial effects of estrogen on CHD risk factors and markers [1-7], much of this new attention has focused on postmenopausal estrogen replacement using natural hormones or selective estrogen receptor modulators (SERMs) designed to distill the best features of estrogen without its potential adverse sequelae (e.g. carcinogenesis in the breast and endometrium). However, recent trials of cholesterol-lowering and other traditional risk factor interventions have also included significant numbers of women. This article reviews the status of clinical trial evidence regarding the primary and secondary prevention of CHD in women as we enter the 21st century.

Postmenopausal Hormone Replacement Therapy (HRT)

It is well known that CHD incidence and mortality rates in women typically lag 15 years or so behind those in men. This fact, combined with the observation that premenopausal women who undergo oophorectomy or natural premature menopause appear to lose some of this relative CHD protection, suggests that estrogen replacement after menopause may be beneficial [1,7]. This supposition is bolstered by the many known positive effects of estrogen observed in clinical studies (Table 1). Estrogen has been shown in many studies to lower low-density (LDL) and raise high-density (HDL) lipoprotein cholesterol levels and thus (in theory) to lower CHD risk [2-4]. Estrogen has also been shown to reduce circulating levels of plasmin activation inhibitor I (PAI-I), a potent inhibitor of thrombolysis [5], and to improve or reverse the paradoxical vasoconstrictive response to acetylcholine in atherosclerotic coronary arteries [6]. Although estrogen has also been shown to raise plasma triglyceride and C-reactive protein levels [8,9], the net effect would still appear to be beneficial.

Table 1. Effects of HRT and SERMs on Lipoproteins and Markers of Thrombosis and Inflammation

Lipoprotein	Tamoxifen [10-12]	Raloxifene [4,13]	HRT [4,13]
LDL	**-16%**	**-12%**	**-14%**
HDL	2%	0%	**10%**
HDL2	2%	**15%**	**33%**
TG	0%	-4%	**20%**
Apo A1	7%	3%	**12%**
Apo B	-7%	**-9%**	-3%
Lp(a)	-32%	-7%	-19%
Fibrinogen	**-24%**	**-10%**	-1%
PAI-1	-15%	8%	**-19%**
Prothrombin fragment 1&2	1%	5%	19%
Fibrinopeptide A	11%	-4%	3%
C-Reactive Protein	-26% [14]	0% [13]	60-80% [8,9]

Statistically significant results are presented in boldface type.

The most powerful evidence suggesting a clinical benefit of estrogen came from several large prospective observational studies reported in the 1980s. Of 18 such studies reviewed in 1991 by Barrett-Connor and Bush, 12 reported at least a 20% reduction in risk of CHD morbidity and mortality associated with estrogen use (generally premarin) relative to untreated postmenopausal women [1]. Seven of these studies showed risk reductions of more than 50%, while only three studies reported a significant increase in risk. While these results were subject to the usual caveats about self-selection and other biases inherent in observational studies, their dramatic reductions in CHD and even all-cause mortality and their remarkable consistency engendered a recognition of HRT as a viable treatment option for clinical CHD in women and a surge in its clinical use.

In the 1990s, randomized clinical trials were undertaken to corroborate the positive results of the observational studies of HRT in a variety of clinical settings. Eleven such trials are summarized in Tables 2 and 3 [15-21]. Seven of the trials were relatively small, short-term trials using imaging methodology such as quantitative coronary angiography (QCA) and carotid ultrasonagrophy to measure progression of atherosclerosis in patients with known lesions. Results from four of these trials (ERA [16], EPAT [17], PHASE [19], and PHOREA [18]) have been reported, while two others (WAVE and WELL-HART) are complete but still undergoing data analysis as of November 2001. Two other completed trials (HERS [15] and WEST [20]) used clinical end points (myocardial infarction and stroke, respectively) in patients with established disease. The last two trials (WHI [21] and WISDOM), whose results are still several years away, are very large long-term trials, in which the majority of participants did not have prior clinical CHD. Of the 6 studies reported to date, only EPAT, a small (199 women) trial examining the effect of estradiol on carotid intima-medial thickness (IMT), reported a benefit of estrogen [17].

Table 2. Randomized Trials of HRT

Type of Trial	Imaging EP	Clinical EP
Primary	EPAT [17] PHOREA [18]	WHI [21] WISDOM
Secondary	ERA [16] PHASE [19] WELL-HART WAVE EAGAR	HERS [15] WEST [20]

Glossary: EAGAR: Estrogen And Graft Atherosclerosis Research; EPAT: Estrogen and Prevention of Atherosclerosis Trial; ERA: Estrogen Replacement and Atherosclerosis; HERS: Heart and Estrogen/progestin Replacement Study; PHASE: Papworth HRT Atherosclerosis Study Enquiry; PHOREA: Postmenopausal Hormone Replacement against Atherosclerosis; WAVE: Women's Angiographic Vitamin and Estrogen trial; WELL-HART: Women's Estrogen-progestin Lipid Lowering Hormone Atherosclerosis Regression Trial; WEST: Women's Estrogen for Stroke Trial; WHI: Women's Health Initiative; WISDOM: Women's International Study of long Duration Oestrogen after the Menopause

The most important clinical trial results reported to date were from the Heart and Estrogen/progestin Replacement Study (HERS) [15]. This large placebo-controlled trial of combined conjugated equine estrogen plus medroxyprogesterone (PremPro) in 2,763 women with prior clinical CHD showed no net difference in the combined incidence of myocardial infarction and CHD death (its primary endpoint) over a mean 4.0 years of follow-up. Women randomized to receive PremPro actually showed a significantly increased rate of CHD events during the first year of the trial, which was offset by a reduced event rate in Years 2-4. Moreover, PremPro-treated women suffered a threefold increase in the incidence of venous thromboembolic events, which only slightly diminished over time. In stark contrast to the observational data, the women in HERS clearly derived no net clinical benefit from their HRT.

Table 3. Results of HRT Trials

Trial	N/Arms	Treatment	End Point	Results
Completed Trials				
ERA [16]	309/3	Premarin PremPro	Coronary QCA	Negative
EPAT [17]	199/2	Estradiol	Carotid IMT	Positive
HERS [15]	2,763/2	PremPro	CHD Events	Negative
PHASE [19]	255/2	Transdermal Estradiol	Coronary QCA	Negative
PHOREA [19]	321/3	Estradiol	Carotid IMT	Negative
WEST [20]	664/2	Estradiol	Recurrent Stroke	Negative
Ongoing Trials				
EAGAR	99/2	Estradiol	Graft occlusion	in 2004
WAVE	423/2	Premarin +/- progestin	Coronary QCA	in 2002
WELL-HART	226/3	Estradiol + /- progestin	Coronary QCA	in 2001
WHI [21]	27,348/2	Premarin + /- progestin	CHD Events	in 2005
WISDOM	34,000/2	Premarin + /- progestin	CHD Events	in 2010

It has been suggested that HERS would have done better to use a pure estrogen (like estradiol) rather than premarin and that the simultaneous use of a progestin may have blunted the anti-atherosclerotic effects of estrogen and introduced deleterious adverse effects of its own. However, most of the favorable observational data in the literature involves use of premarin, and a progestin is clinically required to prevent endometrial cancer in postmenopausal women who still have their uterus. While the progestin (medroxyprogesterone acetate – MPA) used in PremPro does partially offset the estrogen-associated increase in HDL cholesterol, there is no evidence from studies like the ERA trial, which have compared estrogen with and without MPA to placebo, that estrogen alone produces a better result

While the HERS results can be viewed as a straightforward negative trial, the difference between early (adverse) and late (favorable) trends was nominally significant and can be interpreted as suggesting two competing effects of HRT with differing time courses [15]. Thus, one may posit an immediate pro-thrombotic, pro-inflammatory effect that raises risk of myocardial infarction in "susceptible" women, followed by a delayed but sustained anti-atherosclerotic effect due to the favorable changes in lipoprotein profile, endothelial function, etc. Under this scenario, one might have expected to see an eventual net benefit due continuation of the favorable trend of Years 2-4, if only HERS had continued for another year or two.

The operation of opposing early and late effects of HRT could also account for the discrepancy between HERS and the observational epidemiologic studies, since the latter studies had mostly long-term HRT users and few (if any women) who had newly begun treatment. Indeed, two recent reports from observational studies, prompted by the HERS results, have found that women who had used HRT for less than one year did in fact show a 2-fold higher risk of myocardial infarction than longer-term users [22,23]. The recent observation that men treated with high doses of premarin in the Coronary Drug Project also showed an early increase in myocardial infarction rates lends further credence to this formulation [24]. However, efforts to account for mechanisms of the early adverse trends seen in HERS and to identify subgroups of susceptible women have not yet been successful. Also, only one of the four completed trials that measured atherosclerotic lesions directly has shown a beneficial effect of estrogen with or without a progestin on lesion progression. The results of the WHI and WISDOM trials, both of which focus on younger, healthier populations of postmenopausal women, fewer of whom might be susceptible to a CHD event in the first months following the introduction of HRT, and feature an extended duration of treatment and followup, should help clarify these questions.

Selective Estrogen Receptor Modulators (SERMs)

During the 1990s, while clinical trials testing the efficacy of HRT in ameliorating cardiovascular disease were ongoing, considerable progress was being made on another front. New drugs that acted as partial agonists and partial antagonists of estrogen were being developed in the hope of "designing" a therapeutic agent that could capture the benefits of estrogen on cardiovascular risk factors and markers, osteoporosis, and mood and cognition, while avoiding its unwanted stimulatory and potentially carcinogenic effects on the endometrium and breast. Two such drugs – tamoxifen and raloxifene – have been approved by the FDA. Both resemble estrogen in most of their cardiovascular effects (Table 1) [4,10-14], but act as estrogen antagonists in the breast. Indeed, they have been very useful in the treatment of estrogen receptor-positive breast cancer and have been advocated for breast cancer prevention. Raloxifene (but not tamoxifen) also acts as an estrogen antagonist in the uterus, obviating the need for a progestin. However, raloxifene may exacerbate perimenopausal symptoms, and thus is better tolerated in women who are at least a few years postmenopausal.

Although the SERMs represent an exciting development in postmenopausal hormone replacement therapy, it is not yet clear whether the existing SERMs will really perform any better than conventional HRT in preventing or treating cardiovascular disease.

While tamoxifen and raloxifene lower LDL-cholesterol about as much as estrogen, their effect on HDL cholesterol is minimal (Table 1). Also, while the two SERMs (unlike estrogen) have been reported not to increase levels of inflammatory markers like C-reactive protein, neither offers a clear advantage over estrogen with regard to venous thromboembolic complications. Thus, it is uncertain whether these SERMs will perform as well as or better than estrogen in the prevention and treatment of CHD. The Raloxifene Use for The Heart Trial (RUTH), a randomized placebo-controlled trial in 10,101 postmenopausal women, aged 55+, with known cardiovascular disease and/or multiple CHD risk factors, is currently evaluating the efficacy of raloxifene (60 mg) in reducing incidence of invasive breast cancer and CHD events [25].

CHD Prevention in Women

The prevention of CHD in women, of course goes well beyond postmenopausal hormone replacement. Traditional risk factors such as lipids, blood pressure, cigarette smoking, diabetes and the metabolic syndrome, operate in women as in men (more so in some instances), and much evidence exists supporting the clinical benefits of controlling these risk factors. While a detailed review is beyond the scope of this paper, an overview of cholesterol lowering trials is illustrative.

Table 4 summarizes the results of a meta-analysis of randomized, unconfounded, cholesterol-lowering trials, each of at least 2 years duration and with a mean cholesterol difference of at least 4%. Seven such trials have reported subgroup analyses of their results by gender. In these seven trials, there were 4,147 women, in whom 527 CHD events were recorded, and 21,651 men, in whom 3,453 CHD events were recorded. Although none of the seven individual trials were designed with the power to attain statistically significant results in women alone, their composite 34% reduction in CHD event rates in women was highly significant ($P < 0.001$) and virtually identical to the composite 32% reduction in CHD event rates seen among the men in these seven trials. This analysis makes it quite clear that cholesterol lowering is equally efficacious in preventing CHD events in women as in men.

Conclusions

Despite abundant evidence from clinical and epidemiologic studies associating the use of postmenopausal HRT with improvement of CHD risk factors, functional markers, and CHD event rates, the clinical cardiovascular benefits of HRT must at this time be considered unproven. Randomized clinical trials have yet to confirm that HRT reduces CHD event rates, and even suggest that early adverse effects on rates myocardial infarction and venous thromboembolism may result in net harm to women who receive HRT. The results of ongoing HRT trials, particularly two large long-term trials in relatively low-risk women (WHI and WISDOM), should help clarify the usefulness of this treatment. The development of SERMs, which selectively capture the beneficial effects of estrogens, offers a potentially useful alternative to HRT, but until we better understand the adverse effects responsible for the negative results of HERS and other HRT trials, it is not clear that the net cardiovascular impact of the existing SERMs will prove superior to conventional HRT. Finally, we have very strong evidence, with confirmation by randomized clinical trials, that cholesterol lowering and treatment of other traditional CHD risk factors is beneficial in women as in men. Thus, pending the results of ongoing HRT and SERM trials, the best current approach to CHD prevention in women is similar to that in men, and should emphasize control of cholesterol and other known risk factors.

Table 4. Cholesterol Lowering Trials in Women* – Reduction in CHD Event Rates

Trial	N (Women)	%RR (Women)	%RR (Men)
AFCAPS/TexCAPS [26]	996	46%	**37%**
POSCH [27]	78	35%	**43%**
CARE [28]	576	**49%**	**23%**
LIPID [29]	1516	15%	**27%**
PLAC1 [30]	92	59%	**42%**
4S [31]	827	**38%**	**38%**
CCAIT [32]	62	- 8%	34%
Total	4,147	**34% (20 to 45%)**	**32% (26 to 36%)**

* Randomized, unconfounded, duration at least 2 years, cholesterol difference ≥ 4%. Statistically significant results are presented in boldface type.
Glossary: AFCAPS/TexCAPS: Air Force-Texas Coronary Atherosclerosis Prevention Study; **POSCH: Program on the Surgical Control of Hypercholesterolemia**; CARE: Cholesterol and Recurrent Events; LIPID: Long-Term Intervention with Pravastatin in Ischaemic Disease; PLAC I: Pravastatin Limitation of Atherosclerosis in the Coronaries I; 4S: Scandinavian Simvastatin Survival Study; CCAIT: Canadian Coronary Atherosclerosis Intervention Trial.

References

1. Barrett-Connor E, Bush T L. Estrogen and coronary heart disease in women. JAMA 1991; 265:1861-67.
2. The Writing Group for the PEPI trial. Effects of estrogen or Estrogen/Progestin regimens on Heart Disease risk factors in Postmenopausal Women: The Postmenopausal Estrogen/Progestin Interventions (PEPI) Trial. JAMA 1995;273;199-208.
3. Walsh BW, Schiff I, Rosner B, et al. Effects of estrogen replacement on the concentrations and metabolism of plasma lipoproteins. N Engl J Med 1991;325:1196-1204.

4. Walsh BW, Kuller LH, Wild RA, et al. Effects of raloxifene on serum lipids and coagulation factors in healthy postmenopausal women. JAMA 1998;279:1445-51.
5. Cushman M, Meilahn EN, Psaty BM, et al. 1999. Hormone replacement therapy, inflammation, and hemostasis in elderly women. Arterioscler Thromb Vasc Biol 1999;19: 893-99.
6. Koh KK, Cardillo C, Bui MN, et al. 1999. Vascular effects of estrogen and cholesterol-lowering therapies in hypercholesterolemic postmenopausal women. Circulation 1999;99: 354-60.
7. Colditz GA, Willett WC, Stampfer MJ, et al. Menopause and the risk of coronary heart disease in women. N Engl J Med 1987;316:1105-10.
8. Ridker PM, Hennekens CH, Rifai N, et al. Hormone replacement therapy and increased plasma concentration of C-reactive protein. Circulation 1999;100:713-16.
9. Cushman M., Legault C, Barrett-Connor E, et al. Effect of postmenopausal hormones on inflammation-sensitive proteins. The Postmenopausal Estrogen/Progestin Interventions (PEPI) study. Circulation 1999;100:717-22.
10. Grey AB, Stapleton JP, Evans MC, et al. The effect of the anti-estrogen tamoxifen on cardiovascular risk factors in normal postmenopausal women. J Clin Endocrinol Metab 1995;80:3191-95.
11. Mannucci PM, Bettega D, Chantarangkul V, et al. Effect of tamoxifen on measurements of hemostasis in healthy postmenopausal women. Arch Intern Med 1996;156:1806-10.
12. Shewmon DA, Stock JL, Rosen CJ, et al. Tamoxifen and estrogen lower circulating lipoprotein(a) concentrations in healthy postmenopausal women. Arterioscler Thromb 1994;14:1586-93.
13. Walsh BW, Paul S, Wild RA, et al. The effects of hormone replacement therapy and raloxifene on C-reactive protein and homocysteine in healthy postmenopausal women: A randomized, controlled trial. J Clin Endocrinol Metab 2000;85:214-18.
14. Cushman MJ, Costantino P, Tracy RP, et al. Tamoxifen and cardiac risk factor in healthy women: Suggestion of an anti-inflammatory effect. Arterioscler Thromb Vasc Biol 2001; 21:255-61
15. Hulley S, Grady D, Bush T, et al. Randomized trial of estrogen plus progestin for secondary prevention of coronary heart disease in postmenopausal women. JAMA 1998; 280:605-13.
16. Herrington DM, Reboussin, DM, Brosnihan KB, et al. Effects of estrogen replacement on the progression of coronary-artery atherosclerosis. N Engl J Med 2000;343:522-29.
17. Hodis HN, Mack WJ, Lobo RA, et al. Estrogen in the prevention of atherosclerosis trial [abstract]. Circulation 2000: 102(Suppl II): II-837.
18. Angerer P, Stork S, Kothny W, et al. Effect of oral postmenopausal estrogen replacement on progression of atherosclerosis. A randomized, controlled trial. Arterioscler Thromb Vasc Biol 2001;21:262-68.
19. Clarke S, Kelleher J, Lloyd-Jones H, et al. Transdermal hormone replacement therapy for secondary prevention of coronary artery disease in postmenopausal women [abstract]. Eur Heart J 2000;21(Suppl):212.
20. Viscoli CM, Brass LM, Kernan WN, et al. A clinical trial of estrogen-replacement therapy after ischemic stroke. N Engl J Med 345:1243-49.
21. Women's Health Initiative Study Group. Design of the Women's Health Initiative clinical trial and observational study. Control Clin Trials 1998.19:61-109.
22. Heckbert SR, Weiss NS, Psaty BM. Hormone replacement therapy for secondary

prevention of coronary heart disease [letter]. JAMA 1999;281:795-96.
23. Grodstein FJ, Manson E, Stampfer MJ. Postmenopausal hormones and recurrence of coronary events in the Nurses' Health Study [abstract]. Circulation 1999;100: I-871.
24. Wenger NK, Knatterud GL, Canner PJ. Early risks of hormone therapy in patients with coronary heart disease [letter]. JAMA 2000;284:41-43.
25. Mosca L, Barrett-Connor E, Wenger N, et al. Design and methods of the Raloxifene Use For the Heart (RUTH) study. Am J Cardiol 2001; in press.
26. Downs JR, Clearfield M, Weis S, et al for the AFCAPS/TexCAPS Research Group. Primary prevention of acute coronary events with lovastatin in men and women with average cholesterol levels. Results of the AFCAPS/TexCAPS Trial. JAMA 1998;279: 1615-22.
27. Buchwald H, Varco RL, Matts JP, et al, for the POSCH Group. Effect of partial ileal bypass surgery on morbidity and mortality from coronary heart disease in patients with hypercholesterolemia. Report of the Program on the Surgical Control of Hypercholesterolemia (POSCH). N Engl J Med 1990;323:946-55.
28. Sacks FM, Pfeffer MA, Moye LA, et al, for the Cholesterol and Recurrent Events Investigators. The effect of pravastatin on coronary events in patients with average cholesterol levels. N Engl J Med 1996;335:1001-9.
29. The Long-Term Intervention with Pravastatin in Ischaemic Disease (LIPID) Study Group. Prevention of cardiovascular events and death with pravastatin in patients with coronary heart disease and a broad range of initial cholesterol levels. N Engl J Med 1998; 339:1349-57.
30. Pitt B, Mancini GBJ, Ellis SG, et al, for the PLAC I investigators. Pravastatin Limitation of Atherosclerosis in the Coronaries (PLAC I): Reduction in atherosclerosis progression and clinical events. J Am Coll Cardiol 1995;26:1133-39.
31. Scandinavian Simvastatin Survival Study Group. Randomised trial of cholesterol lowering in 4444 patients with coronary heart disease: the Scandinavian Simvastatin Survival Study (4S). Lancet 1994;344:1383-89.
32. Waters D, Higginson L, Gladstone P, et al. Effects of cholesterol lowering on the progression of coronary atherosclerosis in women. A Canadian Coronary Atherosclerosis Intervention Trial (CCAIT) substudy. Circulation 1995;92:2404-10.

BONE AND STATINS

Gregory R. Mundy, I. Ross Garrett, and Gloria Gutierrez

The recent observation that statins stimulate bone formation adds to the list of pleiotropic actions of statins that cannot be accounted for by their effects to lower serum cholesterol. This has led not only to the possibility that statins have an extra therapeutic indication which represents a major market in the aging population, namely established osteoporosis, but also suggests important regulatory mechanisms for the control of osteoclast and osteoblast function. The influence of the mevalonate pathway on osteoclasts and osteoblasts has been emphasized by recent work on the mechanism of action of the nitrogen-containing bisphosphonates. This has led to a flurry of investigation not only on the clinical potential of the statins as stimulators of bone formation, but also on the role of intermediates in the mevalonate pathway as potential targets for drug discovery for osteoporosis.

An ideal anabolic agent for bone would be one that could be taken orally, would have a beneficial effect on restoring substantial amounts of bone mass in trabecular and cortical sites, and have a satisfactory therapeutic-toxic window with relative freedom from adverse effects. While searching for such compounds, we found that the statins, drugs which lower cholesterol and reduce the risk of heart attack, cause substantial increases in bone formation in rodents. The statins increased bone formation by enhancing the expression of the gene bone morphogenetic protein-2 (BMP-2), which is an autocrine-paracrine factor for osteoblast differentiation. The mechanism by which the statins accomplished this was by inhibiting the enzyme HMG Co-A reductase, the rate-limiting step in cholesterol biosynthesis. This effect was unrelated to serum cholesterol, but represents an effect mediated through a different branch of the mevalonate pathway in osteoblastic cells. However, the bulk of evidence suggests that the stimulation of BMP2 is dependent on inhibition of HMG Co-A reductase.

Most of the statins that we tested had this effect to increase bone formation. The most potent of the newer statins both as inhibitors of HMG Co-A reductase and stimulators of bone formation, are atorvastatin and cerivastatin. These compounds were several orders of magnitude more potent in their effects on bone than mevastatin, lovastatin, simvastatin, or fluvastatin. The only statin in which we could not demonstrate an effect was pravastatin, a synthetic compound which does not exist in the pro-drug (closed ring or lactone) form. Pravastatin is less lipophilic than the other statins, and this property may be responsible for its lack of efficacy on bone cells.

The statins were tested in a series of ways. They increase osteoblast proliferation and new bone formation when incubated with organ cultures of neonatal murine calvaria. These effects occur in doses of 0.1 – 1 μM over 4-7 days of bone organ culture. The effect of the statins was even more obvious when there was transient exposure of the bones to the statins for only 6 hours and the cultures were examined 12 days later. There was a marked increase in new bone formation and osteoblast stimulation compared to corresponding control bones which increased over this culture period despite the short time of initial exposure.

The statins also stimulated bone formation *in vivo*. In the first series of experiments, we injected them into the subcutaneous tissue over the murine calvaria, and examined the effects on the underlying bone. There was a 30-60% increase in cortical bone width after only 5 days exposure to lovastatin and simvastatin, similar to the effects we have previously found when we have applied recombinant human BMP-2 and recombinant human FGF-1 in this manner [1].

We also tested their effects on bone following systemic administration to rodents. We examined intact rats, and also rat models of osteoporosis, comprising rats that had been ovariectomized at the time of statin administration, and rats that had been ovariectomized for several months before the statins were administered. The former is a model for the woman who is in the perimenopausal period, and the latter for the older woman with established osteoporosis. In each case, the statins were administered orally for five weeks.

Following 35 days of administration of lovastatin or simvastatin by oral gavage in doses of 5-10 mg/kg body weight/day, there was an increase in trabecular bone area in both intact and ovariectomized rats associated with increases in bone formation and mineral apposition rates. We found similar effects with the statins whether rats were intact or ovariectomized from the time of statin administration. There was also a decrease in osteoclast numbers in the treated animals, suggesting that the statins may have also reduced bone resorption.

We are of course interested in understanding the mechanism by which the statins produce this anabolic effect on bone formation. Our data suggest they do so by increasing the expression of the essential regulatory bone growth factor bone morphogenetic protein 2 (BMP-2). We found that the statins stimulate transcription of the BMP-2 gene by using a bone cell line in which the BMP-2 promoter was linked to firefly luciferase reporter gene [2]. The statins had a selective effect on the BMP-2 promoter, with no apparent effect on the BMP-4 promoter. To confirm that this would lead to an increase in BMP-2 mRNA expression, we examined the effects of the lovastatin and simvastatin on human MG-63 osteoblastic cells and examined BMP-2 and BMP-4 mRNA expression by Northern analysis. Again we found that there was an increase in BMP-2 mRNA using these agents in concentrations of 1-5 μM. This effect again was specific with BMP-2 mRNA with no effect on BMP-4 mRNA. We also examined the effects of these statins on BMP-2 protein production by osteoblastic cells using a sandwich ELISA to BMP-2. We found again there was an increase in BMP-2 protein of 2-3 fold when statins were applied in doses of 1-5 μM. We found that cerivastatin was at least 2 orders of magnitude more potent than earlier statins in these assays.

We also examined the relationship between HMG Co-A reductase and BMP-2 expression. It appears that BMP-2 expression is related to inhibition of HMG Co-A reductase. Firstly, we could reverse the effects of statins on BMP-2 transcription and the biological effects in murine calvaria by adding back mevalonate, the immediate downstream metabolite of HMG Co-A reductase. Secondly, we found that there was a perfect correlation between potency of these compounds on HMG Co-A reductase and their potency as stimulators of bone formation and BMP-2 transcription. Thirdly, we found that biological activity on bone was present only in open ring ester forms of the compounds and not in the closed ring lactone pro-drug forms of the compounds. Taken together, all of this evidence suggests that inhibition of HMG Co-A reductase is responsible ultimately for increasing BMP-2 transcription.

We believe that BMP-2 may be a central growth factor in osteoblast differentiation [3]. BMP-2 belongs to a large family of bone-derived growth factors which include the homologs in the transforming growth factor family as well as other unrelated growth factors such as insulin-like growth factors, the fibroblast growth factor family and the platelet-derived growth factors. All of these growth factors are incorporated into the growth matrix and presumably released in active form when bone is resorbed. The transforming growth factor family is responsible for osteoblast chemotaxis to sites of resorption defects which is required to initiate the process of formation, stimulate proliferation of those osteoblast precursors, and are probably responsible for apoptosis of osteoclasts and cessation of the resorption phase of the remodeling cycle. Bone morphogenetic proteins, in contrast, are responsible for enhancing osteoblast differentiation, including stimulation of expression of the structural proteins of bone such as type-1 collagen and the mineralization of bone matrix [4]. We have found that when BMP-2 is applied to bone surfaces *in vivo*, there is powerful stimulation of new bone formation. Our concept is that BMP-2 is an autocrine factor involved in osteoblast differentiation, is expressed by osteoblasts as they differentiate and further enhances mineralization [4]. Thus, statins, which stimulate transcription of BMP-2, could be expected to further enhance this process of osteoblast differentiation and new bone formation.

Of course, the major question which arises as a consequence of these studies is whether the statins will have similar effects on human bone. It is impossible to answer that question at the present time. However, we have found that the statins increase BMP-2 expression in human osteoblastic cells (MG-63 cells). This is very encouraging that they may produce the same effects on human cells *in vivo*. Based on our findings [5], Bauer and Cummings examined their large databases to determine if there was any previously unrecognized association between statin usage and skeletal status. They found in these databases that there was indeed a possible relationship between statin use, bone mineral density, and subsequent fractures [6]. Since that time, there have been 5 published reports of observational studies suggesting a beneficial effect on fracture rates and bone mineral density [7-11]. On the other hand, several preliminary reports (one from the same data base as a positive published report) suggest no effect [12-14].

In conclusion, these results indicate that statins have the capacity to increase BMP-2 expression and stimulate osteoblast differentiation. However, statins are poorly delivered to bone. All of the statins which are currently on the market have been selected for their capacity to target the liver and decrease cholesterol biosynthesis there. Moreover, many of them are highly subject to first pass metabolism by cytochrome P450 enzymes in the liver and gut wall. As a consequence, the biodistribution of active statin or metabolites to bone and other peripheral tissues is small. This makes it uncertain that current statins will have beneficial effects on bone in humans when they are administered orally. There are several possibilities for improving biodistribution to bone. The more recent potent statins such as cerivastatin or atorvastatin may get past the liver in sufficient amounts to cause beneficial effects on bone, and the animal studies suggest this may be the case. Alternative modes of administration of the statins such as topical application through a skin patch may also solve the problem of poor biodistribution to bone. The third possibility is that there may be other drugs of this class that have not been selected for development as cholesterol-lowering agents because of their relatively greater biodistribution to peripheral tissues. These may be ideal drugs for use as bone-active agents.

Perhaps the most important consequence of these findings is not that the statins themselves may be effective drugs for diseases of bone loss, but rather that these results focus attention on this pathway of cholesterol biosynthesis and its relationship to BMP2 expression and bone formation. This has been further emphasized by recent observations that the nitrogen-containing bisphosphonates, drugs that reduce bone resorption and have a large market for osteoporosis, also target enzymes in this pathway. This may lead to the identification of other potential molecular targets for drug discovery as well as other therapeutic approaches to enhance bone formation and produce the ideal anabolic agent for osteoporosis.

References

1. Dunstan CR, Boyce R, Boyce BF, et al. Systemic administration of acidic fibroblast growth factor (FGF-1) prevents bone loss and increases new bone formation in ovariectomized rats. J Bone Min Res 1999;14:953-59.
2. Ghosh-Choudhury N, Windle JJ, Koop BA, et al. Immortalized murine osteoblasts derived from BMP 2-T-Antigen expressing in transgenic mice. Endocrinology 1996;137:331-39.
3. Mundy GR, Boyce B, Hughes D, et al. The effects of cytokines and growth factors on osteoblastic cells. Bone 1995;17:71S-75S.
4. Harris SE, Bonewald LF, Harris MA, et al. Effects of TGF on bone nodule formation and expression of bone morphogenetic protein-2, osteocalcin, osteopontin, alkaline phosphatase and Type I collagen mRNA in prolonged cultures of fetal rat calvarial osteoblasts. J Bone Miner Res 1994;9:855-63.
5. Mundy G, Garrett R, Harris S, et al. Stimulation of bone formation in vitro and in rodents by statins. Science 1999;286:1946-49.
6. Bauer DC, Mundy GR, Jamal SA, et al. Statin use, bone mass and fracture: An analysis of two prospective studies. J Bone Min Res 1999;14: (Suppl) #1188.
7. Cummings SR, Bauer DC. Do statins prevent both cardiovascular disease and fracture? J Am Med Assoc 2000;283:3255-57.
8. Wang PS, Solomon DH, Mogun H, Zvorn J. HMG-CoA reductase inhibitors and the risk

of hip fractures in elderly patients. J Am Med Assoc 2000;283:3211-16.

9. Meier CR, Schlienger RG, Kraenzlin ME, Schlegel B, Jick H. HMG-CoA reductase inhibitors and the risk of fractures. J Am Med Assoc 2000;283:3205-10.
10. Chan KA, Andrade SE, Boles M, et al. Inhibitors of hydroxymethylglutaryl-coenzyme A reductase and risk of fracture among older women. Lancet 2000;355:2185-88.
11. Edwards CJ, Hart DJ, Spector TD. Oral statins and increased bone-mineral density in postmenopausal women. Lancet 2000;355 (letter).
12. LaCroix AZ, Cauley JA, Jackson R, et al. Does statin use reduce risk of fracture in postmenopausal women? Results from the Women's Health Initiative Observational Study. J Bone Min Res 2000;15:(Suppl) #1066.
13. Van Staa TP, Wegman SLJ, de Vries F, Leufkens HGM, Cooper C. Use of statins and risk of fractures. J Bone Min Res 2000;15:(Suppl) #1067.
14. Cauley JA, Jackson R, Pettinger M, et al. Statin use and bone mineral density (BMD) in older women: The Women's Health Initiative Observational Study (WHI-OS). J Bone Min Res 2000;15:(Suppl) #1068.

SELECTED U.S. GOVERNMENT SPONSORED WOMEN'S HEALTH MENOPAUSE INITIATIVES: SESSION SUMMARY

Vivian W. Pinn, Loretta P. Finnegan, K.M. Brett, Y. Chong, S. Mark, N. Keenan, A. Fugh-Berman, J. Kaczmarczyk, C. Hunter, D. Browne, S.F. Wood, K.A. Hollinger, M.A. Miller, K.K. Chapman, C. M. Clancy, M.L. Gross, C.E. Lewis, J.Y. Groff, R. McKeown, C. Herman, L. Pulley, H. McCreath, C. Cornell, and D. Richter

Introduction

V.W. Pinn and L. P. Finnegan

Issues related to women's health, and particularly to menopause, have been major priorities over the past decade for agencies of the U.S. Department of Health and Human Services (DHHS). In order to prevent morbidity and mortality in perimenopausal and postmenopausal women, an unprecedented concentration of resources and attention has been directed toward menopause. This has included funding of new research to elucidate the menopausal transition and to prevent morbidity, as well as support of studies of associated pharmacological, clinical, and epidemiological aspcets and prevention research.

This session featured presentations describing initiatives undertaken by the Federal government to address the menopausal transition and associated health conditions. The presentations encompassed a study conducted by thc U.S. Centers for Disease Control and Prevention (CDC) through the National Center for Health Statistics (NCHS) and funded by the National Institutes of Health (NIH) Office of Research on Women's Health (ORWH) on women's knowledge and use of hormone replacement therapy (HRT), as well as a talk on women's use of conventional, complementary, and alternative therapies for menopausal symptoms based on a survey by the DHHS Office of Women's Health (OWH). Session participants from the U.S. Food and Drug Administration described that agency's activities to regulate products used by women to treat menopausal symptoms, while representatives of the Agency for Healthcare Research and Quality (AHRQ)discussed their efforts to assess the quality and impact of informed decisionmaking about menopause. Through the community-based ENDOW study of the Women's Health Initiative, representatives of the CDC, NIH, and the University of Alabama at Birmingham considered issues surrounding decisionmaking for hysterectomy and hormone replacement therapy. Identifying methods of effectively disseminating evidence-based information about HRT and menopause to health care providers and women throughout the United States was a common theme in all the presentations.

Hormone Replacement Therapy: Knowledge and Use in the United States
K.M. Brett and Y. Chong

While much has been written about the risks and benefits of hormone replacement therapy (HRT), there is little information on its use in the United States. This presentation highlighted a recently released chart book published by the National Center for Health Statistics (NCHS), which offers researchers, healthcare professionals, and policy makers an inventory of information available about HRT use from recent nationally representative data collected by the NCHS. The data in this chart book came from three U.S. surveys: the Third National Health and Nutrition Examination Survey, 1988-1994; the National Health Interview Survey, 1998; and the National Ambulatory Medical Care Survey and National Hospital Ambulatory Medical Care Survey, 1997-1998. Several findings from the chart book were presented, including the following: 44% of all postmenopausal women in the United States reported having ever used HRT and that while most women started using HRT around the time of menopause, 25% started taking it five or more years after menopause. Factors associated with HRT use included surgical menopause, race, income, and education. There were no substantial differences between HRT users and nonusers in terms of risky health behaviors and self-reported health. Approximately 45% of women 40-60 years of age reported receiving counseling from a physician about HRT, although higher education and white race increased the likelihood of counseling. The surveys found that a prescription for HRT was included in 7.5% of all visits by women 40 years of age and over to office-based physicians and hospital out-patient departments. Only 8.8% of visits to primary care physicians and clinics included an HRT prescription, compared with 25.6% of visits to obstetrics/gynecology physicians and clinics.

Use of Conventional, Complementary and Alternative Therapies for Menopausal Symptoms
S. Mark, N. Keenan, A. Fugh-Berman, J. Kaczmarczyk, C. Hunter and D. Browne

The Conventional, Complementary and Alternative Menopausal Practices Survey (CAMPS) provides unique prevalence data on the use of conventional and complementary and alternative (CAM) therapies for menopausal symptoms. CAMPS, a telephone survey of 2,602 women aged 45 years or older who were residents of Florida, Minnesota, or Tennessee in the United States in 1997-98, included items on menopausal status and symptoms, and on the use of conventional and CAM health care providers, noncontraceptive hormones, and CAM therapies in relation to menopause. The reported prevalence for menopausal symptoms ranged from 62.9% for hot flashes to 21.1% for heavy vaginal bleeding. The therapies with the highest prevalence of use were estrogen (41.4%), vitamins and minerals (36.4%), progestins (13.7%), increasing the amount of physical activity (11.5%), and herbal remedies (9.5%). When grouped into mutually exclusive categories based on the type of therapy used, 18.7% of the respondents used only conventional therapies, 20.8% used only CAM, 25.2% used both conventional and CAM therapies, and 35.3% reported that they had not used any of the therapies asked about in the survey.

Food and Drug Administration (FDA) Activities on Regulated Products Related to Menopause
S.F. Wood, K.A. Hollinger, M.A. Miller, and K.K. Chapman

Although natural menopause is medically defined as the cessation of menses resulting from declining estrogen levels and is related to changes accompanying decreased hormone levels, the term is also used to describe changes considered consequences of aging. Many medicinal, herbal, and diagnostic products have been developed to ameliorate these health problems and conditions. The source, mandate, and stringency of oversight of FDA regulatory authority varies greatly among these products. The presentation provided an overview of products used to treat, prevent, and diagnose menopausal associated conditions and described the standards of safety and use for these products. The products and devices used for menopausal related conditions are classified as drugs, foods, devises, and dietary supplements. The FDA ensures the following: 1) that drugs are safe, effective, and accurately labeled; 2) that foods are safe, wholesome, unadulterated, and truthfully labeled; 3) that dietary supplements are safe and truthfully labeled; and 4) that devices are safe and effective for their intended use. The monitoring of products for safety and truthful labeling extends from the premarketing phase of development to the postmarketing phase of a product's life. Products that are imported into the United States must meet the same standards through equivalence reviews. Through assurance that industry is in compliance with the laws and regulations pertaining to products, the FDA protects the public health of women using these products to improve their health and quality of life.

Assessing the Quality and Impact of Informed Decision Making About Menopause
C.M. Clancy, and M.L. Gross

The scientific evidence regarding the appropriate use of hormone replacement therapy (HRT) or other interventions to relieve menopausal symptoms, prevent osteoporosis, and reduce the risk of cardiovascular disease is far from resolved. The science needed to inform clinical decisions is further complicated by controversies regarding the risks and benefits of HRT, proliferation of new therapeutic options to address specific health issues related to menopause, publication of studies with apparently conflicting results, and inconsistent media coverage. Yet women beginning menopause must make decisions based on their personal preferences and values and the best information available. Since existing evidence does not support a single strategy for all women, an alternative approach to assessing quality of care for menopausal women that examines the content and quality of communication between women and clinicians was developed. In 2000, the National Committee on Quality Assurance, a private organization that accredits managed care in the

United States, included a new measure for health plan accreditation that asks women if their plan or a health professional provided information about menopause; if the response is "yes," women are asked about specific content domains, whether the information is tailored to their personal circumstances, and whether it is provided in a respectful fashion. Results are reported as the percentage of women who report exposure to information, who report adequate breadth (risks, benefits, and alternatives to HRT) of information, and who report adequate personalization (whether counseling considered personal and family history and individual concerns). While a majority of women report exposure to information (66-78%; 10th and 90th percentiles), smaller proportions of exposed women report sufficient breadth of information (41-58%) or adequate personalization of information (37.9-55.6%). The results are similar to those documented in other surveys, including the Commonwealth Fund 1998 Survey on Women's Health, indicating that further research is needed to improve patient-physician communication on menopause and other key health issues for women. Studies are needed to examine the factors (clinical and organizational) which determine the quality of patient-provider interactions, and to assess how multi-dimension medical decisions can be presented to patients most effectively.

Decision-Making for Hysterectomy: The Ethnicity, Needs and Decisions of Women (ENDOW) Study
C.E. Lewis, J.Y. Groff, R. McKeown, C. Herman, L. Pulley, H. McCreath, C. Cornell, and D. Richter

Hysterectomy is extremely common, and is most often performed electively. Previous research on hysterectomy has included few data on ethnic minority groups, and little on women's decision-making, preferences, and values related to hysterectomy. The ENDOW program was designed to explore ethnic, geographic, cultural/acculturation variations in attitudes and decision making concerning hysterectomy, and to develop and pilot test materials appropriate for different sociocultural groups in order to enhance women's decision-making. The ENDOW planners described how they developed a survey using previous research, theory, and focus group information from 480 women, and implemented it in four communities; approximately 3,500 African-American (30%), Hispanic (19%), Navajo (11%) and non-Hispanic white women (39%) responded. Data from the information-seeking and decision-making subscales of the autonomy preference index showed that women desire involvement in medical decisions, more and better information on hysterectomy and other health issues, and improved communication with doctors. Although the planners found that education was associated with preferences for involvement, demographic factors explained little of the variance in these measures. Therefore, providers should not presume to know women's preferences based solely on race, ethnicity, education, or SES. The data were then used to develop intervention methods and strategies to facilitate women's decision-making. Materials developed included a video, brochures, and a decision-making guide. The materials and dissemination strategies were then pilot tested with these data showing that the interventions were valuable.

Conclusion

V. W. Pinn and L. P. Finnegan

Although there has been a virtual explosion in new information related to menopause in recent years, many clinical and scientific questions remain Many of the questions most commonly asked by women approaching menopause are related to the risks and benefits of hormone replacement therapy, and/or about alternatives to HRT, including complementary or alternative therapies. Some questions center on hysterectomy, especially when it results in premature menopause. Other questions center on the ways in which women of diverse backgrounds experience menopause, as well as the factors that influence women's decisionmaking concerning menopause. Through the programs, policies, and data presented during this session, Federal agencies are endeavoring to find answers to these questions and to supply women and their health care providers with scientifically sound data.

INDEX

1. A.M. Gotto, C. Lenfant, R. Paoletti (eds.) and M. Soma (ass. ed.): *Multiple Risk Factors in Cardiovascular Disease.* 1992 ISBN 0-7923-1938-9
2. A.L. Catapano, A.M. Gotto, Jr., L.C. Smith and R. Paoletti (eds.): *Drugs Affecting Lipid Metabolism.* 1993 ISBN 0-7923-2232-0
3. T.Godfraind,S.Govoni, R. Paoletti and P.M. Vanhoutte (eds.):*Calcium Antagonists. Pharmacology and Clinical Research.* 1993 ISBN 0-7923-2259-2
4. D. Galmarini, L.R. Fassati, R. Paoletti and S. Sherlock (eds.): *Drugs and the Liver: High Risk Patients and Transplantation.* 1993 ISBN 0-7923-2307-6
5. P.M. Vanhoutte, P.R. Saxena, R. Paoletti, N. Brunello (eds.) and A.S. Jackson (ass.ed.): *Serotonin. From Cell Biology to Pharmacology and Therapeutics.* 1993 ISBN 0-7923-2518-4
6. A.G. Dalgleish, A. Albertini and R. Paoletti (eds.): *The Impact of Biotechnology on Autoimmunity.* 1994 ISBN 0-7923-2724-1
7. P.G. Crosignani, R. Paoletti, P.M. Sarrel, N.K. Wenger (eds.), M. Meschia and M. Soma (ass.eds.):*Women's Health in Menopause.Behaviour, Cancer, Cardiovascular Disease, Hormone Replacement Therapy.* 1994 ISBN 0-7923-3068-4
8. A.M. Gotto Jr., C. Lenfant, A.L. Catapano and R. Paoletti (eds.): *Multiple Risk Factors in Cardiovascular Disease.* 1995 ISBN 0-7923-3503-1
9. T. Godfraind, G. Mancia, M.P. Abbracchio, L. Aguilar-Bryan and S. Govoni (eds.): *Pharmacological Control of Calcium and Potassium Homeostasis. Biological,* Therapeutical, and Clinical Aspects. 1995 ISBN 0-7923-3604-6
10. A.M Gotto Jr., R. Paoletti, L.C. Smith, A.L. Catapano and A.S. Jackson (eds.): *Drugs Affecting Lipid Metabolism. Risk Factors and Future Directions.* 1996 ISBN 0-7923-4167-8
11. R. Paoletti, P.G. Crosignani, P. Kenemans, G. Samsioe, M. Soma and A.S. Jackson (eds.): *Women's Health and Menopause.* Risk Reduction Strategies. 1997 ISBN 0-7923-4697-1
12. A.M. Gotto Jr., C. Lenfant, R. Paoletti, A.L. Catapano and A.S. Jackson (eds.): *Multiple Risk Factors in Cardiovascular Disease.* Strategies of Prevention of Coronary Heart Disease, Cardiac Failure. 1998 ISBN 0-7923-5023-5
13. R. Paoletti, P.G. Crosignani, P. Kenemans, N.K. Wenger and A.S. Jackson (eds.): *Women's Health and Menopause.* Risk Reduction Strategies – Improved Quality of Health. 1999 ISBN 0-7923-5906-2
14. R. Paoletti, A. Poli and A.S. Jackson (eds.): *Creatine.* From Basic Science to Clinical Application. 2000 ISBN 0-7923-6118-0
15. R. Paoletti, A.L. Klatsky, A. Poli, S. Zakhari (eds.): *Moderate Alcohol Consumption and Cardiovascular Disease.* 2000 ISBN 0-7923-6572-0
16. B. Samuelsson, R. Paoletti, G.C. Folco, E. Granström and S. Nicosia (eds.): *Advances in Prostaglandin and Leukotriene Research: Basic Science and New Clinical Applications.* 2001 ISBN 1-4020-0146-0
17. R.A. Lobo, P.G. Crosignani, R. Paoletti (eds.) and F. Bruschi (ass.ed.): *Women's Health and Menopause.* New Strategies – Improved Quality of Life. 2002 ISBN 1-4020-7149-3

KLUWER ACADEMIC PUBLISHERS – DORDRECHT / BOSTON / LONDON

www.ingramcontent.com/pod-product-compliance
Ingram Content Group UK Ltd.
Pitfield, Milton Keynes, MK11 3LW, UK
UKHW020134160926
475607UK00003B/34

9781402071492